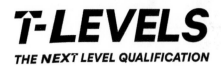

T-LEVELS
THE NEXT LEVEL QUALIFICATION

D1380217

HEALTH

CORE

Stephen Hoare, Judith Adams, Mary Riley

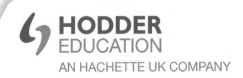

HODDER EDUCATION
AN HACHETTE UK COMPANY

'T Level' is a registered trade mark of the Institute for Apprenticeships and Technical Education. The T Level Technical Qualification is a qualification approved and managed by the Institute for Apprenticeships and Technical Education.

Every effort has been made to trace all copyright holders, but if any have been inadvertently overlooked, the Publishers will be pleased to make the necessary arrangements at the first opportunity.

Although every effort has been made to ensure that website addresses are correct at time of going to press, Hodder Education cannot be held responsible for the content of any website mentioned in this book. It is sometimes possible to find a relocated web page by typing in the address of the home page for a website in the URL window of your browser.

Hachette UK's policy is to use papers that are natural, renewable and recyclable products and made from wood grown in well-managed forests and other controlled sources. The logging and manufacturing processes are expected to conform to the environmental regulations of the country of origin.

Orders: please contact Hachette UK Distribution, Hely Hutchinson Centre, Milton Road, Didcot, Oxfordshire, OX11 7HH. Telephone: +44 (0)1235 827827. Email education@hachette.co.uk Lines are open from 9 a.m. to 5 p.m., Monday to Friday.

You can also order through our website: www.hoddereducation.co.uk

ISBN: 978-1-3983-4740-3

© Stephen Hoare, Judith Adams and Mary Riley 2022

First published in 2022 by
Hodder Education,
An Hachette UK Company
Carmelite House
50 Victoria Embankment
London EC4Y 0DZ

www.hoddereducation.co.uk

Impression number 10 9 8 7 6 5 4 3 2

Year   2026 2025 2024 2023 2022

Cover photo © E+/SDI Productions/Getty Images

Illustrations by Integra Software Services Pvt. Ltd., Pondicherry, India.

Typeset in India by Integra Software Services Pvt. Ltd.

Printed and bound by CPI Group (UK) Ltd, Croydon, CR0 4YY

A catalogue record for this title is available from the British Library.

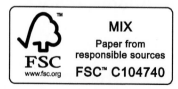

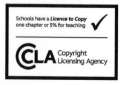

Contents

Answers can be found online at: www.hoddereducation.co.uk/subjects/health-social-care/products/t-level/health-t-level-core

Acknowledgements

Stephen Hoare

I would like to thank my wife, Janet, for her patience and forbearance during all the hours I was tied to the computer. Also to Rachel and her colleagues at Hodder Education for their support. Finally, to the NCFE reviewers for their helpful and constructive criticisms and suggestions.

Judith Adams

Thank you to Ruth Murphy, Rachel Edge and the team at Hodder for their huge support, advice and editorial guidance. I would also like to thank my friend and co-author Mary for her support during this project.

A special thank you to Paul for kindly sharing his experience of health implants – it was invaluable.

Love and thanks to Tony for the endless cups of coffee and for always being there.

Mary Riley

I would like to thank Ruth Murphy, Rachel Edge and Emma Coopshon for all their expert help as well as their patience throughout this process.

Also a big thank you to my husband, Ian, for his constant support and forbearance.

Photo credits

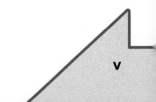

Guide to the book

The following features can be found in this book.

Learning outcomes

Core knowledge outcomes that you must understand and learn. These are presented at the start of every chapter.

Key term

Definitions to help you understand important terms.

Reflect

Tasks and questions providing an opportunity to reflect on the knowledge learned.

Test yourself

A knowledge consolidation feature containing short questions and tasks to aid understanding and guide you to think about a topic in detail.

Research

Research-based activities – either stretch and challenge activities, enabling you to go beyond the course, or industry placement-based activities, encouraging you to discover more about your placement.

Practice points

Helpful tips and guidelines to help develop professional skills during the industry placement.

Case study

Placing knowledge into a fictionalised, real-life context. Useful to introduce problem-solving and dilemmas.

Health and safety

Important points to ensure safety in the workplace.

Project practice

Short scenarios and 1–3 focused activities, at the end of each chapter, reflecting one or more of the tasks that you will need to undertake during completion of the ESP. These support the development of the four core skills required.

Assessment practice

Core content containing knowledge-based practice questions at the end of each chapter.

Answers can be found online at: www.hoddereducation.co.uk/subjects/health-social-care/products/t-level/health-t-level-core

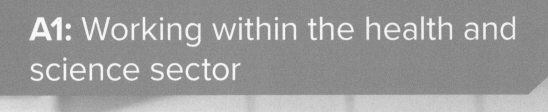

A1: Working within the health and science sector

Introduction

The health and science sector covers a wide range of organisations and employers as well as a wide range of jobs. Despite this variety, all well-run organisations usually have a common approach based around:

▶ policies and procedures
▶ quality
▶ ethics
▶ professionalism
▶ investment in the development and progression of their employees.

We will cover these aspects in this chapter and will expand on some points in future chapters.

Learning outcomes

The core knowledge outcomes that you must understand and learn:

A1.1 the purpose of organisational policies and procedures in the health and science sector

A1.2 the importance of adhering to quality standards, quality management and audit processes within the health and science sector

A1.3 the key principles of ethical practice in the health and science sector

A1.4 the purpose of following professional codes of conduct

A1.5 the difference between technical, higher technical and professional occupations in health, healthcare science and science, as defined by the Institute for Apprenticeships and Technical Education occupational maps

A1.6 opportunities to support progression within the health and science sector.

A1.1 The purpose of organisational policies and procedures in the health and science sector

In our professional lives we must maintain high standards out of respect for ourselves, our colleagues and those who require our services – customers, patients, etc. It is not enough to have good intentions; we need policies to consult and procedures to follow so that we know we are always working to the highest standards.

Equality, diversity and inclusion policy

Sometimes we can act in a way that is discriminatory without even realising it. If we stop and put ourselves in the other person's place, we might realise the effect our actions would have. Even if we do that, we may still have room to improve. That is why we have policies that cover equality, diversity and inclusion in the workplace which make it clear how to behave (Figure 1.1).

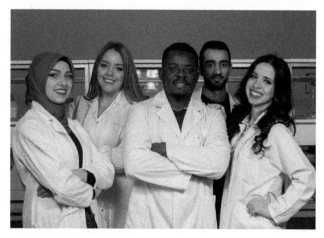

▲ Figure 1.1 Equality, diversity and inclusion should be central to our professional lives

Complying with legislation

One very good reason for having policies that cover equality, diversity and inclusion is to ensure that we comply with the relevant legislation. The main piece of legislation in the UK is the **Equality Act 2010**.

This gives legal protection from discrimination in the workplace and in wider society. Before this **law** came into force, there were several laws that covered discrimination, including:

► Sex Discrimination Act 1975
► Race Relations Act 1976
► Disability Discrimination Act 1995.

Replacing these and other laws with a single Act made the law easier to understand and gave increased protection in some areas. The Act sets out the different ways in which it is unlawful to treat someone. The Equality Act 2010 is administered by the **Government Equalities Office**, which has produced an easy-to-read publication called 'The Equality Act – making equality real'. You can find this by carrying out an internet search using this title.

Key term

Laws (legislation): passed by Parliament. They state the rights and entitlements of individuals and provide legal rules that have to be followed. The law is upheld through the courts. If an individual or care setting breaks the law by, for example, inappropriately sharing or inaccurately recording information, they can, in certain circumstances, be fined, dismissed or given a prison sentence.

Ensuring equality

The Equality Act places responsibility on employers, providers of goods and services, caregivers, public sector bodies, private clubs and associations, voluntary organisations and many others not to discriminate on the basis of:

► age
► disability
► gender reassignment
► pregnancy and maternity
► race – this includes ethnic or national origins, colour and nationality
► religion or belief
► sex
► sexual orientation.

Eliminating discrimination

These are called **protected characteristics**. By having policies in place to cover these aspects of equality, and promoting diversity and inclusion, organisations can ensure that they comply with the law and also benefit from treating everyone fairly and equally.

We should also be aware of **indirect discrimination**. This is where there is a practice, policy or rule that applies to everyone in the same way but could have a worse effect on some people than others. Here are two examples of indirect discrimination:

▶ A woman has been on maternity leave. On return to work, she makes a flexible working request so that she can reduce her hours and look after her child instead of using childcare. Her manager refuses her request and says everyone doing that job must work full-time. This could be indirect sex discrimination.

▶ A Jewish woman works in a large store. She is told that because of a change in shifts, she now must work one Saturday a month. She explains that, as an observant Jew, she cannot work on Saturdays (the Sabbath). Her manager tells her that it would be unfair to everyone else if she were allowed not to work on Saturdays. This could be indirect religious discrimination.

Safeguarding policies

Safeguarding means ensuring individuals are protected from harm. The NHS England website is a useful source of information about safeguarding in the context of healthcare. Its definition of safeguarding is worth consulting:

> 'Safeguarding means protecting a citizen's health, wellbeing and human rights; enabling them to live free from harm, abuse and neglect. It is an integral part of providing high-quality health care. Safeguarding children, young people and adults is a collective responsibility.'
>
> Source: www.england.nhs.uk/safeguarding/about/

Note that the policy specifies 'children, young people and adults' – basically, everyone. We probably think of children and young people as being in greater need of protection. However, adults can also be vulnerable and require protection, such as people with learning difficulties or those with a physical or mental disability.

That is why safeguarding policies are required in all organisations, not just in those dealing with children, young people or the elderly. Organisations in the science sector also require proper safeguarding policies covering employees, customers and others they come into contact with, including visitors.

Chapter A11 covers safeguarding in more detail (see pages 196–228).

DBS checks

There are many situations where you might be working with children or vulnerable adults, such as in healthcare, childcare, education or a voluntary organisation such as Scouts or a youth club. In such situations, the employer or organisation is responsible for checking whether you have a criminal record. This is done through the Disclosure and Barring Service (hence the term DBS check – previously known as CRB). Different levels of DBS check are available, depending on how sensitive the job or role is:

▶ A basic check just shows any unspent convictions and conditional cautions. Convictions become 'spent' (i.e. they no longer appear on your criminal record) after a period of time, depending on age and length of sentence (if any).

▶ A standard check shows spent *and* unspent convictions, cautions, reprimands and final warnings.

▶ An enhanced check shows, in addition to the standard check, any information held by local police that is considered relevant to the role.

▶ An enhanced check with barred lists shows the same as an enhanced check plus whether the applicant is on the list of people barred from doing the role, e.g. someone on the sex offenders register.

You can only request a basic check yourself. For more information, search gov.uk for 'DBS'. Take care, because if you just do an internet search for 'DBS' the top results will be for commercial organisations that want to sell you a DBS check.

Employment contracts

Every employee has an employment contract with their employer. The contract does not have to be written down – in fact, as soon as someone accepts a job offer, they have a contract with their employer. This means that if either side backs out (for example, the employer withdraws the job offer or the employee decides to take a different job), they could risk legal action for compensation. The employment contract is an agreement that sets out:

▶ employment conditions
▶ rights
▶ responsibilities
▶ duties.

Both employer and employee must stick to the terms of the contract until it ends. That will happen when either side gives notice, i.e. when the employee announces they will be leaving, or the employer decides to end their employment (for example, through redundancy), or an employee is dismissed (they lose their job). The terms of the contract can be changed, usually by agreement between both sides.

Do not confuse an employment contract with a 'contract to provide services', such as when you agree with someone that they will paint your house or mow your lawn. In those circumstances, the decorator or gardener does not become your employee.

The legal parts of a contract are known as the **terms**; these are legally binding on both parties. Contract terms can take different forms:

▶ a written contract or statement of employment
▶ a verbal agreement
▶ in an offer letter from the employer
▶ in an employee handbook, on a company noticeboard or intranet.

Some terms are required by law, such as the requirement to pay at least the National Minimum Wage to all employees over 18 years of age (and the rate called the National Living Wage for people aged 23 and over), or the right to a minimum of paid holiday.

Practice point

You can find the minimum wage for your age group on the Gov.uk website:
www.gov.uk/national-minimum-wage-rates

Some contracts are based on **collective agreements**. This is where the employer or employers negotiate agreements with trade unions or staff associations which represent a group of employees.

Some terms might be **implied** rather than clearly agreed. Examples include:

▶ Employees should not steal from their employer.
▶ Your employer must provide a safe and secure working environment.
▶ If a job provides a company car, the employee needs a valid driving licence.
▶ Something that has been done regularly over a long period of time, such as paying an annual bonus or certain days off.

When you start a job, your employer is obliged to give you a **written statement of employment particulars**. This is not an employment contract. There are two statements of employment particulars. The **principal statement** must be provided on the first day of work

and covers things such as:

▶ the employer's name, the employee's name, job title (or description of work) and start date
▶ how much and how often you will be paid
▶ your hours and days of work and how they might change – as well as if you are expected to work Sundays, nights or overtime
▶ how long the job is expected to last (or, if permanent, that it is indefinite), and the end date if it is a fixed-term contract
▶ if there is a probation period, how long it will last and what its conditions are, e.g. to achieve satisfactory performance
▶ other benefits, such as childcare vouchers or free lunches
▶ any obligatory training.

As well as this, on day one an employer must give the employee information about:

▶ sick pay and procedures
▶ other paid leave, such as maternity and paternity leave
▶ notice periods, both from the employer and the employee (they may be different).

Within two months of starting work, the employer must give a **wider written statement** that covers:

▶ pensions and pension schemes
▶ any collective agreements (see above) that might be in place
▶ any right to other (non-compulsory) training provided by (or on behalf of) the employer
▶ disciplinary and grievance procedures (see page 5).

Performance reviews

How do you know that you are doing a good job? You might think you are doing well, but does your employer agree? That is why organisations usually have regular performance reviews for staff. However, this is not just a one-way process.

Performance reviews have several objectives:

▶ Evaluating work performance against standards and expectations: you might have been given targets to achieve or, if you work in a highly regulated sector, you might have formal standards to maintain or strive for.
▶ Giving feedback: a performance review gives your line manager (the person who manages you directly, i.e. your boss) the opportunity to help you improve your performance. You should expect feedback to be supportive and encouraging.

▶ Providing opportunities to raise concerns or issues: performance reviews are not simply about the organisation evaluating your performance, you can also raise any concerns or issues that you have. Try to be non-confrontational – telling your manager exactly what they do wrong and how you could do it so much better might be a career-limiting move!

▶ Contributing to continuing professional development (CPD): this might mean identifying areas where you need more training or education so that you can develop in your work.

Disciplinary policy

If your employer has concerns about your work, conduct or absence from work (including sickness absence), initially they should raise these concerns in an informal way. However, they can go straight to formal **disciplinary** or even dismissal procedures. A disciplinary procedure is a formal way for an employer to deal with an employee's unacceptable or improper behaviour (this is known as misconduct) or their performance (lack of capability).

Part of this process is that the employer should set and maintain expected standards of work and conduct. You need to know what is expected of you before you can be disciplined for not achieving it!

The disciplinary policy should also ensure consistent and fair treatment of all employees; there should be no favouritism, nor should individual employees feel picked on or bullied.

There should be a process for disciplinary action. This will be part of the disciplinary policy that all employers must have. You should have been given details of this process as part of the wider written statement of employment particulars that you receive within two months of starting work. This should say what performance and behaviour might lead to disciplinary action and what action your employer might take. It should also include the name of someone that you can speak to if you do not agree with your employer's decision.

Your employer's disciplinary procedure should include the following steps:

▶ A letter setting out the disciplinary issue.

▶ A meeting to discuss the issue; the employee should have the right to be accompanied by a colleague or trade union representative at this meeting. Some employers may have a policy of allowing a wider range of people to accompany you, such as a friend or relative.

▶ A decision about the disciplinary issue. This might result in no further action, a first or final written warning, dismissal (i.e. losing your job) or some other sanction.

▶ A chance to appeal the decision.

Grievance policy

In a well-run organisation, there will be open communication and consultation between managers and their staff. This means that problems and concerns can be raised quickly and settled as part of the normal working relationship.

However, anyone working in an organisation may have problems or concerns about their work or working conditions; they may have problems in their relationships with colleagues. These are all **grievances** that employees want to be addressed and, if possible, resolved. As well as this, the management will want to resolve any problems before they develop into major difficulties.

> **Key term**
>
> *Grievance:* any concern, problem or complaint you may have at work. If you take this up with your employer, it is called 'raising a grievance'.

Issues that may cause grievances include:
▶ terms and conditions of employment
▶ health and safety issues and concerns (see Chapter A3)
▶ relationships with colleagues and management
▶ bullying and harassment
▶ working practices, particularly when new practices are introduced
▶ the working environment
▶ changes in the organisation
▶ discrimination – or perceived discrimination.

However, there may be occasions where an employee has a grievance against their line manager and this needs a different approach.

As with disciplinary procedures, all employers should have a written grievance procedure. This should explain what to do if you have a grievance and what happens at each stage in the process. It should provide opportunities for employees to confidentially raise and address grievances. There should be a sequence for raising and resolving grievances. This will usually involve a meeting to discuss the issue. As with disciplinary procedures, you can appeal if you do not agree with your employer's decision.

Key term

Employment tribunals: responsible for hearing claims from people who think an employer has treated them unlawfully, for example, through unfair dismissal or discrimination.

A1.2 The importance of adhering to quality standards, quality management and audit processes

Adhering to quality standards should be central to any organisation's way of working. Those standards may be national or international standards such as British Standard or ISO (the International Organization for Standardization) or the organisation's own internal quality standards. In the health and science sector, quality standards help improve the quality of care or service provided.

Ensuring consistency

One reason for adhering to quality standards is to ensure **consistency** – always obtaining the same, high-quality outcome.

Reflect

Quality and consistency are terms you will encounter a lot, both in this book and in your working life. Think about how we should always strive for both quality and consistency. If you go to a restaurant, you want the food to be consistently good. If it is consistently bad, you probably will not want to go. But what about a restaurant that is inconsistent? You might occasionally get a good meal, but is it worth a gamble? An organisation should always strive to achieve consistently high quality.

Maintaining health and safety

You will learn, in subsequent chapters, how adhering to proper procedures can help avoid (or at least reduce) accidents and harm to employees, service or care receivers or the general public.

This is covered in most detail in Chapter A3 Health, safety and environmental regulations in the health and science sector.

Monitoring processes and procedures

It is not good enough to intend to do something properly, you must do it. This applies to doing a favour for a friend but is even more important in the workplace. That is why there will often be a check sheet on the wall of a public toilet showing that it has been cleaned according to the required schedule.

This will be covered in more detail in Chapter A7 Good scientific and clinical practice.

Case study

In the summer of 2015, the Smiler roller coaster at the Alton Towers theme park crashed, causing life-altering injuries to four riders (two teenagers had to undergo amputations). The Health & Safety Executive (HSE) report found that there were no mechanical failings in the track, the cars or the system designed to keep the cars separate. The investigation identified a number of human errors that led to the crash. However, the HSE investigators found that Merlin Entertainments (the operator of the theme park) had multiple failings in not performing an adequate risk assessment and not having proper procedures to prevent a series of errors by staff, leading to harm to the public. As a result, Merlin Attractions was fined £5 million.

Do you think 'human error' is ever a valid defence or excuse when harm is caused to employees, patients, care-receivers or members of the public?

Facilitating continuous improvement

Continuous improvement means making many, often small, improvements over time. The success of the GB Olympic cycling team in recent years has been due, in part, to an approach that looks for many tiny performance improvements – in athlete training, equipment or clothing, for example. Each one might shave a hundredth or even a thousandth of a second off a lap time. Cumulatively, they have contributed to many gold medals being won.

We can take the same approach in a science, health or healthcare environment. It starts with adopting quality standards and adhering to them, monitoring performance against those standards and then looking for ways to improve performance.

Facilitating objective, independent review

Audit processes might be a legal requirement – see Chapter A7 for examples. But an audit really means asking the question: 'Did we achieve what we set out to achieve?' We need to have processes that ensure we ask that question in an objective and independent way so that we get useful answers. If we did not achieve our objective, what can we do to achieve it in future? If we did achieve our objective, are there ways we can improve further?

Practice points

Quality control (QC) means the testing of a product to ensure that it meets required standards. The QC department in an organisation will be responsible for testing products before they are sold. Any product that fails QC tests will have to be reworked or scrapped.

Quality assurance (QA) means having procedures in place that ensure that the product will always meet the required standards.

Which do you think is more important, QC or QA?

A1.3 The key principles of ethical practice in the health and science sector

We are probably all aware of medical ethics – the need for medical professionals to adhere to a set of values or moral principles. This provides a framework for analysing a situation and deciding on the best course of action to take. We will expand upon that in this section. However, aspects of ethical practice are important in all areas of health and science, as we will see.

Beneficence

Put simply, **beneficence** means 'doing good'. All healthcare professionals need to follow the course of action that they believe to be in the best interest of their patient. However, 'doing good' is often too simple in the real world. It is better to think of beneficence as ranking the possible options for a patient, from best to worst, taking account of:
- Will the option resolve the medical problem?
- Is it proportionate to the scale of the problem?
- Is it compatible with the patient's individual circumstances?
- Are the option and its outcomes in line with the patient's expectations?

Several of these points are related to the patient's circumstances or expectations. This forms the basis of patient-centred or person-centred care. This will be expanded on in Chapter A8: Providing person-centred care.

Nonmaleficence

If you have seen the 2014 Disney movie 'Maleficent' you can probably work out that **maleficence** means 'doing harm', so **nonmaleficence** must mean 'not doing harm'. In that sense, beneficence (doing good) and nonmaleficence (not doing harm) go together. In the science and healthcare sector we all have a duty of both beneficence and nonmaleficence to those we are responsible for.

You can think of nonmaleficence as a threshold for treatment. In other words, if a treatment causes more harm than good then we should not consider it. That is different to beneficence, where we consider all the valid treatment options and then rank them in order of preference or benefit to the patient. A treatment could still be the most beneficial and cause more harm than good.

Another difference is that we usually think of beneficence in response to a specific situation – what is the best treatment for a patient? However, nonmaleficence is something that should always be considered in a healthcare setting. If you see someone collapse, you have a duty to provide (or seek) help for that person. Because we must try to prevent harm, it will be better for that person to receive medical attention than to be left there. Even if you are not qualified or able to help, you can at least make sure that help is given or called for (e.g. by calling 999).

We have described beneficence and nonmaleficence in the context of a doctor providing medical treatment. However, the same principles apply to all health workers who are providing care.

Reflect

Here are some factors to consider in the context of nonmaleficence:
▶ What are the risks associated with intervening or not intervening?
▶ Do I have the skills necessary to help this person or carry out this action?
▶ Are any other factors (staff shortages, lack of resources, etc.) putting the person at risk?
▶ Is this person being treated with dignity and respect?

Autonomy and informed consent

Autonomy means that everyone has the right to make the final decision about their care or treatment. That means that, as caregivers, we cannot impose care or treatment on any individual, with some limited exceptions (see below).

This has not always been the case – there have been many instances of 'doctor knows best' in the past and some people might still feel the need to defer to what they see as an authority figure.

Informed consent means that before making that final decision, a person receiving care or treatment has the right to be given all the relevant information about the care or treatment. This might include the benefits, the potential risks and what might happen if the care or treatment is not given.

In some cases, the person may not have the **capacity** to give informed consent. To have capacity, the person must be able to:
▶ understand the information they are given
▶ retain that information long enough to make a decision
▶ weigh up or assess the information to make a decision
▶ communicate their decision.

If the person does not have capacity to give informed consent, the principles of beneficence and nonmaleficence should be applied. In some cases, for example, with children, the parent or guardian would have to give consent.

According to UK law, adults are over 18 years. However, 16- and 17-year-olds are considered able to give informed consent without the need for a parent. Children under 16 can also give informed consent, provided they have sufficient capacity – intelligence, competence and understanding.

In some cases, the beliefs of a parent (e.g. religious beliefs) may lead them to oppose a course of treatment that healthcare staff believe to be in the interests of the child. In such cases it might be necessary to obtain a court order to overrule the parent's wishes. Of course, this might not be possible in an emergency. In such cases, the principles of beneficence and nonmaleficence should be applied. However, this might result in the parent taking legal action. Ethical issues are not always straightforward!

Truthfulness and confidentiality

Confidentiality is central to the relationship between patients, care-receivers or the general public on the one hand and science and healthcare staff on the other. Lack of confidentiality may lead to loss of trust; if a patient feels their confidential information may be disclosed without their consent, they may withhold necessary information or even avoid seeking treatment – either way, they are less likely to receive appropriate treatment.

Truthfulness is an obligation on the part of science and healthcare staff. We have an obligation to be truthful, whether that is answering a patient's questions or reporting the results of experiments or analysis. Being truthful with patients is important, even if it might lead to them deciding against a course of action or treatment that we think will be beneficial for them. This is a consequence of informed consent that healthcare staff must accept.

Reflect

How would you apply the principles we have covered to help you deal with the following situations?
- A colleague has told you that they have a drink problem, but that it does not affect their work. You, however, are not sure because you have noticed that they are not always fully attentive and even show signs of being drunk on duty.
- A friend has asked if you can access their partner's medical records as they believe the partner is having an affair and they are worried about STIs (sexually transmitted infections).
- A patient tells you that they have been using illegal drugs.

Justice

Justice can mean fairness, equality and respect for all. Therefore, when we decide whether something is ethical or not, we must think about:
- Is it legal or compatible with the law?
- Is it fair?
- Does it respect the person's right and equality?
- Does it show respect for all concerned?

A1.4 The purpose of following professional codes of conduct

Whatever area of science, health or healthcare we work in, it is likely that we will be expected to follow specific professional **codes of conduct**. It is not enough to have good intentions; we need to achieve good outcomes – codes of conduct are one way to help ensure that.

Professional codes of conduct may be written by professional societies or organisations. Some examples, covering a diverse range of professions, include:
- The Nursing and Midwifery Council (NMC)
- The Royal College of Nursing (RCN)
- The Health Care Compliance Association (HCCA)
- The Royal Society of Chemistry (RSC)
- The Institute of Food Science & Technology (IFST)
- The Science Council
- The Royal Society of Biology (RSB)
- The Society of Radiographers (SoR)
- The Health and Care Professions Council (HCPC)
- The British Association of Sport and Exercise Sciences (BASES)
- The Institute of Biomedical Science (IBMS).

There are many more. Members of these societies or organisations are expected to follow the code of conduct.

In addition, many organisations in the science, health and healthcare sectors have their own codes of conduct:
- Government agencies, such as Public Health England.
- Private companies, such as HCA Healthcare UK.
- Employer-led bodies such as the Sector Skills Councils, including Skills for Care and Skills for Health.

Professional codes of conduct will usually follow the same format:
- They clarify the missions (aims) of the organisation and its values and principles.
- They clarify the standards that everyone must adhere to.
- They outline expected professional behaviours and attitudes.
- They outline rules and responsibilities within organisations.
- They promote confidence in the organisation and profession.

A1.5 The difference between technical, higher technical and professional occupations in health, healthcare science and science, as defined by the IfATE occupational maps

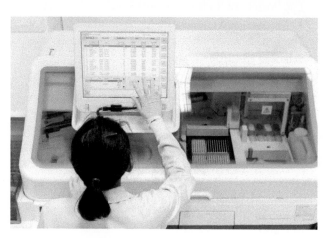

▲ Figure 1.2 Modern laboratory equipment needs qualified and highly trained staff

The Institute for Apprenticeships and Technical Education (IfATE) is an employer-led organisation sponsored by the Department for Education. A key element in the work of the Institute is to support employer groups in developing apprenticeships.

The Institute also maintains the **occupational maps** that underpin technical education. These occupational maps show where technical education can lead. They group occupations that have related knowledge, skills and behaviours into **pathways** so that it is easier to see opportunities for career progression within a particular route. Within each pathway, occupations at the same **level** are grouped into clusters to show how skills you have learned can be applied to other related occupations (Figure 1.2).

This is a small selection of the qualifications available at each level:
▶ Level 1 qualifications:
  – GCSE grades 3 to 1 or D to G
  – Level 1 NVQ.
▶ Level 2 qualifications:
  – GCSE grades 9 to 4 or A* to C
  – Intermediate apprenticeship
  – Level 2 award, certificate or diploma.
▶ Level 3 qualifications:
  – AS/A Level
  – T Level
  – Advanced apprenticeship.
▶ Level 4 qualifications:
  – Higher apprenticeship
  – Higher national certificate (HNC).
▶ Level 5 qualifications:
  – Foundation degree
  – Diploma of higher education (DipHE)
  – Higher national diploma (HND).
▶ Level 6 qualifications:
  – Ordinary or honours degree, e.g. BA, BSc.
▶ Level 7 qualifications:
  – Master's degree, e.g. MA, MSc, MChem, Meng.
▶ Level 8 qualifications:
  – Doctorate, e.g. PhD or DPhil.

For a full list, visit **www.gov.uk** and search for 'What qualification levels mean'.

Technical

These are skilled occupations that a college leaver or an apprentice would be entering, typically requiring qualifications at levels 2/3. Examples include:
▶ adult care worker/lead care worker
▶ healthcare support worker

- dental nurse
- food technologist
- laboratory technician.

Higher technical

These are occupations that require more knowledge and skills. This could be acquired through experience in the workplace or further technical education. They typically require qualifications at levels 4/5. Examples include:

- lead practitioner in adult care
- healthcare assistant practitioner
- nursing associate
- dental technician
- food testing/laboratory manager
- technician scientist.

Professional

These are all occupations where there is a clear career progression from higher technical occupations, as well as occupations where a degree apprenticeship exists (level 6). Examples include:

- social worker
- healthcare science practitioner
- registered nurse or midwife .
- biochemist/biologist/chemist/physicist
- research scientist.

> **Research**
>
> You can view the latest occupational maps on the Institute for Apprenticeships & Technical Education website (**www.instituteforapprenticeships.org/about/occupational-maps**) or search online for 'Institute for Apprenticeships occupational maps'.
>
> Were you able to find relevant information? Will this be a useful resource to help you to plan your career?

A1.6 Opportunities to support progression within the health and science sector

When you were a child, what did you want to be when you grew up? Is that still what you want to do? Some people seem able to plan their careers and then pursue their objectives with single-minded determination. Others may move from job to job without any clear plan. The former group is usually, but not always, more successful than the latter. Whichever category you fall into, the end of your T Level course is just the beginning. It helps if you have a plan as to how you can

progress in your career. Even if you are not sure where you want to go, at the very least you should be aware of the opportunities that are available.

> **Research**
>
> Although it is more relevant to the science sector than health or healthcare sectors, the Royal Society of Chemistry offers a 'careers toolkit' of online resources to its members.
>
> Other professional bodies in your field may offer something similar. You should use all the resources and sources of advice and information available to you. Look at the professional bodies listed in section A1.4. Are any of those relevant to your chosen field of work? If so, their website might have useful resources. Make a list of sources of help and information about how to progress your career.

Undertaking further/higher education programmes

As you come to finish your T Level, it is a good idea to have already planned your next move. You will have achieved a level 3 qualification, so you should normally consider moving on to a level 4 or level 5 qualification, unless you decide to change track – in which case there will be a range of other level 3 qualifications that might be suitable.

If you plan to remain in the science, health or healthcare sector, you will probably consider a level 4 or level 5 qualification appropriate to your chosen field of work, such as Higher Technical Qualifications. In some cases this will mean that you have to become registered with a statutory regulator, such as the Nursing and Midwifery Council or the General Dental Council.

Your T Level will be worth UCAS points, so you can continue into higher education (level 5 or 6) at university or with another education provider if you wish.

Undertaking apprenticeship/degree apprenticeship

An **apprenticeship** is a job with training to industry standards and should involve entry into a recognised occupation. Apprenticeships are employer-led, so employers will:

- set the standards the apprentices need to meet
- create the demand for apprentices to meet their skills needs
- fund the apprenticeship, i.e. pay for training

- employ the apprentice, i.e. pay them and give them work
- be responsible for training the apprentice on the job.

The needs of the apprentice are also important. Apprentices are not meant to be simply a source of cheap labour. The apprentice must be able to achieve competence in a skilled occupation. Not only that, but they should also acquire skills that are transferable and offer the possibility of long-term earnings potential, greater security and the ability to progress in the workplace.

A higher apprenticeship (level 4) might lead on naturally from a level 3 T Level, but entry to a level 6 or level 7 degree apprenticeship is also possible. Degree apprenticeships combine working for an employer with studying at a university. Study periods can be on a day-to-day basis or in blocks, depending on the programme and the needs of the employer.

More information about degree apprenticeships is available on the UCAS website (www.ucas.com) or the Institute for Apprenticeships and Technical Education website (www.instituteforapprenticeships.org).

Undertaking continuing professional development (CPD)

Continuing professional development can take many forms. It is a way in which professionals use different learning activities to maintain, develop and enhance their abilities, skills and knowledge. CPD combines different methods of learning, such as:

- conferences and events
- training workshops
- e-learning programmes
- best practice techniques
- ideas sharing
- shadowing a more experienced professional in the field.

CPD programmes are often run by employers or professional bodies such as those described in section A1.4.

Joining professional bodies

Professional bodies fulfil a number of important functions. As well as being the guardians of professional codes of conduct in their area of expertise, they offer CPD programmes.

In some occupations in the science, health and healthcare sectors you need to be registered with a statutory body, such as one of the professional bodies.

Some professional bodies offer **chartered** status. As well as indicating an in-depth knowledge of the field, chartered status is required in some regulated activities that have to be supervised by a **qualified person**, such as production of pharmaceuticals (see section A7.3 for more information). Examples include:

- Chartered Chemist (CChem) administered by the Royal Society of Chemistry
- Chartered Biologist (CBiol) administered by the Royal Society of Biology
- Chartered Physicist (CPhys) administered by the Institute of Physics
- Chartered Scientist (CSci) administered by the Science Council.

Undertaking an internship

Internships can offer valuable experience in a real work environment – particularly if you have not gained this through an apprenticeship. Internships are usually relatively short and often take place during the summer months, as many are designed for university students. Placements are similar, but generally last longer. Internships and placements are usually offered by large companies, such as GSK (which manufactures pharmaceuticals) or Unilever (consumer products). In some cases, you will be paid at least the UK National Living Wage, but in others it can be much higher than this – though some internships are not paid at all. Bursaries are often available to cover your costs in an unpaid internship. Many of the professional bodies already mentioned will offer help with internships, placements or bursaries. Their websites are the best place to look for advice and information.

Undertaking a scholarship

As well as help with bursaries, many of the professional bodies can offer help with scholarships. These are usually available to help with the costs of obtaining higher qualifications, usually at level 6 or level 7. Educational institutions that offer these qualifications may also offer scholarships or can give guidance on what scholarships and other sources of funding are available.

Project practice

You are working in a science/health/healthcare organisation (choose one according to your own area of work). You have been asked to produce materials to help new apprentices understand the importance of the working practices of the organisation, as well as to inform them about the ways in which their careers might develop.

1   Prepare a summary of the organisation policies that you are aware of in your organisation, or ones that you know should be in place. Give explanations for the relevance and importance of these.

2   Research the professional codes of practice relevant to your area of work. This might require you to use the websites of any relevant professional bodies to gather information.

3   Prepare a list of the types of CPD that are available or recommended in your organisation.

4   Finally, outline the additional ways in which apprentices can progress in their careers.

You should present the information in the form of a poster or short written document, such as an employee handbook.

Assessment practice

1   What piece of legislation covers the requirement for diversity and inclusion for people with certain characteristics?

2   Who is responsible for obtaining a DBS check for work?

3   What is the name for the legal parts of an employment contract?

4   What are collective agreements?

5   Your employer has a disciplinary policy that includes informal and formal written warnings. You have been found stealing and dismissed. You feel that you have been treated unfairly because you were not given any warnings or a notice period. Are you correct?

6   Give **two** reasons why an organisation needs an equality, diversity and inclusion policy.

7   Explain, using an example, what is meant by safeguarding.

8   Give **two** reasons why organisations adhere to quality standards.

9   During the early stages of the COVID-19 pandemic, there were serious concerns that NHS hospitals would be overwhelmed and unable to treat patients. Therefore, hospitals were instructed by the government to discharge any patients who could be transferred back to their care homes. In many cases this led to the introduction of COVID-19 into care homes from hospitals because patients were not tested for COVID-19 or were known to be infected.

Evaluate this instruction, considering the key principles of ethical practice.

Your response should demonstrate:
 –   reasoned judgements
 –   informed conclusions.

A2: The healthcare sector

Introduction

This unit gives an overview of the healthcare sector, its historical context and development over time. We will discuss the diverse nature of services provided, where they fit into the national framework and how they are funded.

Many areas of healthcare now use advanced technology to deliver care and monitor patients. Some of these advances, such as using a health app on your phone, you may have tried out; others including artificial intelligence and assistive computer technology, you may not have experienced. Use of technological innovations is explored and their benefits for patient care and treatment evaluated.

Job descriptions and career pathways in the healthcare sector are covered along with the benefits of evidence-based practice and multidisciplinary team working. The importance of following national, organisational and departmental policies and the consequences of not doing so are examined.

Public health is concerned with protecting, and improving, the health of the population rather than focusing on the health of the individual. The final part of the unit focuses on the public health approach to healthcare and how this benefits regional and national population health through prevention and improvement initiatives.

Learning outcomes

The core knowledge outcomes that you must understand and learn:

A2.1 the diversity of employers and organisations within the healthcare sector

A2.2 the characteristics of primary, secondary and tertiary healthcare tiers

A2.3 the diverse range of personal factors that would dictate the services accessed by an individual including barrier to service access

A2.4 how the use of different developments in technology supports the healthcare sector

A2.5 the origins of the healthcare sector and how this has developed into the healthcare sector we have today

A2.6 the potential impacts of future developments in the healthcare sector in relation to care provision

A2.7 the importance of adhering to national, organisational and departmental policies in the healthcare sector including the possible consequences of not following policy

A2.8 the different ways in which the sectors are funded

A2.9 the meaning of evidence-based practice, its application and how it benefits and improves the healthcare sector

A2.10 the different types of organisational structures within the healthcare sector and the resulting job roles

A2.11 the importance of job descriptions and person specifications and how this defines roles and responsibilities

A2.12 the career pathway opportunities for employment and progression within the healthcare sector as defined by the Institute for Apprenticeships and Technical Education occupational maps

A2.13 the potential impact of external factors on the activities of the healthcare sector

A2.14 the role of public health approaches and how this benefits regional and national population health through prevention and improvement initiatives.

A2.1 The diversity of employers and organisations within the healthcare sector

A wide range of local and national healthcare provision is in place to meet the diverse needs of individuals in society.

NHS

The National Health Service is provided by the state, funded by the taxpayer, with the government (UK, Scottish and Welsh) responsible for making decisions about funding allocation and policy. It provides healthcare, free at the point of use (other than some prescription and dental charges) throughout the United Kingdom.

NHS England, the body responsible for managing national health provision in England, aims to improve the population's quality of life by providing the care, support and treatment needed. Prevention of ill-health and the promotion of healthy living lifestyles are also key aspects of national health and social care provision. Clinical **commissioning** groups (CCGs) provide services needed by the client groups in a local area, matching the services provided to the needs of the local population. For example, some areas have a large elderly population, whereas others have more families. These groups will require different combinations or balances of services.

The organisations making up the NHS include:
▶ national bodies that oversee and regulate NHS services
▶ CCGs that plan and commission care for local populations
▶ healthcare provider organisations:
  – primary care organisations – independent businesses offering NHS services, including GP practices, dental practices, opticians
  – acute (hospital) trusts – providers of hospital-based NHS services
  – mental health trusts – organisations offering mental health and social care services
  – community trusts – providers of community-based services, such as district nursing, physiotherapy and speech and language therapy

  – ambulance trusts – organisations offering NHS transportation services, emergency and non-emergency care
  – charities and social enterprises – organisations providing support services to the NHS.

As you can see, the NHS is actually made up of multiple organisations. Also, the NHS does not just have clinical roles – it has more than 350 different roles available in a wide variety of areas, not just in healthcare. Each individual organisation has its own recruitment team and list of vacancies.

Private healthcare

Private healthcare services are not owned or run by the government but by private individuals or corporations. Private care providers usually charge a fee for their services. They are businesses and work to make a profit. Examples include private residential care homes, BUPA and Nuffield Health Hospitals, non-NHS dentists, and opticians. Some of the services private organisations provide may not be available from the state sector, i.e. provided by the NHS; examples include some cosmetic surgery, cosmetic dental procedures, pharmacists and **IVF**.

Private/non-profit organisations

A **non-profit organisation** is a business whose aim is not to make money for directors, owners or shareholders; rather, its purpose is to provide a benefit to society, usually in the form of help and support for individuals in need.

Key terms

Commissioning: the process of planning and agreeing health services that are needed in a local area.

IVF: in vitro fertilisation. A fertility treatment in which an egg is fertilised by sperm in a test tube and then the fertilised egg is implanted in the uterus.

Third sector: also called the voluntary sector. An umbrella term for **non-profit making organisations** and other organisations that are not public (i.e. state-run) or private, such as non-governmental organisations (NGOs) and charities.

Charities have a distinct aim to provide a benefit to society and are funded by donations from the community. Not-for-profit organisations and charities are sometimes referred to as **third sector** organisations. Although some staff will be paid to lead and manage the organisation (usually from income received in the form of donations or grants), services are mainly provided by volunteers who do not get paid and who give their time for free. These are private organisations in that their services are not run by the government and they do not have a duty to provide services; instead they provide healthcare and other services because they see a need for them.

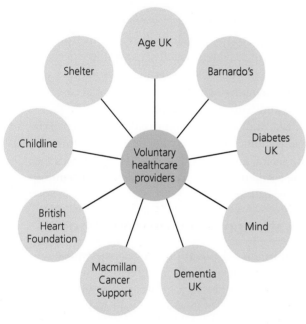

▲ Figure 2.1 Examples of non-profit healthcare providers

Research

Look at the websites of three of the voluntary organisations shown in Figure 2.1. Read about the types of physical and mental health services care and support they can provide.

Find out about the current health-related campaigns they are running.

Working environments

Health services are delivered in a wide range of settings and environments, including in people's own homes as well as in community clinics, community centres and schools, not to mention services delivered in hospitals, GP surgeries and nursing homes.

Beyond NHS services, a much wider network delivers care and support to people in their homes and communities. This includes pharmacies, hospices, nursing homes, home care agencies, voluntary sector services and carers.

Community health services provide support across a range of needs and age groups but are most often used by children, older people, those living with frailty or chronic conditions, and people who are near the end of their life. Community services often support people with multiple, complex health needs who depend on many health and social care services to meet those needs. Health visitors, home care assistants, chiropody, heart failure nurse, occupational therapy, palliative care nursing and school nurses are examples of services provided in the community. This can be, for example, in people's own homes, in residential homes, in schools or at the local GP surgery. The increasing number of people living longer and with long-term conditions means that more people are likely to need support from community health services in the future.

Judicial healthcare ensures that detainees in custody and prisoners get the same healthcare and treatment as anyone outside of prison or custody. Treatment is provided by the NHS and is free of charge but has to be approved by a prison doctor or member of the healthcare team.

Key term

Judicial healthcare: healthcare provided for those individuals detained in prison and detainees who are kept in police custody before being charged with an offence. Also involves the Youth Offending Team which aims to engage young people in health education, and reduce drugs and alcohol misuse in the local area.

Most problems are dealt with by the prison healthcare team. If they cannot do this, the prison may:

▶ ask an expert/specialist to visit the prison
▶ arrange for treatment in an outside hospital.

Prisoners and custody detainees are offered specialist support, for example, if they have:

▶ drug addiction problems
▶ alcohol problems
▶ a disability
▶ a learning difficulty.

A prisoner or detainee has the right to refuse medical treatment. However, the healthcare team may follow procedures that enable them to give treatment if the prisoner is not judged capable of making decisions themselves (for example, if they have a mental health condition). Wherever possible, the healthcare team will discuss this with the prisoner's family first.

Case study

Healthcare in custody

John is arrested by the police and is taken to the custody suite – a large, specialised building that contains cells where individuals who have been arrested have to stay until they have been questioned and charged with a crime or released. On arrival at the custody suite, the sergeant asks John for his personal details and medical history: name, address, current and past health issues, any medication used, any drug dependencies and/or any history of self-harm.

John says he has taken drugs and alcohol in the hours before his arrest, due to feeling anxious and upset about his treatment of his partner. John says he has had a huge and violent argument with his partner, which he now regrets. This argument has led to his arrest. The sergeant uses this information to inform a **risk assessment** for John and it is the basis for deciding the level of care appropriate for John during his stay in custody. As John has taken drugs and been drinking, the sergeant introduces the custody suite's **healthcare professional (HCP)** to John.

The HCP wants to carry out an assessment of John's mental and physical health before he is locked in a cell on his own, and so asks John if he would like to have a private chat in the medical room when the sergeant has finished booking him into custody. John agrees to having a chat with the HCP.

Following the chat, the HCP recommends to the sergeant that John is placed in a camera cell so that he can be observed, and that he should be personally checked by a custody officer regularly until he has sobered up. The HCP has given John some information to read through about counselling services and alcohol/drug support groups. The HCP has also promised to pop in and see John a bit later to see how he is feeling.

▶ Why do you think the HCP has recommended a camera cell and regular checks?
▶ How can the HCP encourage John to reduce his alcohol intake and drug taking?
▶ Can you think of any other aspects of the HCP role in a custody suite?

Key terms

Risk assessment: the process of evaluating the likelihood of a hazard actually causing harm.

Healthcare professional (HCP): someone who looks after the health and welfare of individuals who have been arrested and are kept in custody.

Test yourself

1 Briefly explain three roles within the NHS.
2 Give three examples of private healthcare services.
3 Explain what is meant by a 'non-profit' organisation. Give an example.
4 Other than hospitals, list three examples of healthcare working environments.
5 State two environments where judicial care is provided.

A2.2 The characteristics of primary, secondary and tertiary healthcare tiers

Care provision in the healthcare sector is classified as **primary care**, **secondary care** and **tertiary care**.

Primary care

Primary care (see Figure 2.2) is where an individual has made a first contact with a medical practitioner, usually a **GP**, for advice or treatment. As a result of this first contact the patient will be questioned, probably examined, and may be treated by the GP or referred on to a specialist for further care.

> **Key term**
>
> **GP:** general practitioner. This is the doctor in the local community and is usually based in a health centre or surgery. GPs deliver primary care and will provide initial diagnosis and treatment or will refer the individual to a specialist.

Examples of primary care providers are:
- GP surgery
- dentist
- optician
- walk-in centre
- A&E (accident and emergency department of a hospital)
- NHS 111 telephone service – this is a free service, available 24/7, for people with medical concerns where patients are uncertain about their severity or who to consult. It can save attending A&E unnecessarily and can provide reassuring advice from a professional who will direct patients to call 999 if emergency treatment is required
- community health services such as health visitors and school nurses.

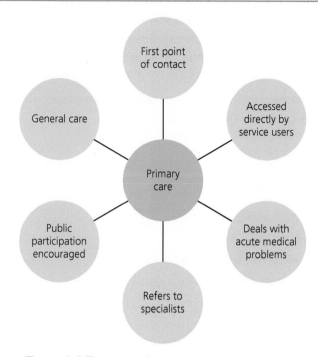

▲ Figure 2.2 Features of primary care

People who need, use and care about healthcare services are encouraged to get involved in providing feedback on local area services. For example, all GP practices must have a **PPG** (**Patient Participation Group**) made up of patients from their practice. These groups regularly meet with staff and talk about how to improve services and promote health for people who use the practice. This public participation can help to influence the provision of services so that they are the most appropriate to meet local needs.

> **Research**
>
> To find out more about the different opportunities for public participation in healthcare provision, use the following links:
>
> www.england.nhs.uk/get-involved – the NHS England website provides a vast library of information for individuals who would like to participate in some way in the work of NHS England.
>
> www.healthwatch.co.uk/your-local-healthwatch/list – local 'Healthwatch' groups give the opportunity for the public to have an input into the type of healthcare services provided in the local area.

Secondary care

Secondary care involves, for example, hospital services where individuals have to attend as **inpatients** or **outpatients**. This could be for investigations, tests or treatment for an illness or condition. It also includes maternity services.

Features of secondary care include:
▶ healthcare services which individuals are referred to, usually by their GP
▶ planned care treating a specific illness, condition or injury, such as carrying out an operation, for example, a hip replacement or removal of tonsils
▶ specialised care, for example, at a clinic that specialises in the illness or condition. This could be a series of appointments with a physiotherapist to help with a sports injury, for example.

Tertiary care

This includes care provided in residential nursing homes, in **hospices**, through mental health services and in the individual's own home.

Features of tertiary care include:
▶ care is often long term
▶ is highly specialised
▶ can be used as respite for families
▶ includes end of life care (**palliative care**).

Tertiary care refers to specialist medical attention provided by practitioners who focus on particular diseases or **anatomical** (body) systems. People typically access this level of treatment through a referral from another care provider. For example, when a GP identifies cancer in a patient, they will be referred to an **oncologist** (a cancer specialist) for a course of chemotherapy, after surgery, for the treatment of the cancer. Another example is where someone is referred for treatment by a specialist burns unit if they have suffered a severe burn injury.

Respite care (also known as short break care) provides specialist care that enables families and carers to have a short break from looking after the person they are caring for. This may be an individual with learning or physical disabilities who needs care and support with daily living tasks. Provision of specialist short breaks care helps and supports carers to take time out to focus on their own needs and helps stop them becoming run down and exhausted by the demands of providing continuing care.

End of life care is personalised care provided by specialist teams of professionals such as community nurses, Macmillan nurses and sometimes also volunteers. It supports the person to live as well as possible until they die. Alongside taking care of the ill individual's physical needs, end of life care takes a **holistic approach**, helping with their emotional, spiritual and social needs. The team will also support carers, family members and close friends of the individual.

End of life care can be provided by hospices. These are specialist care settings that can provide a range of services to support individuals. Some hospice care is provided by charitable organisations such as Marie Curie Cancer Care and Sue Ryder services.

Key terms

Hospice: provides support and end of life care to individuals and their families. Hospice care can be provided where individuals choose, for example, at home, in a hospice room at a hospital, in a nursing home or at a Marie Curie hospice.

Palliative care: aims to achieve the best quality of life possible, as actively as possible, until the individual's death from a terminal illness. It is a holistic approach and supports the individual and their family.

Respite care: offers a break for carers from caring responsibilities, while the person they care for is looked after by someone else. Increasingly known as 'short breaks' care because of negative implications of 'respite', i.e. that the cared-for person is a burden.

Holistic approach: a way of approaching the delivery of healthcare that considers the whole person, not just the part that requires physical treatment. It also takes into account an individual's intellectual, emotional and social needs.

Inpatient: patient who receives medical treatment, tests, etc. while staying in hospital.

Outpatient: patient who visits a hospital or clinic to have treatment, tests and investigations, but does not have to stay there.

Case study

Read the following case study about young people using a local short break service:

www.longtermplan.nhs.uk/case-studies/youngsters-in-ealing-benefitting-from-anintensive-therapeutic-and-short-break-service/

▶ Discuss the benefits for the young people and their parents of the intensive therapeutic and short break service.

▶ Identify the benefits for the NHS of delivering the service in this way.

Research

Produce a list of healthcare settings or organisations that you know of in your local area.

Classify the care settings/organisations as primary, secondary or tertiary providers.

Practice point

Which type of care does your placement organisation provide?

Give reasons to explain your answer, including:

▶ whether it is a primary, secondary or tertiary care provider

▶ features of the type of care provided.

Reflect

Dr Richard Berman FRCP is NHS England's National Clinical Lead for Enhanced Supportive Care, and a Consultant in Supportive & Palliative Care based at the Christie NHS Foundation Trust:

www.rcplondon.ac.uk/education-practice/interview/specialty-career-profile-palliative-medicine

▶ Read Dr Berman's profile and blog and consider his approach to end of life care:
www.england.nhs.uk/blog/richard-berman/

▶ Discuss with a partner the importance of team working and communication skills in Dr Berman's work.

Test yourself

1 Define the term 'primary care'.
2 Give four examples where primary care would be provided.
3 What does 'public participation' in primary care mean?
4 Explain the features of secondary care.
5 List three features of tertiary care.

A2.3 The diverse range of personal factors that would dictate the services accessed by an individual including barrier to service access

Range of personal factors

Personal factor	Examples of how it affects the services required
Pre-existing health condition such as diabetes	Diabetes management (blood tests at the GP surgery every three months to monitor glucose levels, checks of any wounds as they can heal slowly and cause ulcers, regular eye checks as vision can be affected by diabetes)
Physical disabilities, such as multiple sclerosis	Ongoing support with managing specific symptoms

Physical disabilities are wide-ranging and each may require different types of care and support, whether help with mobility, such as needing walking aids or physiotherapy, for example |
| Mental health disorders – such as anxiety, depression, panic disorder, OCD (obsessive compulsive disorder) | Psychological therapies such as **Cognitive behaviour therapies (CBT)** are often offered by the NHS before prescribing medication. CBT aims to help and enable individuals to change their negative thought patterns by looking at practical ways to improve their state of mind. More detail about mental health therapies can be found on the NHS website: www.nhs.uk/mental-health/talking-therapies-medicine-treatments/talking-therapies-and-counselling |

Personal factor	Examples of how it affects the services required
	Conditions such as anxiety and post-traumatic stress disorder may require antidepressant medication, which is sometimes used to treat people coping with long-term pain. The medication increases the level of certain chemicals in the brain, which can help to relieve their symptoms. Panic disorder is a severe type of anxiety where individuals can feel worried and fearful, which causes them to have panic attacks. Talking therapies and medication are the main treatments (see the NHS website), but treatment will depend on the symptoms being experienced. Obsessive compulsive disorder (OCD) results in repetitive behaviours, such as repetitive cleaning, checking locks or repeatedly checking a baby is breathing. CBT is often used as treatment to help individuals to face their fears. Antidepressant medications can also be given.
Learning difficulties	Annual health checks People with a learning disability sometimes have poor physical and mental health due to health issues not being recognised or conditions not being noticed. This is why the NHS encourages individuals, aged 14 and over, who are on their GP's learning disability register to have an annual health check. Full details of the physical and other checks, and how the check is made accessible for individuals with learning disabilities, can be found on the NHS website using this link: www.nhs.uk/conditions/learning-disabilities/annual-health-checks/
Different ages – infancy, childhood, adulthood, senior years	Common children's illnesses, ageing process Personal factors at different life stages, such as common childhood illnesses and ageing affect the types of services required. See section A8.4 for detailed information about support and services required at different ages in the lifespan

Barriers to accessing healthcare services

There are countless potential reasons why individuals may not access services, but some of the most common types are given in the table. It is important that all healthcare practitioners consider these potential barriers and take responsibility for doing their bit to help individuals overcome them.

Barrier	Examples
Socioeconomic	• Live in a deprived area, unemployed/low income • Can't afford cost of some services, e.g. dentist • Cost of public transport to get there/expensive parking • Don't want to/can't afford to take time off work • Unaware of services/poor education • Unfamiliar with/don't understand medical terminology/jargon
Psychological	• Fear of diagnosis • Embarrassed about their problem • May feel there is a stigma in using the service • Scared, e.g. of dentists
Physical	• Lack of access – no ramps, lifts or disabled parking/toilets • Health services not available at convenient times – e.g. after work or early morning • Sensory impairments not catered for: information not available in Braille or large print, staff not trained in BSL
Cultural and language	• Staff only speaking English • Information only available in English • Service ethnocentric, practitioners not aware of cultural differences • No female staff • Some treatments not acceptable to some cultures
Geographical	• No local services • Lack of transport to get there, e.g. not on a bus route • Waiting lists – may be a long wait for services in some areas

Key term

Cognitive behaviour therapy (CBT): talking and listening therapy which examines how an individual behaves and thinks in order to help change the behaviour that is an issue and ultimately improve mental health.

Test yourself

1 Identify four personal factors that would require access to healthcare services.
2 Give an example for each of the following barriers to accessing healthcare services:
   ▶ socioeconomic
   ▶ psychological
   ▶ physical
   ▶ cultural and language
   ▶ geographical.
3 Describe how **two** different personal factors would influence the services required by an individual.

A2.4 How the use of different developments in technology supports the healthcare sector

Health applications

Evergreen Life

Evergreen Life is an NHS-assured provider of GP online services. The app (Figure 2.3) can be downloaded for free and is designed to enable individuals to build an accurate, up-to-date personal health and wellness record. It also provides a quick way to access GP services and various measures of health. Based on the individual's answers to clinically-reviewed wellbeing questions, the app generates their 'Wellness Score' out of 100 that helps them to see if they're doing all they can to be healthy. It provides practical tips on how to improve their health and wellbeing and monitor personal health goals.

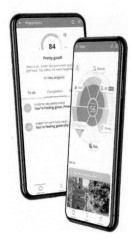

▲ Figure 2.3 Personal health and wellbeing app Evergreen Life

The Evergreen Life app:

▶ helps users to monitor their health goals
▶ connects to their GP – they can order repeat prescriptions, book appointments and view their GP record
▶ enables users to set medication reminders
▶ keeps track of vaccination records
▶ stores and tracks body measurements – for instance, blood pressure and glucose (sugar) levels.

Research

Visit the Evergreen app web page:
www.evergreen-life.co.uk/what-we-do/app-features

Explore what the app can do.
▶ Do you think the app is useful? Give reasons for your answer.
▶ Are there any disadvantages for some people in using an app such as Evergreen Life?

NHS app

The NHS app (**www.nhs.uk/nhs-app/about-the-nhs-app/**) is another app developed for and run by the NHS which allows users (who must be over the age of 13 and registered with a GP in England) access to a variety of common services.

You can also use the NHS app to:

▶ order repeat prescriptions – see your available medicines, request a new repeat prescription and choose a pharmacy for your prescriptions to be sent to
▶ book appointments – search for, book and cancel appointments at your GP surgery, see details of your upcoming and past appointments
▶ get health advice – search trusted NHS information and advice on hundreds of conditions and treatments. You can also answer questions to get instant advice and medical help near you
▶ view your health record – securely access your GP health record to see information like your allergies and your current and past medicines. If your GP surgery has given you access to your detailed medical record, you can also see information such as test results and details of your consultations
▶ register to be an organ donor – choose to donate some or all of your organs and check your registered decision
▶ find out how the NHS uses your data – choose whether data from your health records is shared for research and planning.

After you have downloaded the app, you will need to set up an NHS login and prove who you are. The app then securely connects to information from your GP surgery.

If your device supports fingerprint detection or facial recognition, you can use it to log into the NHS app each time instead of using a password and security code.

> ### Research
>
> Use the link below to find out more about how a range of individuals use the NHS app:
>
> **www.youtube.com/watch?v=I-ubImf5wJs**
>
> Do you think the NHS app would be useful for your own needs?

My Diabetes My Way

My Diabetes My Way is an interactive diabetes website from NHS (Scotland) to help support people who have diabetes and their family and friends.

The website includes content such as:
- information useful for newly diagnosed patients and family members of people with diabetes
- guidance on diet and activity
- information about physical and psychological complications
- how to monitor glucose levels and what they mean
- information about diabetes treatments
- help with managing diabetes during pregnancy and in children and young adults
- personal stories of patients living with diabetes.

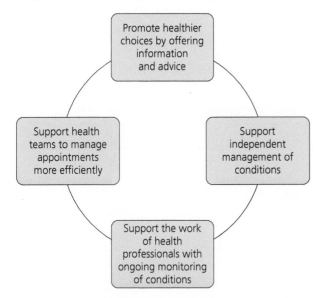

▲ Figure 2.4 Benefits of using health apps

Using health apps has benefits for the individual as well as for the NHS and health professionals (see Figure 2.4). Their use promotes healthy choices and lifestyles, raising awareness of how individuals can independently take control of their health.

Some apps also enable remote monitoring and so can be more convenient for a **practice nurse** or GP to regularly monitor patients without having to make an appointment to visit the surgery, thus reducing the demand on GP services.

> ### Key term
>
> ***Practice nurse:*** based at the GP surgery, offers a range of services including immunisations, diabetes monitoring, cervical smears and general health checks.

Assistive computer technology

Assistive computer technology can be beneficial in that it provides support for healthcare practitioners, enabling them to treat or manage conditions more efficiently. It also provides solutions and treatments that may not have been available previously, such as remote monitoring of heart conditions, 3D printing of prosthetic limbs and robotic surgery, in order to offer improved support and treatment for many health conditions.

CAD/CAM/3D printing

3D printing is the creation of a physical object from a three-dimensional digital **CAD** model. The object is constructed with appropriate material that is joined together layer after layer to create a new version of the design. Although perhaps associated more with engineering, it has been used in a variety of industries, including medicine. Here, imaging techniques such as CT scans, X-rays and ultrasounds can be used to produce a digital model for an object to be printed.

Source: https://medicaldevicescommunity.com/md_news/3d-printing-in-the-medical-field-four-major-applications-revolutionising-the-industry/

> ### Key terms
>
> ***CAD/CAM:*** computer-aided design/computer-aided manufacture.
>
> ***Prosthetics:*** artificial replacements for missing limbs such as a leg, foot, hand or arm.

In the healthcare and medical fields there are currently four main applications of 3D printing.

Surgery preparation assisted by the use of 3D printed models

3D printing can provide an exact copy of a patient's organ. The surgeon can then practise on the model and plan the best way to operate before actually performing a complicated surgery. Benefits of doing this are that it can reduce the time the operation takes because the procedure has been practised and so may lead to fewer complications and a shorter, better recovery for the patient.

Custom-made prosthetics

Traditional **prosthetic** limbs can be very expensive and can often cause discomfort for the amputee. They can also take weeks or months to be produced. 3D printing can produce prosthetics that are customised to the individual much more speedily and at a much cheaper cost. This is especially useful for children, who regularly need replacements as they quickly outgrow their prosthetic limbs. Scanning can be used to design prosthetics that have a more natural fit and match more closely to the appearance of the other limbs.

3D printing of surgical instruments

Personalised surgical instruments, such as forceps and scalpels, can be produced using 3D printers. Custom-made tools make a surgeon more accurate, which in turn supports better surgical outcomes. Another benefit is that the instruments can be produced much less expensively than traditionally manufactured surgical instruments.

Bioprinting tissues and organs

Bioprinting is in its early stages but has great potential. Rather than printing using metal or plastic, bioprinters use a computer-guided pipette to layer living cells, known as 'bio-ink', on top of one another to create artificial living tissue in a laboratory. These 'organoids' can be used for medical research as they mimic body organs (Figure 2.5). They are being researched as potential alternatives to transplants of human organs such as the liver or kidney. Research is also looking at printing skin grafts that can be directly applied to burns victims or tissue to repair muscle damage.

Source: https://medicaldevicescommunity.com/md_news/3d-printing-in-the-medical-field-four-major-applications-revolutionising-the-industry/

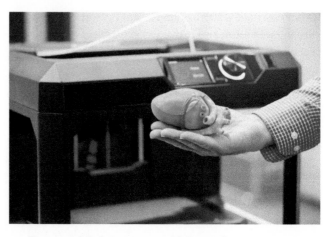

▲ Figure 2.5 Is bioprinting the future?

Reflect

Read the article: www.theguardian.com/artanddesign/architecture-design-blog/2015/aug/05/the-first-3d-printed-pill-opens-up-a-world-of-downloadable-medicine

▶ What do you think is the most useful benefit in producing pills in the way described?
▶ How soon do you think we will see some of these uses of 3D printing?

Health implants

Health implants are devices that are placed inside the human body for medical purposes. They can be used to treat or monitor health conditions or to restore body function, such as regulating the heart rate or glucose levels.

Health implants can be used to deliver medication such as for pain relief or for monitoring diabetes. They can regulate body functions such as an individual's heart rate by actively interacting with the body, for example, a pacemaker defibrillator sending out electric shocks in response to changes in heart rhythm (Figure 2.6).

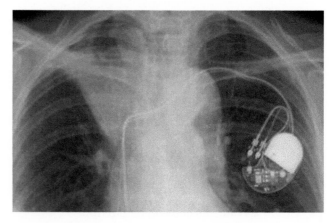

▲ Figure 2.6 X-ray of a pacemaker implant

The development of connected implants opens up possibilities for improving patient care by allowing health data to be gathered remotely, which enables monitoring and accurate analysis of how best to treat the patient. Some implants are 'smart' – they can communicate with external devices where readings are monitored and treatment is delivered in response to readings received. Heart pacemakers and defibrillator implants often work like this, collecting, processing and transmitting data from the patient, who is at home, to the hospital for analysis.

Case study

Interview with Paul

I often felt breathless and had difficulty walking even a short distance. On holiday with my family, I had to stay in the car while they went for a walk – I just couldn't keep up, 50 metres was really hard work. I couldn't sleep due to feeling breathless. I realised I couldn't go on like this so went to see my GP. He sent me for blood tests, an ECG and x-rays. 'I don't like the look of that' was his reaction to my ECG! I was sent to a cardiac specialist who diagnosed me with heart failure.

As a result of this diagnosis, I had to have a pacemaker and a defibrillator implant to help my heart pump more effectively. I also take various different kinds of medication such as beta blockers, tablets that slow down my heart. The implant was fitted in hospital, but I was able to go home the same day. My implant was fitted by a surgeon but it was programmed by a team using laptops to set it up.

The implant was supplied with a monitor (see Figure 2.7). I just move the mouse over my implant, the mouse downloads the information to the monitor, which sends it to the hospital 'pacing team'. This data informs them about the performance of my heart and the effectiveness of my medication, so they know if anything needs changing. It monitors my heart rate and fluid levels; an alarm is triggered if these are not within the correct range. I can then download the information to the hospital straight away using the monitor and they can start analysing the data. This means when I go to a hospital appointment, they have already seen the information and worked out any treatment changes that are needed. I don't have to go to the hospital that often because they will know if all is ok when I download my information, and they don't need to see me.

My implant really does provide reassurance as I am continually monitored. If I don't feel well, I can use the mouse to do a scan of my implant, which I can then send to the pacing team. The same if the alarm goes off – I just do a scan with the mouse and download the data to the pacing team. Since having my implant, my symptoms of breathlessness and the constant tiredness have more or less disappeared. Now I can be more active, I can go for a walk and keep up with my family, I don't have to keep sitting down and resting.

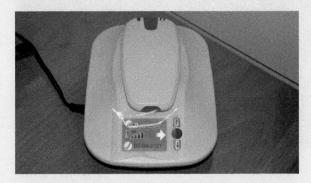

▲ Figure 2.7 Remote heart monitoring

▶ Use the NHS website to find out the meaning of 'ECG', 'heart failure' and 'beta blockers'.
▶ Using information from Paul's experience, write about the benefits for an individual and their quality of life while having a pacemaker and defibrillator implant.
▶ Discuss the benefits for the NHS of using this type of technology.

Research

Find out how a pacemaker works.

You can use the NHS link below or any other reputable source.

www.nhs.uk/conditions/pacemaker-implantation/

Read the articles below and answer the questions.

www.fiercebiotech.com/medtech/nih-backed-device-first-to-offer-long-term-wireless-monitoring-parkinson-s-patients-brain

https://parkinsonslife.eu/ai-rory-cellan-jones-parkinsons-disease/

▶ What activity does Rory Cellan-Jones do each day while wearing a medical device?
▶ How will wireless monitoring implants potentially help individuals with Parkinson's?

Robotic surgery

Robotic or robot-assisted surgery combines computer technology with the experience of skilled surgeons. This technology provides the surgeon with a magnification of 10×, high-definition, 3D-image of the operation site. The surgeon uses controls in a console (see Figure 2.8) to manipulate special surgical instruments that are smaller, as well as more flexible and movable, than the human hand. The robot replicates the surgeon's hand movements while also reducing hand tremors. This means that the surgeon can operate with improved accuracy, dexterity and control, even during the most complicated of procedures.

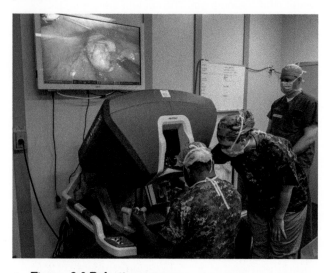

▲ Figure 2.8 Robotic surgery

Benefits for patients of having robotic surgery include:
▶ a smaller **incision**
▶ less damage to healthy tissue
▶ less pain
▶ shorter hospital stay
▶ less visible scars
▶ faster recovery and return to normal activities.

The benefits are interrelated, for example, less damage to the healthy tissue will result in quicker healing, possibly less pain and a shorter hospital stay. A smaller incision will usually result in less scarring and a faster return to normal activities.

> **Key term**
>
> **Incision:** a cut made through the skin and soft tissue for a surgical procedure.

Artificial intelligence technologies

Artificial intelligence technologies have a range of applications that make them useful tools in healthcare.

The use of **AI** can:
▶ support health teams by giving them access to more expansive data across a wider geographical area
▶ help health professionals with staying informed about trends in conditions and responses to treatment from a wider pool of individuals
▶ support diagnosis through the use of patient data/images and complex algorithms.

All of these benefits save time and human labour and help to ensure that patients are diagnosed quicker and treated more effectively, leading to better outcomes.

Machine learning radiology

Radiology is a branch of medicine that uses medical imaging – for example, X-rays, CT and MRI scans – to diagnose and treat diseases within the body. **Machine learning** is becoming increasingly important for making computer-aided diagnoses. It uses **algorithms** based on large data sets from scans taken in a wide range of geographical areas of the country. Averages from lots of patient data are used to work out whether there is anything unusual and thus likely an issue with a specific patient. Algorithms can highlight patterns and trends based on huge data sets, which was not previously possible. Many of the tasks that are currently considered mainstream radiology tasks, for example, abnormality detection in images and classification of images, will, in a few years, be performed by machine. Complex cases will be identified and passed on to specialist **radiologists**.

> **Key terms**
>
> **AI:** stands for artificial intelligence.
>
> **Machine learning:** the study of computer algorithms that improve in validity automatically through experience over time and by the use of huge amounts of data. Machine learning algorithms build a model based on sample data, known as 'training data', in order to make predictions or decisions without being explicitly programmed to do so.
>
> **Algorithm:** a computer process that dictates a way of doing things or a set of rules to follow.
>
> **Radiologist:** a medical practitioner who diagnoses, using X-rays, CT and MRI scans, and treats illness or injury with therapeutic radiography.

Machine learning identifies complex patterns and enables automatic detection and diagnosis that some say is comparable to that of a well-trained and experienced radiologist.

Test yourself

1 State two benefits for an individual of using a health app.
2 State two benefits for healthcare services of individuals using a health app.
3 List four functions of the NHS app.
4 Identify four potential main applications for 3D printing in healthcare.
5 Explain the benefits for patients of having robotic surgery rather than conventional surgery.

A2.5 The origins of the healthcare sector and how this has developed into the healthcare sector we have today

Origins of the healthcare sector in the UK

The creation of the NHS was the result of many years of debate and discussion from the early 1900s onwards. In 1942 Sir William Beveridge, former Liberal MP, produced what has become known as The Beveridge Report. In it he outlined what he described as five evils in society: 'want' (poverty), 'disease', 'ignorance' (lack of education), 'squalor' (poor housing) and 'unemployment'. Among his proposals to deal with these social problems was the suggestion to set up a National Health Service.

Before the creation of the NHS, patients who found themselves needing a doctor or medical facilities generally had to pay for those treatments and healthcare was very expensive. Many people could not afford to pay for treatment, which had serious health consequences – lower infant survival rates, death from diseases which could be treated but the cost was too expensive, and poor dental health, for example.

In 1945 Aneurin Bevan became Health Minister. He campaigned to bring about the NHS in the form we are now familiar with. Bevan said the NHS should be based on the essential principles that:
▶ everyone should be entitled to use it
▶ healthcare provided should be free of charge (at the point of use)
▶ it should be based on need rather than the ability to pay for it.

The NHS launched on 5 July 1948 and it was the world's first completely free healthcare service. Bevan's NHS was funded under the National Insurance Act of 1911 and it was set up to be funded by taxpayers, who paid a small amount from their wages each week. A leaflet was sent to every household in June 1948 which explained that:

> It will provide you with all medical, dental and nursing care. Everyone — rich or poor, man, woman or child — can use it or any part of it. There are no charges, except for a few special items. There are no insurance qualifications. But it is not a 'charity'. You are all paying for it, mainly as taxpayers, and it will relieve your money worries in time of illness.

Source: www.sochealth.co.uk/national-health-service/the-sma-and-the-foundation-of-the-national-health-service-dr-leslie-hilliard-1980/the-start-of-the-nhs-1948/

How the healthcare sector has developed since 1945

5 July 1948
The first NHS hospital, Park Hospital, treats the first ever NHS patient.

1952
As most hospitals are now funded by the NHS, the amount of money required to run the service has increased. A prescription charge of one shilling is introduced. This charge is removed in 1965, but reinstated in 1968.

1958
Vaccines against diseases such as polio and diphtheria are introduced to prevent the spread of disease, but also to reduce the cost of treatment for the NHS.

1959
The Mental Health Act allows people with a mental disorder to be treated, for the first time,in the same way as those with physical illnesses. The Act abolished the divide between psychiatric 'asylums' and hospitals. Instead of being treated for 'mental deficiency', it promised individuals they would no longer be kept out of sight but appropriately treated in hospitals or in the community wherever possible.

1960
Edinburgh Royal Infirmary carries out the first ever kidney transplant.

1961
The contraceptive pill is introduced but until 1967 is available to married women only.

1962
A large hospital building programme is carried out, so that all areas with a population above 125,000 have their own NHS hospital.

1972
CT scanners are used in the NHS for the first time. Godfrey Newbold Hounsfield wins a Nobel Prize for the design.

1978
Thanks to NHS funding and research, Louise Brown becomes the first child to be conceived by in vitro fertilisation (IVF).

1980–88
There is a period of scientific advancement, seeing the introduction of keyhole surgery and the invention of the MRI scanner. The NHS introduces free mammograms (breast screening) for women over 50, to help reduce the risk of breast cancer.

1990
The Community Care Act introduces the NHS 'internal market', meaning that health authorities are given their own budgets to buy care from hospitals for local populations.

1998
NHS Direct provides a telephone service as a more efficient way to handle health concerns that are less urgent and do not merit a 999 call. (This is replaced in 2010 by NHS 111.)

2006
A smoking ban is brought in for public areas in England and begins to successfully reduce second-hand smoke damage to patients.

2020–21
The NHS treats more than 1 million patients every 36 hours. There are now 1.2 million people employed by the NHS Hospital and Community Health Service (source: https://digital.nhs.uk/data-and-information/publications/statistical/nhs-workforce-statistics/march-2021). However, the COVID-19 pandemic poses the greatest challenge yet.

▲ Figure 2.9 NHS timeline

The NHS has undergone many changes, updates and reorganisations (see Figure 2.9). As medicine advances, health needs change and society develops, the NHS has to move forward so that the service continues to function for the future.

In response to increasing costs and expenditure to meet the demand for healthcare and the need to keep up with health innovations, some services now incur charges, for example:

▶ prescription changes in England – £9.35 at the time of writing
▶ most hospital trusts now limit the number of free IVF attempts
▶ only medications and treatments verified by NICE (National Institute for Health and Care Excellence) as 'value for money and cost effective' are funded by the NHS
▶ there are charges for some dental work (with exemptions for children, pregnant/nursing individuals) and opticians.

The numbers working for the NHS have increased significantly over the years. There are now more than 1.2 million people working for the NHS. For example, in 1948 11,700 doctors worked for the NHS, now there are over 200,000.

Source: https://digital.nhs.uk/data-and-information/publications/statistical/nhs-workforce-statistics/february-2021

Job roles have also changed – for instance, the basic personal care that nurses used to provide is now more likely to be provided by healthcare assistants. Nursing is now a degree-level profession and nurses are involved in providing more complex care that was historically given by doctors.

There are now four times fewer beds, approximately 120,000 instead of 480,000. One reason for this is due to more care being provided in the community. Patients' recovery time is also generally shorter thanks to improving methods of treatment, such as keyhole surgery, which enables patients to be treated as 'day cases' instead of being in hospital for a week. Women used to spend a week in hospital after giving birth, now they are typically able to leave on the same day or the day after, assuming no complications.

The NHS has had an enormous impact on the nation's health. Statistically, people now live on average 13 years longer than they did 70 years ago, thanks to access to good healthcare. Improved healthcare and immunisations have changed the conditions that people are dying of, with infectious diseases, strokes and heart attacks no longer the cause of as many deaths as previously. People are more likely to be living with a long-term condition that does not have (as yet) a cure – dementia, motor neurone disease or Parkinson's are examples.

To help address the future demands for services, the government has produced the 'NHS Long Term Plan' to prepare the NHS for meeting the challenges of providing healthcare for the nation. This features more care in the community, promoting overall wellbeing and preventing rather than only treating illness, and strategies to challenge health inequalities and deprivation in society.

Reflect

Find out more about the NHS Long Term Plan by visiting www.longtermplan.nhs.uk/wp-content/uploads/2019/01/the-nhs-long-term-plansummary.pdf

Read the summary.
▶ Which aspects of the plan do you think are the most important to achieve? Why?
▶ Discuss with others in your class. Do they agree?

Private sector healthcare (see section A2.1 above) has developed in parallel with the NHS, often providing the same type of treatment and care, but at a cost to the patient.

Private sector healthcare:

▶ is funded through private medical insurance or individual payments for treatment or care
▶ continues to expand – sometimes to avoid NHS waiting times, for example, hip replacement has long waiting times on the NHS but can be done much sooner at a private hospital.

Sometimes the NHS will buy in private treatment in order to shorten the wait time for individuals as the local NHS trust hospital may have a lack of available beds but a local private hospital has beds available.

Many charities have developed services to support health and wellbeing and provide healthcare, for example, Marie Curie Hospices, Macmillan Cancer Support, Mind, Diabetes UK and Age UK. (See also section A2.1 and Figure 2.1 on page 16.)

Test yourself

1 State the three essential principles of the NHS.
2 When were prescription charges brought in?
3 Describe two ways the role of a nurse has changed since the NHS was introduced.
4 List three ways the NHS Long Term Plan is helping prepare the NHS to meet future demands.
5 State two features of the private sector.

A2.6 The potential impacts of future developments in the healthcare sector in relation to care provision

Developments	Potential impacts on healthcare provision
Artificial intelligence (AI)	• Improved diagnostic process • Improved triage system – individual enters symptoms onto an online portal and is directed to appropriate services
Technological infrastructure	• Remote access for all healthcare professionals • Hardware and software need to be available • Collaboration across services is required
Regenerative medicine	• Ability to restore function to damaged organs or tissues (for example, bioprinting to repair scar tissue)
Biomarkers	• Will assist in identifying early onset of cardiovascular disease • Increase success rate of drug development programmes • Accelerate the availability of new therapeutics (see Figure 2.10)
Remote care	• Online clinics and virtual consultations • Mobile clinics and screening • Remote monitoring and downloading of health data
Patient self-management	• Use of personal digital health monitors • Use of personal health apps

Funding of services	• Stretched funding as:
	  • more people access the services
	  • more innovative treatments become available

Private healthcare provision	• More services available to users • More service users as a result • Shorter wait time for individuals to be treated • Potential of the NHS buying in private healthcare to meet increased demand (see above)
Changes in patient/service user demographics	• Changes in life expectancy – increased numbers of older people • Increase in complex care needs • Increase in rates of obesity and related conditions • All will result in increasing the need for health services

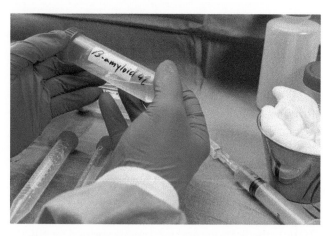

▲ Figure 2.10 Combining biomarkers from cerebrospinal fluid is helping researchers identify and distinguish between dementia with Lewy bodies and Alzheimer's disease

See also section A2.4 for details about and examples of future developments.

Key terms

Triage: screening of individuals by a medical professional to decide the order in which patients are treated, or the type of care required, depending on the urgency and nature of symptoms, wounds or illness.

Biomarkers: found by laboratory testing of blood, other body fluids or tissue, provide a measurable indicator of a biological state or condition, e.g. indicating the progress of a disease. They can help to determine the most effective therapy for a condition and establish the likelihood of recurrence of a condition such as cancer.

Therapeutics: the different treatments for symptoms, a disease or condition.

Demographics: the study of the changing characteristics of populations over time, for example, the proportion in each age group, gender balance.

A2.7 The importance of adhering to national, organisational and departmental policies in the healthcare sector including the possible consequences of not following policy

Importance of adhering to national, organisational and departmental policies

Following policies and procedures is a requirement of the healthcare worker role. Most policies and procedures are in place to protect both service providers and service users from harm and to protect their rights. Some examples of policies are shown in Figure 2.11.

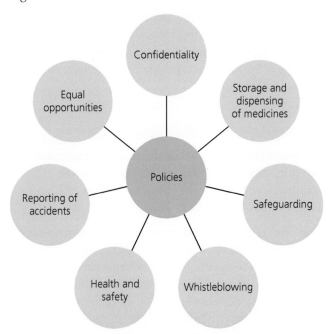

▲ Figure 2.11 Examples of policies in healthcare

Policies and procedures vary from one care setting to another because they reflect the type of care provided. Some policies exist to put into practice national **legislation** such as the Equality Act 2010 (equal opportunities policies) or the Health and Safety at Work Act 1974 (health and safety policy). Data protection legislation is another important example (see section A5.3, page 76). All care services are also required to have **safeguarding** policies in place and arrangements for **whistleblowing** (see Chapter A11 for more on both).

Organisational policies will set out steps to be taken to support the organisation's purpose and the services that it provides, i.e. what staff will need to do and be aware of in the course of their work, for example, a **manual handling** policy, **confidentiality** policy or disposal of hazardous waste policy.

A **departmental policy** will be very specific about tasks and work that is carried out in a particular department, such as a manual handling policy or policies around the storage and dispensing of medication.

Practice point

▶ Name four policies which you must adhere to in your placement.
▶ Write a summary about what each policy covers and how it affects your work.

Key terms

Legislation: a collection of laws passed by Parliament which state the rights and entitlements of the individual. Law is upheld through the courts.

Safeguarding: actions taken to protect individuals, reduce the risks of harm and abuse, and provide a safe and healthy environment.

Whistleblowing: when someone reveals serious wrongdoing within an organisation to an outside authority such as the Care Quality Commission, so that it can be investigated.

Manual handling: using the correct procedures when physically moving any load by lifting, putting down, pushing or pulling.

Confidentiality: limits access or places restrictions on sharing certain types of sensitive information, such as medical records, so that it is kept private and available only to those who need to be aware of it.

Reasons for the importance of adhering to national, organisational and departmental policies

▶ To provide quality standardised care for all patients and service users.
▶ To ensure safety of all service users – following health and safety policies and instructions is a legal requirement and is essential to ensure a safe workplace for everyone.
▶ To prevent errors – a set of clear instructions for tasks ensures that errors are minimised.

- To provide consistency – all staff doing the same thing in the same way ensures the same standard and quality of patient care.
- To promote health and wellbeing – people know what to expect, it improves practitioners' job satisfaction, knowing what is expected of them and how to achieve it.
- To ensure safety and wellbeing for practitioners – following appropriate policies, such as wearing of PPE, dispensing of medication procedures, ensures safety standards are high.

Health and safety

Whenever you are dealing with medication, you need to be aware of the main points of agreed procedures about handling medication.
- Read through the medicines policy in Figure 2.12.
- For each step of the policy, explain why it is important. Use the six 'Reasons for the importance of adhering to policies' to help.

Medicines Policy

Ordering: the process should be quick and efficient.

Receiving: a list of medication ordered should be checked against that received.

Storing: controlled drugs (CDs) must be stored in a locked cupboard or might be kept by the individual if self-administering.

Administering: ensure the right person receives the right dose of the right medication at the right time.

Recording: use the medicine administration record (MAR), which charts the administration of drugs. Make sure the records are clear.

Transfer: medication has to stay with the individual as it is their property, so if they are transferred to another care setting, the medication goes with them. ('Staying with' includes being kept in a locked cupboard if necessary.)

Disposal: return unwanted medication to a pharmacy. Care homes must use a licensed waste management company.

▲ Figure 2.12 Medicines policy

Source: *The Care Certificate Workbook Standard 13*, page 9

Possible consequences of not following policy

If healthcare settings do not meet their legal responsibilities, there can be severe consequences for employers, employees, individuals who require care and support and their families, and visitors to the care organisation.

Health and safety risks
- Poor standards of care; neglect; abuse.
- Causing harm.
- Injury, death of residents, patients, staff or visitors.

Harm to self and the individual
- Examples could be fractured limbs, food poisoning, disease, exposure to infection, burns.
- Illness, disease getting worse.

Termination of employment
- Dismissal of those responsible.
- Instigation of disciplinary procedures: verbal warning, first written warning, final written warning, suspension, dismissal.
- May find it difficult to obtain another job, will have poor references.

Negative media coverage
- Bad publicity about the service.
- Poor reputation for the setting.
- Unfavourable information causes lack of confidence in the care provider.
- Loss of business for a private care provider; could result in closure.
- Could lead to difficulties recruiting staff.

Implications for inspection/grading

If policies are not followed and an organisation does not fulfil its legal responsibilities and follow the required standard of care, the organisation could fail Care Quality Commission (CQC) inspections.

The CQC registers and licenses care services to ensure essential standards of quality and safety are met. It also publishes inspection reports which rate care settings from 'outstanding' to 'inadequate'. It has the power to issue warning notices and fines if standards are not met. This might also lead to increased monitoring of the setting, e.g. CQC, local authority inspections and re-inspections. There will also be a requirement for individuals working for the organisation to undergo further training/retraining to ensure that lessons are learned and issues do not reoccur.

Deregistration for registered practitioners

Individuals can be 'struck off' their professional register due to 'fitness to practise' concerns. The fitness to practise process is designed to protect the public from registrants who should not be licensed to practise, i.e. where there are concerns about their ability to practise safely and effectively. This could be due to, for example, dishonesty, violence or harm to service users. Removal from professional registers can involve:

► being 'struck off' and not allowed to practise at all
► restriction of practice – they may be limited in what they are allowed to do
► loss of professional status and reputation.

The Nursing and Midwifery Council, for example, is the regulator for nurses, midwives and specialist community public health nurses eligible to practise within the UK. This body deals with allegations against or issues reported with any of these professionals. (See page 119 for more on regulators.)

Potential criminal prosecution or civil legal action against employer or individual

In civil law, someone is sued for compensation.

Criminal law could result in:
► prosecution for breaching regulations if serious injury or death has occurred, and in cases of negligence
► a custodial sentence in very serious cases
► fines, or paying out compensation.

Practice point

Refer to three of the policies used in your placement. Explain the possible consequences of not following each of the policies:
► for yourself
► for the service users
► for the placement organisation.

Find out who updates each of the three policies and how staff are informed of the changes.

Test yourself

1 Name four examples of policies that would be used in a healthcare setting.
2 Give three reasons why staff should adhere to policies in the workplace.
3 Describe two possible consequences for service users of a health and safety policy not being adhered to.
4 State three actions that the CQC can take if the services of a healthcare provider are found to be below the required standard.
5 Explain what is meant by 'deregistration' for a care practitioner.

A2.8 The different ways in which the sectors are funded

Public sector

The government sets up, manages and leads the public sector services. They are paid for from working people's taxes (national insurance) based on their income (Figure 2.13). Most hospitals and GP surgeries are examples of public sector services.

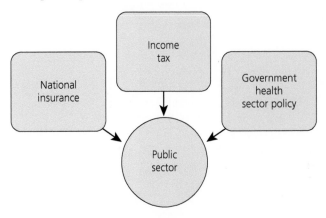

▲ Figure 2.13 How the public sector is funded

Private sector

Private sector services are owned or run by private individuals rather than by the government. Private care providers charge fees for their services as they are businesses and need to make a profit. Examples include private nursing homes, Nuffield Health Hospitals and non-NHS dental services. Service users will pay for treatment or may have private health insurance that covers the cost (Figure 2.14). Sometimes the NHS may refer patients to private services or beds, usually to reduce waiting lists, in which case the cost will be covered by the NHS, not the patient.

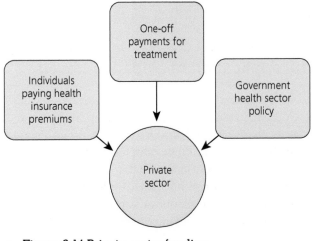

▲ Figure 2.14 Private sector funding

Voluntary/charity sector

These are not-for-profit organisations and charities. Their services are mainly provided by volunteers who do not get paid. To cover the cost of providing their services, they rely on donations from members of the public, running campaigns to raise funds, and sometimes government grants which they receive if there is a specific need for their services that the NHS is unable to offer (Figure 2.15).

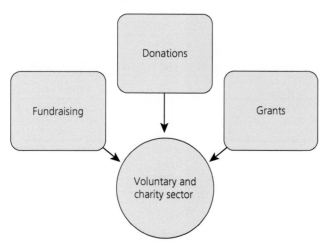

▲ Figure 2.15 Funding the voluntary and charity sector

A2.9 The meaning of evidence-based practice, its application and how it benefits and improves the healthcare sector

Meaning of evidence-based practice

Evidence-based practice is an approach of making decisions and providing the best standard of care by considering all the available facts, knowledge, data, statistics, etc. and using them as a basis for making a decision.

The application of evidence-based practice

▶ Combines research findings with clinical expertise and professional judgement.
▶ Assesses all the findings from research, including validity of information and data.
▶ Draws conclusions and applies findings to improve practice or introduce innovations.
▶ Reviews the impact of improvements or innovations.

Evidence-based practice involves healthcare practitioners and providers in being able to justify and give a clear account of their practice, why they provided care in the way that they did. They must be able to give a sound rationale for why they provided care in a particular way. Just to say 'I was told to do this' or 'we have always done it this way' is not sufficient.

When organisations and practitioners look critically at existing methods and practice, they can use this reflection to improve care. An example of a GP surgery applying evidence-based practice is given below. By using data to 'risk profile' patients, the GPs were able to identify individuals who were most likely to have falls. This enabled the practice to provide more appropriate home support and so the numbers of emergency admissions to hospital were reduced.

> **Case study**
>
> ### GP example: Using evidence-based guidance
>
> E1: Are people's needs assessed and care and treatment delivered in line with current legislation, standards and evidence-based guidance?
>
> **An urban practice with over 16,000 patients**
> The practice had a clear proactive approach to seeking out and embedding new ways of providing care and treatment to improve outcomes for its patients. It used innovative IT systems to drive improved patient care. For example, it used 'risk profiling' to identify patients who were most at risk of admission to hospital. This helped the practice reduce the rate of emergency admissions from 92 per 1000 patients in 2013/14 to 67 per 1000 patients in 2015/16. This allowed the practice to offer more support to patients at risk and care for more patients at home.
>
> Source: extract from www.cqc.org.uk/guidance-providers/gps/gp-example-using-evidence-based-guidance

A 'menu' of evidence-based interventions and approaches for addressing and reducing health inequalities has been developed as part of the government's Long Term Plan for the NHS (visit **www.england.nhs.uk/ltphimenu/**).

Examples include:
▶ the 'Small c' campaign: increasing public awareness and early diagnosis of breast and lung cancer in East London using social media (**www.england.nhs.uk/ltphimenu/cancer/the-small-c-campaign/**)

- early intervention programmes for supporting children and young people's mental health and wellbeing listed as part of the EIF Guidebook (**www.england.nhs.uk/ltphimenu/mental-health/better-care-for-major-conditions-improving-mental-health-children-and-young-peoples-mental-health/**)
- intervention – improved access to the NHS Health Check in high-risk groups (**www.england.nhs.uk/ltphimenu/cvd/nhs-health-checks/**)
- falls prevention – in accordance with NICE CG 161 (**www.england.nhs.uk/ltphimenu/integrated-care-for-older-people/long-term-conditions-including-frailty-cognitive-disorder-and-multimorbidity/**).

The government carried out a review in 2019/20 of the current and available evidence-based interventions that can support local healthcare providers to begin to address health inequalities in local area plans. The aim was to capture as many interventions as possible and share them nationally, with a view to reduce inequalities and improve healthcare in all areas.

> **Reflect**
>
> Have you used evidence-based practice on your placement?
>
> Describe what you did or suggest an example of what could be done.

How evidence-based practice benefits and improves the healthcare sector

For the population:
- facilitates improvements in person-centred care
- improves outcomes for individuals
- improves safety
- promotes equality in provision
- informs health promotion requirements.

For the healthcare sector:
- encourages quality provision
- improves cost effectiveness
- improves capability and competency of the workforce.

For the healthcare practitioner:
- brings job satisfaction
- gives empowerment
- offers continuous professional development.

> **Research**
>
> Choose one of the examples listed above of NHS evidence-based practice from the NHS Long Term Plan. Explain how it benefits the population, the healthcare sector and healthcare practitioners.

> **Test yourself**
>
> 1 Write a definition of evidence-based practice.
> 2 List three benefits of evidence-based practice for the population as a whole.
> 3 Identify two benefits of evidence-based practice for the healthcare sector.

A2.10 The different types of organisational structures within the healthcare sector and the resulting job roles

Flat structure

A horizontal or flat organisational structure involves few or no levels of middle management, with employees reporting directly to executives. This suits organisations with few levels between upper management and staff-level employees. Many small businesses use a horizontal structure before they grow large enough to build out different departments, but some organisations maintain this structure since it encourages fewer levels of managerial supervision and more involvement from all employees.

Pros:
- Gives employees more responsibility.
- Fosters more open communication.
- Improves co-ordination and speed of implementing new ideas.

Cons:
- Can create confusion if employees do not have a clear supervisor to report to.
- Can produce employees with more generalised skills and knowledge.
- Can be difficult to maintain once the organisation grows.

Health&Care @ Home

Health&Care @ Home is a private care agency.

Our Mission is to provide evidence-based and compassionately caring service to those in our care.

We provide personal care, help with housework, escorts to and from day centres, hospitals and shopping.

Our care teams comprise of a Care Co-ordinator and a small team of carers split across the three service areas. This flat organisation structure [Figure 2.16] means we can quickly react to increases in workload either within a team or across teams.

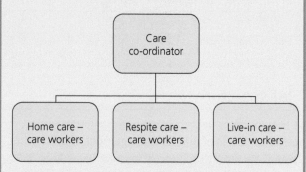

▲ Figure 2.16 Using a flat organisation structure

▶ How many **management roles** does Health&Care @ Home have?
▶ Describe the three types of **caring roles** provided.
▶ What are the benefits of this type of flat organisation structure?
▶ Can you think of any additional **ancillary roles** at Health&Care @ Home?

Management roles: involve the leadership, monitoring and supervision of staff and the organisation.

Caring roles: directly involved in providing care for individuals, roles such as nursing, midwifery, GP or a surgeon.

Ancillary roles: roles not specific to the care sector and not involving the provision of direct care. However, they are vital to providing a high-quality service to service users. Roles within the ancillary category may include administration staff, domestic/housekeeping/cleaning staff, catering assistant/cook/chef, driver/transport manager, maintenance worker/gardener.

Tiered hierarchical structure

The NHS is an example of a tiered hierarchical organisation structure. The chain of command and responsibility goes from the top downwards to entry-level employees. To see the structure visit: **www.nuffieldtrust.org.uk/chart/the-structure-of-the-health-and-social-system-in-england**

Advantages:
▶ Better defines levels of authority and responsibility.
▶ Shows who each person reports to or who to talk to about specific projects.
▶ Motivates employees with clear career paths and chances for promotion.
▶ Gives each employee a specialty.

Disadvantages:
▶ Can slow down innovation or important changes due to increased bureaucracy.
▶ Can cause employees to act in the interests of the department instead of the organisation as a whole.
▶ Can make lower-level employees feel as though they have less ownership and can't express their ideas for the organisation.

Watch the video 'How does the NHS in England work?' from thinktank The King's Fund to find out more about the current structure of the NHS:

www.youtube.com/watch?v=DEARD4I3xtE&t=13s

External agencies

External agencies are not necessarily part of the NHS, they could be private businesses such as care homes, private hospitals, social care agencies or charities that, for example, provide hospice care. NHS Supply Chain (NHSSC) is an external agency that provides the NHS with medical supplies. This term can also apply to external agencies such as the police or social care services provision and quality assurance organisations such as the Care Quality Commission, which inspects care settings.

External agencies tend to fulfil the following three types of job roles in the NHS:

▶ functions within the sector – complementing or supporting NHS care services or providing continuing care. An example would be agencies providing domiciliary care

▶ contractors/contracting roles – services purchased for a set period of time to do a specific task, for example, local pharmacies delivering COVID-19 vaccinations

▶ providing **integrated care**. This gives people the support they need across local councils, the NHS and other partners. The idea is that barriers between GPs, hospitals and council services are removed so that people receive continuity in their care.

> **Research**
>
> Visit www.healthcareers.nhs.uk
>
> Find examples for each of the following types of job roles in the NHS:
> ▶ management roles
> ▶ caring roles
> ▶ ancillary roles.
>
> Which of the holders of these job roles would be NHS employees and which could be working for external agencies?

Multidisciplinary team working within healthcare organisations

> **Research**
>
> Watch the YouTube video 'What are multidisciplinary teams? (Integrated care)' from the Social Care Institute for Excellence (SCIE): https://youtu.be/bENp2lmh0Rw
>
> Write your own definition of a multidisciplinary team.

How multidisciplinary teams work together effectively as part of organisational structures

Multidisciplinary teams (MDTs) often consist of individuals who have different roles, for example, caring roles working alongside those with management roles.

Features of multidisciplinary teams:

▶ provide respect for colleagues – they value each other's area of expertise and what it can offer and contribute

▶ build rapport and positive relationships – this is important for a successful team, people need to operate with respect for others' roles

▶ take ownership of own job role and responsibilities – be professional and take responsibility for your tasks, act in a timely and organised way

▶ take on board feedback and contribute to discussions to support problem solving

▶ actively listen to colleagues' contributions – develop good communication between the team members, value others' opinions and contributions

▶ share relevant information and collaborate to support the continuity of care – working together sharing information on a need-to-know basis to support the team and service user.

The MDT will be working in partnership with other healthcare professionals, for example, therapists, dieticians, doctors and dentists, to ensure effective nutrition and hydration of an individual.

Read the case study to understand more about multidisciplinary teamwork in action.

Multidisciplinary team working in Manchester

Central Manchester CCG developed 'practice integrated care teams' (PICTs). These included general practitioners, social workers, practice and community health practitioners, such as district nurses, and case managers. Specialist teams were called upon as necessary, depending on the needs of the individuals and families concerned.

The PICTs had clear principles to guide their work – people would feel more in control of their lives; they would be seen as a whole person; health and social care would work together; and care would be planned ahead. To aid co-ordination of care, a key worker was identified and electronic care plans were accessible to all team members.

By including all relevant professionals in a single patient-centred approach to care, the aim is to deliver high-quality care, improve the patient experience and ultimately avoid unnecessary hospital admissions.

One example of the impact that the neighbourhood teams can have is Eileen. She is 89 and had lost her confidence after a fall while out shopping. She was only able to get out of the house if assisted in a wheelchair, and experienced long days by herself. Reducing Eileen's social isolation was a key priority for the MDT.

The care navigator took the lead and began visiting Eileen to build rapport and find out more about her individual situation and interests. Eileen was helped with day-to-day chores by friends and family but did not have any opportunities to take part in different and stimulating social activities or interactions. Volunteers from Didsbury Good Neighbours arranged for Eileen to attend a regular local coffee morning and also engaged a local befriender who now visits once a month for a cup of tea and a chat.

Source: Extract from: SCIE (Social Care Institute for Excellence), 'Delivering integrated care: the role of the multidisciplinary team', SCIE Highlights No 4, July 2018, (scie.org.uk)

▶ Discuss the roles of those involved in the multidisciplinary team, listing the 'caring' roles and the 'management' roles.
▶ Identify which features of multidisciplinary teams (from the features list above) are demonstrated by the case study.

A2.11 The importance of job descriptions and person specifications and how this defines roles and responsibilities

Job description

A job description sets out all the specific responsibilities of a job role and includes detailed information about:

▶ the scope of the role – the tasks and activities involved in the job
▶ the purpose of the role – main focus of the role, e.g. administration, managing, caring
▶ responsibilities – e.g. keep accurate and up-to-date records; monitor progress; carry out observations
▶ reporting lines – who is your supervisor, i.e. the person you report to
▶ accountabilities – details of what precisely you are in charge of and responsible for.

Reflect on your placement role. What are you expected to do? What are your responsibilities? Are there any restrictions on what tasks you are not allowed to do within the setting?

Write a person specification for your role.

Research and find a job description for a future role you are interested in.

List the information provided relating to the following:
▶ the scope of the role
▶ the purpose of the role
▶ responsibilities
▶ reporting lines
▶ accountabilities.

Person specification

The following terms may be used in job descriptions to explain the role:

▶ Experience required – any tasks, jobs or activities you should have done previously and are familiar with.

▶ Essential and desirable skills – essential: the ability and knowledge the person must have to do a specific task or type of work; desirable: other skills that would be useful extra skills but are not compulsory.

▶ Attributes required – a quality or a characteristic that someone needs to do the job, for example, confidence, cheerfulness, trustworthiness, a willingness to learn.

▶ Qualifications required – proof that you are trained and have been assessed as being able to do specific tasks or types of work. This may need to be confirmed by producing the certificates received when you were awarded them.

▶ Mandatory training and continuing professional development required; reflective practice – you must be willing to attend training sessions and keep up to date with best practice. Reflective practice means you must be in the habit of contemplating the effectiveness of your current practice and learn new ways of working throughout the role.

▶ Registration requirements – health professionals such as nurses, midwives, doctors, teachers and social workers have to be 'registered' in order to be allowed to practise (see pages 119 and 222). They can be 'struck off' their professional register due to 'fitness to practise' concerns such as dishonesty or harm to service users.

Case study

Healthcare Assistant: person specification

	Essential	Desirable
Academic or vocational qualifications	• Health Studies (or similar) • Level 2/3	• A commitment to professional development
Experience	• Working within a nursing team • Dealing with vulnerable patients	
Knowledge and skills	• Blood pressure monitoring • Carrying out new patient medicals • Injections • Suture/stitch removal • Simple wound care • Testing and processing of specimens • Excellent communication skills	• Experience of smoking cessation clinics • Vascular health checks • Assisting with minor surgery procedures
Qualities and attributes	• Ability to work without direct supervision • Can determine own workload priorities • Ability to work as part of a multi-skilled team • Ability to work under pressure • Ability to use initiative • Confident and outgoing personality	
Other	• Flexibility of working hours to cover colleagues	• Evidence of continuing professional development

1 Divide a sheet of paper into three columns: 'Skills', 'Attributes' and 'Experience'.
2 Read the person specification and in the appropriate column list the skills, behaviours and attributes required for a healthcare assistant.

A2.12 The career pathway opportunities for employment and progression within the healthcare sector as defined by the IfATE occupational maps

You will probably have taken this course because you are interested in a particular role in the healthcare sector. Do you know what is required for this role and how to get there?

As part of the Health T Level, there are different occupational specialisms that you can choose to learn about alongside the core content in this book. This section includes links to details of routes into certain roles.

Career pathways as per the occupational maps

The Institute for Apprenticeships and Technical Education (IfATE) website shows where technical qualifications like this one can lead – see www.instituteforapprenticeships.org/occupational-maps

Scroll down to 'Health and Science' and click on the job titles under the heading 'Health Pathway' (see Figure 2.17).

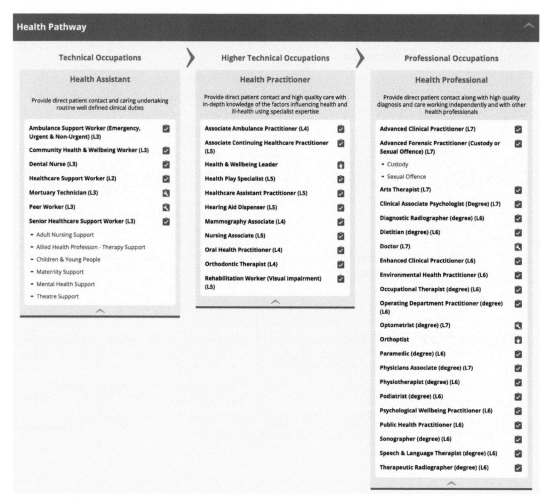

▲ Figure 2.17 Health pathway

A2.13 The potential impact of external factors on the activities of the healthcare sector

Factors

Outside of normal levels of healthcare required, certain things can have an effect on people's health and wellbeing and thus the healthcare sector.

▶ Pandemic – the worldwide spread of an infectious disease. Examples include the influenza pandemic (known as Spanish Flu) of 1918–19 and the current COVID-19 pandemic. Pandemics have devastating effects on populations and can put severe pressure on healthcare provision, with long-term effects.

▶ Epidemic – a widespread outbreak of an infectious disease in a number of people at the same time. This can have a huge impact on healthcare systems in affected areas and/or populations – for instance, the Ebola virus several times in the 2010s, or the Zika virus in 2015–16.

▶ Endemic diseases – diseases or conditions regularly found, and very common, among a particular group or in a particular area. For example, malaria is endemic in many of the hotter regions of the world where mosquitoes are prevalent, such as Africa, South America and Asia.

▶ Extreme weather – exceptionally cold or hot weather, or very serious, intense storms, etc. The bushfires in Australia in January 2020 destroyed lives, homes and wildlife. These now occur regularly in the summer in Australia. In the UK, very hot weather can cause individuals, particularly older people and those with conditions such as heart disease, to become seriously ill if they do not keep cool and well hydrated. Extreme cold weather can increase the risk of hypothermia, which can be fatal. A recent increase in extreme weather events around the world is believed to be a result of climate change, so this challenge will likely only become more significant in the future.

▶ Infrastructure – the basic systems and structures needed and used by a society or organisation in order to function effectively. It includes roads, transportation and other services. In a healthcare sense, buildings and maintenance of older hospitals may cause limitations on the services offered. Certain types of care or treatment may not be available in all areas because of a lack of facilities. Power failures and water shortages could result in care settings having to be evacuated. Major incidents such as a train crash or motorway accident could affect hundreds of people, and a lack of infrastructure can inhibit or prevent the movement of supplies or people in many regions.

▶ Geographical events – may involve fire and floods which can affect the operation of local care services. Certain areas of the UK are becoming more at risk of flooding, resulting in families having to be rescued from their homes and treated for injuries or hypothermia, for example. Also, disasters that happen in specific geographical locations can have a sudden and significant impact, for example, the eruption of the Mount Nyiragongo volcano in the Congo in May 2021 when thousands of people had to leave their homes.

Impacts

The impacts of external factors on the provision of healthcare services can be significant (see Figure 2.18).

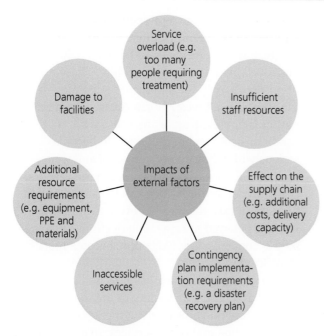

▲ Figure 2.18 Impacts of external factors on healthcare services

During a disaster situation, hospitals and other healthcare settings must continue to provide essential medical care to their communities. Any incident that causes loss of infrastructure or a patient surge, such as a natural disaster, terrorist act, or chemical, biological or explosive hazard, requires a response and recovery plan which enables the continuing provision of healthcare. Without appropriate emergency planning, local health systems can easily become overwhelmed in attempting to provide care during a critical event. Limited resources, a surge in demand for medical services, and the disruption of communication and supply lines create a significant barrier to the provision of healthcare.

The impact of the COVID-19 pandemic in 2020–21 on the NHS was significant. BBC News reported that waiting lists at nearly one in three hospitals in the UK increased hugely (over a year without treatment for 10 per cent of patients), including major disruption to cancer services and worries around fewer people being referred or screened for cancer as a result of pressure on the health service.

Source: www.bbc.co.uk/news/health-57092797

To ensure health facilities' readiness to cope with the challenges of a disaster, hospitals and other healthcare organisations have to be well prepared and should have a **disaster recovery plan**.

A disaster recovery plan for a hospital may cover:
▶ communications: how will the hospital be notified of an external disaster and how will this be communicated throughout the hospital? Consider how this might be done if the usual infrastructure is damaged, e.g. if electricity is down
▶ resources and equipment: extra supplies should be kept in case of emergency, so that essential activity can continue and patients can be protected
▶ safety and security: the police may become involved in the event of a disaster, and internal security measures need to be maintained to ensure, for instance, that people entering and leaving the hospital can still be controlled.

Staff responsibilities:
▶ All staff in the hospital must have received training so that they know what to do in a disaster situation, who will be in charge (chain of command) and any other relevant preparation to keep the system functioning.

Utilities:
▶ In the event of a disaster, water, fuel and electricity supplies may be disrupted. How will the hospital ensure there is enough oxygen and that generators will kick in to maintain essential systems?

Testing and evaluation of the disaster plan

The hospital should regularly test its disaster plan and note areas for improvement:
▶ Was it possible to effectively communicate within the hospital and throughout the community?
▶ Were there enough necessary resources and supplies?
▶ Was it possible to provide for the safety of the patients and staff?
▶ Were staff aware of their responsibilities during an external disaster situation?
▶ Was the hospital able to maintain proper patient care throughout?

Test yourself

1 Identify three external factors that can potentially impact the activities of the healthcare sector.
2 Describe two examples of the long-term impact of the COVID-19 pandemic on the NHS that have already become evident.
3 What is the purpose of a disaster recovery plan?
4 Give three examples of what a disaster recovery plan should cover.

A2.14 The role of public health approaches and how this benefits regional and national population health through prevention and improvement initiatives

The role of public health approaches

Public health protection involves protecting the nation from public health hazards by preparing for and responding to public health emergencies. It also involves improving the health of the whole population by sharing information and expertise and by identifying and preparing for future public health challenges.

World Health Organization (WHO)

Better health for everyone, everywhere

We are building a better, healthier future for people all over the world.

Working with 194 Member States, across six regions, and from more than 150 offices, WHO staff are united in a shared commitment to achieve better health for everyone, everywhere.

Together we strive to combat diseases – communicable diseases like influenza and HIV, and noncommunicable diseases like cancer and heart disease.

We help mothers and children survive and thrive so they can look forward to a healthy old age. We ensure the safety of the air people breathe, the food they eat, the water they drink – and the medicines and vaccines they need.

Source: www.who.int/about

The WHO was founded on 7 April 1948 – a date now celebrated every year as World Health Day. Today it consists of more than 7000 people working in 150 country offices, in six regional offices and at its headquarters in Geneva, Switzerland.

The organisation's major role is to direct and co-ordinate international health within the United Nations system. The main areas of work are health systems; health through the life-course; non-communicable and communicable diseases; preparedness, surveillance and response.

In addition to medical doctors, public health specialists, scientists and epidemiologists, WHO staff include people trained to manage administrative, financial and information systems, as well as experts in the fields of health statistics, economics and emergency relief. Working together, they aim to help achieve health objectives by supporting national health policies and strategies.

Research

Explore the WHO using the links below. Choose a health topic you are interested in (for example, air pollution or children's health) and then research the topic using the WHO resources.
- The WHO work in international emergencies: **www.who.int/emergencies/overview**
- Facts in pictures: **www.who.int/news-room/facts-in-pictures**
- Factsheets covering all aspects of health and healthcare: **www.who.int/news-room/fact-sheets**

Based on the information you have collected, produce a presentation for your group, including:
- an introduction to the topic
- key facts
- the WHO response (i.e. what the WHO is doing about it).

The UK Health Security Agency (UKHSA)

To give the UK the best chance of beating COVID-19, and to continue to monitor, identify and be ready to respond to other health threats, now and in the future, the UK government created a new organisation to support public health protection. The organisation began operating from 1 April 2021. The UKHSA brings together Public Health England (PHE), NHS Test and Trace and Joint **Biosecurity** Centre (JBC) and the National Institute for Health Protection (NIHP).

The UKHSA will be responsible for planning, preventing and responding to external health threats, and providing intellectual, scientific and operational leadership at national and local level, as well as on the global stage. The UKHSA will ensure the nation can respond quickly and at greater scale to deal with pandemics and future threats.

Key term

Biosecurity: refers to procedures or measures designed to protect the population against harmful biological or biochemical substances.

Research

Use the link below to find out more about the work of the UK Health Security Agency:

www.gov.uk/government/news/dr-jenny-harries-marks-official-launch-of-uk-health-security-agency

Write a summary of the planned role of the new UKHSA.

The UKHSA will use a rigorous science-led approach to public health protection. It will boost the UK's ability to deal with and recover from COVID-19 and meet the health challenges of the future. An example of its work is described in the case study 'Analysing waste water'.

Case study

Analysing waste water

Scientists discovered early in the pandemic that genetic fragments of the COVID-19 virus could be detected in sewage. Samples were taken at waste water treatment plants throughout the UK and sent to a new lab in Exeter.

Using the link below, read about this scientific approach to monitoring the spread of COVID-19:

www.bbc.co.uk/news/science-environment-57205126

Write an explanation detailing how the research is being carried out and the benefits of the results for public health. Use the following headings:
- Which locations are the samples taken from and how often?
- What are the benefits of sampling at community level?
- Why will this sampling be continued after the pandemic is over?

Responsibilities of the UKHSA include:
- local health protection teams to deal with infections and other threats
- support and resources for local authorities to manage local outbreaks

- the COVID-19 testing programme
- contact tracing
- the Joint Biosecurity Centre
- emergency response and preparedness to deal with the most severe incidents at national and local level
- research laboratories and associated services
- specialist epidemiology and surveillance of all infectious diseases
- global health security
- providing specialistic scientific advice on immunisation and countermeasures.

The overall role of the WHO and the UKHSA is to identify, through evidence collection, health issues affecting or threatening the population. This determines the extent of the issue, who it impacts and its effects. Protecting the population from COVID-19, improving the nation's health and prevention of ill-health are priorities. This is along with the government's ambition to give children the best start in life, tackle risk factors such as obesity and smoking, and reduce health inequalities.

The organisations have a clear focus on:
- providing evidence and support for national and local government on policy decisions for health improvement and protection
- providing expert advice, support and assurance on vital health services in the NHS and local government, including screening and immunisation programmes
- delivering health interventions in the form of social marketing campaigns to support individuals to take control of their health.

The benefit of public health approaches to regional and national health

Public health is concerned with protecting, and improving, the health of the population rather than focusing on the health of each individual. Promoting public health and wellbeing benefits society as a whole and aims to reduce health inequalities.

An approach which addresses the wider influences on health, namely people's living conditions, can have a big impact on improving the health of the population overall (Figure 2.19). This is unlike a **disease-oriented approach**, which focuses on interventions for a single condition, often at one particular point in an individual's life rather than throughout. Government strategies to tackle inequalities and how the environments where people live and work affect them can make a difference across their lifespan and beyond; future generations also benefit. Public health approaches are therefore holistic ways to reduce the need for health interventions, saving lives and preventing harm to health that would have needed treatment.

Some of the benefits of the public health approach for regional and national health are shown in Figure 2.20.

> See also Chapter A9 for details of the 'prevention agenda' approach to healthcare.

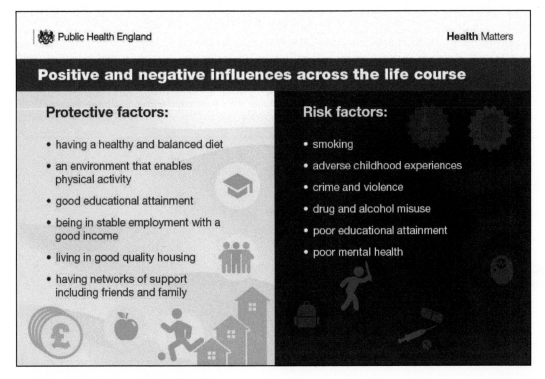

▲ Figure 2.19 Influences on health

Source: www.gov.uk/government/publications/health-matters-life-course-approach-to-prevention/health-matters-prevention-a-life-course-approach

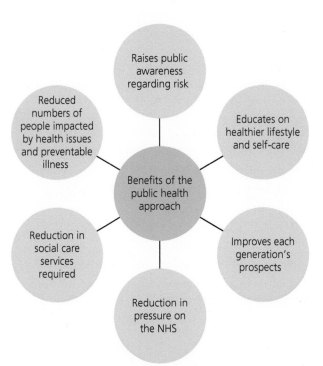

▲ Figure 2.20 Benefits of the public health approach

Project practice

Arrange an interview with an individual who has a health condition that requires taking medication and/or involves regularly monitoring their condition. Examples could include diabetes or heart failure. You can use a case study if necessary.

1   Ask the individual about how they manage their condition. Establish what is going well, but also whether they have any difficulties, e.g. forgetting medication or monitoring weight or glucose levels.

2   Following the interview, consider how the use of a health app such as Evergreen Life, the NHS app or My Diabetes My Way could help the individual to manage their condition. Produce a leaflet that explains how an app could be used to help them. Cover features of the app, how it can help them and how to use it.

3   At a follow-up meeting, present your leaflet and discuss how the health app could help the individual.

4   If possible, return for an evaluation meeting. Discuss with the individual the pros and cons of using the app, then write up an evaluation.

Assessment practice

1   Describe the role of community health services.

2   Give an example for each of the following barriers to seeking healthcare services and explain why they are a barrier.

Barrier	Example
Socioeconomic	
Psychological	
Geographical	

3   Evaluate the use of 'public health' and 'disease-oriented' approaches to national health. Your answer should demonstrate:
   ▶ a comparison of the two approaches
   ▶ a reasoned conclusion.

4   Explain how charity organisations play an important role within the healthcare sector.

5   State **four** benefits of robotic surgery.

6   Identify whether each of the following care services are primary care, secondary care or tertiary care:
   ▶ GP surgery
   ▶ hospice
   ▶ hospital maternity department
   ▶ optician
   ▶ physiotherapy clinic
   ▶ residential nursing home.

7   Discuss the benefits of remotely monitored health implants (for example, a pacemaker) for the individual and for the NHS. Your response should demonstrate:
   ▶ reasoned judgements
   ▶ conclusions about the benefits for the individual and for the NHS.

8   (a) Identify **two** policies that would be followed in a healthcare setting.
   (b) Explain why it is important to adhere to organisational policies.

9   Give a definition of evidence-based practice.

10 Explain why it is necessary for healthcare settings to have a disaster recovery plan.

A3: Health, safety and environmental regulations in the health and science sector

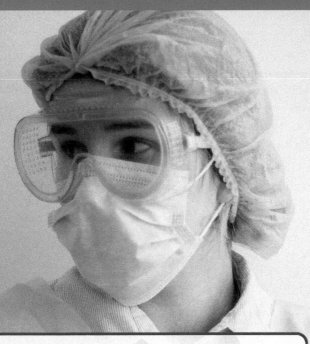

Introduction

When you work in the health and science sector you should feel safe. Your employer must make sure that you have a safe working environment and are not exposed to any unnecessary risks – we say that they owe you a **duty of care**. However, it is also the duty of every employee to play their part. You will need to be aware of the legislation and regulations that help to keep you and your colleagues safe, and to understand your rights, duties and responsibilities.

Laboratory and industrial processes can cause harm to the wider public and to the environment. So, you also need to be aware of your responsibility to help in eliminating (as far as possible) such harm.

This chapter covers the relevant legislation and regulations while Chapter A4 will cover how these are applied in the workplace.

Learning outcomes

The core knowledge outcomes that you must understand and learn:

A3.1 the purpose of legislation and regulations in the health and science sector

A3.2 how to assess and minimise potential hazards and risks, including specific levels of risk, by using the Health and Safety Executive's 5 Steps to Risk Assessment

A3.3 how health and safety at work is promoted

A3.4 how to deal with situations that can occur in a health or science environment that could cause harm to self or others (for example, spillage of hazardous material).

A3.1 The purpose of legislation and regulations in the health and science sector

Health and Safety at Work etc. Act 1974

The Health and Safety at Work etc. Act 1974 (sometimes referred to as HSWA 1974 or HASAWA) sets out the duties of employers and employees to ensure the health of anyone at work or who may be affected by work activities. Under HSWA 1974, the employer must ensure, as far as is reasonably possible, the health, safety and welfare of all employees while they are at work.

The employer's specific duties include the following:
▶ providing and maintaining **plant** and systems of work that are safe and without risks to health
▶ arrangements for ensuring safety and absence of risks to health in the use, handling, storage and transport of articles and substances
▶ giving the information, instruction, training and supervision necessary to ensure the health and safety at work of employees
▶ maintaining any place of work in a condition that is safe and without risks to health
▶ providing and maintaining all means of entry and exit (i.e. doorways, corridors, walkways, etc.) that are safe and without such risks
▶ providing and maintaining a working environment for employees that is safe, without risks to health, and adequate as regards facilities and arrangements for their welfare at work.

The legislation recognises that it is impossible to avoid all risk and so all of the above duties are to be carried out 'so far as is reasonably practicable'.

Key term

Plant: any equipment used in the workplace, e.g. laboratory equipment.

Health and safety is not the sole responsibility of the employer. Employees must play their part. HSWA 1974 states that it is the duty of every employee:
▶ to take reasonable care for the health and safety of themselves and of others who may be affected by what they do, or don't do, at work
▶ to cooperate with the employer to enable the employer to perform their duty under the legislation.

Reflect

HSWA 1974 means that employees have a duty to themselves and to their co-workers. You should not do anything that could cause harm. But not doing something you should have done can also affect health and safety in the workplace. The act says that employees must co-operate with the employer in ensuring safe working practices are carried out. Think about how health and safety in the workplace is a partnership between the employer and the employee – how can you play your part in how you work? Is there anything that you are doing that you should not be doing? Is there anything that you are not doing that you should be doing?

HSWA 1974 is an enabling act – that means that the government can introduce regulations at any time to modify the act or to establish up-to-date standards. Many regulations have been introduced under HSWA 1974. The ones that are most relevant to work within the health and science sectors are covered in the following sections.

Research

The Health and Safety Executive (HSE) is responsible for enforcement of HSWA 1974 and associated regulations. It has a website that is an excellent source of information about all matters related to health and safety in the workplace: **www.hse.gov.uk**

The COVID-19 pandemic meant there was an increase in the number of people working alone (**lone working**). This includes people working from home as well as those more likely to be alone in the workplace because of COVID-safe practices. Find out what the HSE recommends that lone workers should do to protect their health and safety.

Management of Health and Safety at Work Regulations 1999

These regulations aim to reduce the number and severity of accidents in the workplace, through assessing and managing risks. They make good health and safety management a legal requirement for, and impose duties on, both the employer and the employee. The main duty of the employer is to assess risks to health and safety in the workplace as they affect both employees and any others present (e.g. members of the public, visitors, etc.). The employer must then ensure effective planning, organisation, control, monitoring and review of measures taken to prevent or protect against risk. The employer must also appoint one or more 'competent persons' to assist in carrying out these legal responsibilities – this could be the employer themselves or employees appointed to the role.

The duties of employees under the regulations are to use machinery, equipment, dangerous substances, transport equipment and safety devices in accordance with their training and instructions. Also, employees have a duty to inform their employer and other employees of any dangers or shortcomings in the arrangements.

Practice points

As we have seen, there is a legal requirement for employers to manage health and safety through assessment and management of risk. Good employers will always take this responsibility seriously. However, there will always be some employers who do not do this. When you apply for a job, it is worth considering a prospective employer's approach to health and safety in the workplace.

Similarly, it is your responsibility to abide by the letter and the spirit of these regulations – for both your own health and safety and that of your colleagues. Be prepared to demonstrate to an employer that you understand these responsibilities and can be trusted to follow the regulations.

Control of Substances Hazardous to Health (COSHH) Regulations 1994 and subsequent amendments 2002

COSHH is designed to protect people against risks to health arising from work-related exposure to hazardous substances. It requires assessment and control of risks before any work takes place.

Anyone in charge of, or working in, a laboratory should be familiar with COSHH and actively involved in implementing it. The steps involved are shown in the table.

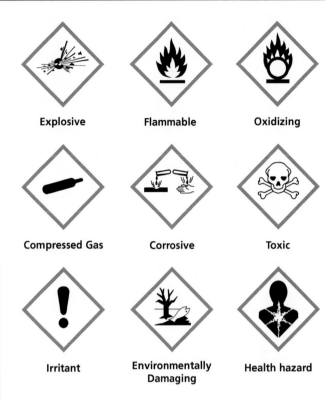

Explosive   Flammable   Oxidizing

Compressed Gas   Corrosive   Toxic

Irritant   Environmentally Damaging   Health hazard

▲ Figure 3.1 The GHS hazard pictograms

Carry out an assessment of the tasks in the laboratory:
- Record the scope of assessment (who the tasks are carried out by, what is being assessed, when the tasks are carried out).
- List significant laboratory tasks.
- List substances involved.

Assess the factors that decide the appropriate control approach:
- What are the hazard categories associated with each task?
- What degree of exposure is likely? (This depends on the quantity handled as well as the nature of the substance.)

Determine the control approach:
- None: open bench working (i.e. not in a fume cupboard or other containment) with general ventilation.
- Intermediate: fume cupboard or other exhaust ventilation.
- High: glove box or similar containment.
- Special: purpose-designed facility.
- Use of personal protective equipment (PPE) for eyes and skin where there is a risk from skin contact or for inhalational protection.

Implement and review:
- Assess other tasks and related risks.
- Planning (how it will be implemented and resources needed).
- Consider safety and environmental risks.
- Consider other aspects of COSHH – monitoring, health surveillance and training.
- Use and maintenance of control measures (including regular checks and reporting defects).
- Set up proper record-keeping and review procedures.

Research

The Royal Society of Chemistry website has a great deal of information about COSHH in chemical laboratories, although this is applicable to many types of workplace in the health and science sectors. Visit **www.rsc.org** and search for 'COSHH in laboratories'.

Personal Protective Equipment (Enforcement) Regulations (1992; updated 2018)

Managing and reducing risk is always the priority. If a factory roof leaks, it is better to repair it than to issue every member of staff with their own umbrella. Use of PPE should be considered only after everything else has been done to reduce risk. However, in most workplaces in the health and science sectors, some level of PPE will always be necessary. These regulations define employers' responsibilities to provide appropriate PPE to reduce harm to employees, visitors and clients. This can include providing safety helmets, masks, goggles and gloves.

Health and safety

PPE is not always convenient or comfortable. Healthcare staff have spoken about the discomfort of wearing full PPE throughout shifts lasting eight hours or longer during the COVID-19 pandemic. That is one reason why all other steps to remove or reduce risk should be taken before considering the use of PPE. However, the pandemic also illustrated the importance of appropriate PPE when faced with an invisible and potentially life-threatening risk.

Reporting of Injuries, Diseases and Dangerous Occurrences Regulations 2013 (RIDDOR)

The purpose of RIDDOR is to define employers' duties to report serious workplace accidents, occupational diseases and specified dangerous occurrences ('near misses').

RIDDOR puts duties on employers, the self-employed and people in control of work premises (the **Responsible Person**) to report certain serious workplace **accidents**, occupational diseases and specified dangerous occurrences as well as **reportable injuries**.

Reportable accidents are those that result in death, major injury, or being absent from work or unable to do normal work for more than seven days. Accidents that result in absence from work for more than three days but less than seven days must be recorded but do not need to be reported unless they are reportable injuries.

RIDDOR requires employers and self-employed workers to report cases of occupational cancer and any disease or acute illness caused by **work-related** exposure to a biological agent (e.g. bacteria, viruses or toxins). This may take place because of identifiable events or unidentified events.

Key terms

The following terms have a specific meaning in terms of RIDDOR:

Accident: a separate, identifiable, unintended incident, which causes physical injury. This specifically includes acts of violence to people at work.

Reportable injuries: the following injuries are reportable under RIDDOR when they result from a work-related accident:
- the death of any person
- specified injuries to workers (see the HSE website for more information)
- injuries to workers which result in them being unable to work for more than seven days
- injuries to non-workers which result in them being taken directly to hospital for treatment, or specified injuries to non-workers which occur on the premises.

Work-related: an accident in the workplace does not always mean that the accident is work-related – the work activity itself must contribute to the accident. An accident is 'work-related' if any of the following played a significant role: the way the work was carried out; any machinery, plant, substances or equipment used for the work; the condition of the site or premises where the accident happened.

Case study

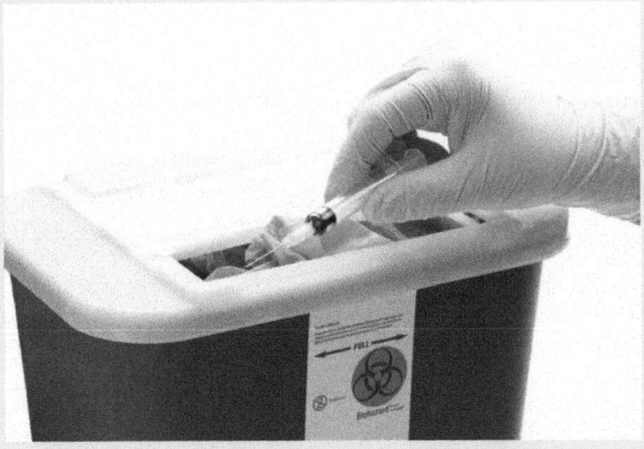

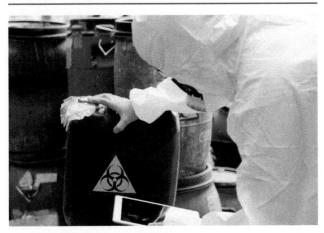

▲ Figure 3.2 Safe disposal of contaminated syringe needles, 'sharps'

Samah made a list of identifiable events in her workplace, including accidental breakage of a laboratory flask, accidental injury with a contaminated syringe needle (Figure 3.2) or an animal bite. She found it harder to think of unidentified events.

▶ Samah read that an unidentified event could be when a worker is exposed to legionella bacteria while conducting routine maintenance on a hot water service system. What other unidentified events could be present in your workplace?

▶ Do you think laboratory workers are more likely to be exposed to identifiable or unidentified events?

Environmental Protection Act (EPA) 1990

▲ Figure 3.3 Hazardous waste can be harmful to the environment

The EPA aims to improve control of pollution to the air, water and land by regulating the management of waste and the control of emissions.

▶ The EPA enables the Secretary of State to make any process or substance subject to strict controls and to set limits on its emissions into the environment. Carrying out such processes requires approval and there are criminal sanctions against offenders.

▶ The EPA also covers regulation and licensing of the disposal of controlled waste – this has a very broad meaning and includes any household, industrial or commercial waste.

▶ The way in which the EPA is enforced is quite complex. The Environment Agency (EA) or, in Scotland, the Scottish Environment Protection Agency (SEPA), together with local authorities, are responsible for control of processes specified by the EPA.

▶ Local authorities are responsible for the collection of some controlled waste, such as household waste.

▶ Local authorities also regulate and license the disposal of controlled waste from industrial or commercial premises such as shops, offices, laboratories, hospitals, GP surgeries, care homes, etc.

Thus, the EPA 1990 applies equally to the contents of your wheelie bin and to waste or emissions in the workplace.

Other legislation

The table lists some of the other legislation relevant to the health and science sectors and explains the relevance of each.

Special Waste Regulations 1996

Measures relating to:
- the regulation and control of the transit, import and export of waste (including recyclable materials)
- the prevention, reduction and elimination of pollution caused by waste
- the requirement for assessing the impact on the environment of projects likely to have significant effects on the environment.

Hazardous Waste Regulations 2005

Controls the storage, transport and disposal of hazardous waste to ensure it is appropriately managed and any risks are minimised.

Waste Electrical and Electronic Equipment Regulations (WEEE) 2012/19/EU

Aims to reduce the amount of electronic and electrical equipment incinerated or sent to landfill sites. Places onus on all businesses to correctly store and transport electrical waste.

Regulatory Reform (Fire Safety) Order (RRO) 2005

Aims to reduce death, damage and injury caused by fire, by placing legal responsibilities on employers to carry out a fire risk assessment. Because of this, all organisations are required to have procedures for evacuation in the event of a fire.

Manual Handling Operations Regulations 1992 (as amended)

Requires employers to assess and minimise the risk to health of employees involved in the manual handling, moving and positioning of an object, person or animal. It also covers workplace ergonomics, i.e. ensuring furniture is suitable and adaptable to different body sizes and types.

Health and Safety (Display Screen Equipment) Regulations 1992

Defines employers' responsibilities in carrying out risk assessments of workstations used by employees, including the use of display screen equipment, to minimise identified risks, such as:
- tiredness caused by poorly designed or adjusted workstations
- repetitive strain injury (RSI) and carpal tunnel syndrome
- eye strain leading to headaches, fatigue and sore eyes.

Test yourself

1 Which act (rather than regulations) listed above controls the disposal of waste in the workplace?
2 Name two sets of regulations that cover accidents in the workplace.
3 Name three sets of regulations that cover hazardous substances.
4 How does RIDDOR define a work-related accident?
5 What is a reportable injury under RIDDOR?
6 Who is responsible for safety in the workplace – the employer or the employee?

A3.2 How to assess and minimise potential hazards and risks

Minimising risk is extremely important in reducing harm in the workplace. Before we can minimise risk, we must first identify the risks. This is generally done by carrying out a risk assessment.

Risk assessment is a part of the risk management process and involves identifying a **hazard** and then deciding on the likelihood of exposure to that hazard (the **risk**). You need to decide:
- how likely a hazard is to actually cause harm
- the severity of that harm – just how serious the consequences could be.

This means that if a highly dangerous substance (i.e. the hazard) is contained so effectively that there is almost no possibility of coming into contact with it, the risk will be low. However, the probability of exposure to a less hazardous substance might be much higher and could pose a greater risk.

The Health and Safety Executive's 5 Steps to Risk Assessment are outlined in the following sections.

Key terms

Hazard: something that has the potential to cause harm.

Risk: how likely a hazard is to cause that harm.

Step 1: Identifying the hazards

Look around your workplace and think about what hazards there are. It is easy to overlook some hazards when you work in a place every day, so it is useful to follow some guidelines:
- Check manufacturers' instructions, particularly data sheets for chemicals and equipment.
- Look at accident or sickness records to see what has caused issues before.
- Think about non-routine activities such as changes in procedures or maintenance and cleaning, for example, when equipment is taken out of service.
- Consider long-term hazards to health, such as high levels of noise or exposure to harmful substances.

Step 2: Deciding who might be harmed and how

Once you have identified the hazards, you can then think about how employees (and others, such as visitors and contractors) might be harmed. That means you identify groups of people that might be at risk, including those with particular requirements (e.g. new employees, young workers, people with disabilities, visitors or temporary workers).

Step 3: Evaluating the risks and deciding on precautions

Risk is a part of our everyday lives and it is impossible to eliminate all risks. What you must do is identify the main risks and what action you need to take to manage those risks. An employer must do everything reasonable to protect people from harm. This means there is a balance between the level of risk and the measures needed to control the real risk.

You need to ask:
▶ Can the hazard be eliminated?
▶ If not, what can be done to control the risks so that they are unlikely to cause harm?

Once you have evaluated the risks, you can consider some suitable precautions:
▶ Try a safer way of doing things.
▶ Restrict access to the hazards.
▶ Organise the work so that it reduces exposure to the hazard.
▶ Finally, once all other precautions have been taken, use PPE.

It is important that all employees are involved in this stage, to make sure that any course of action will work in practice.

Step 4: Recording findings and implementing them, including completing risk assessment documentation

This is important: remember, to be effective, documentation should be simple and focus on the controls needed. The key points that should be recorded are:
▶ A proper check was carried out.
▶ Everyone who might be affected has been consulted.
▶ All the obvious significant hazards were dealt with.
▶ Reasonable precautions were put in place and any remaining risk was low.
▶ Employees, or their representatives, were involved in the process.

Step 5: Reviewing your assessment and updating if necessary

Workplaces change and evolve; new equipment is brought in or new substances and procedures are used. This means that a risk assessment has to be reviewed regularly to answer some key questions:
▶ Have there been any significant changes?
▶ Are there any improvements that could be made?
▶ Have any employees noticed any problems?
▶ Have there been any accidents or near misses that you could learn from?

Research

The HSE website is a great source of advice and information about many aspects of safety in the workplace. You can read more about risk assessment in its guide – download a copy from **www.hse.gov.uk/pubns/indg163.pdf** or visit **www.hse.gov.uk** and search for 'risk assessment'. The HSE also produces a risk assessment template in Word or PDF format as well as examples of risk assessments, although these are not so relevant to the health and science sectors.

Test yourself

1 What is meant by a hazard?
2 What are the five steps in a risk assessment?

A3.3 How health and safety at work is promoted

So far, we have seen how health and safety in the workplace depends on everyone playing their part. This is made clear in HSWA 1974 and other legislation, but it should be obvious: an employer must provide a safe working environment, but employees must do all they can to take care of their own safety and that of their colleagues.

Therefore, a good approach to health and safety must become engrained in the workplace. It must become part of the culture, not just something added on or viewed reluctantly or simply as rules to be followed.

For this reason, health and safety must be promoted by providing a framework of good practice and getting everyone to pull together in ensuring a safe working environment. This section will look at ways that can be achieved. Some of this involves following organisational policies and standard operating procedures (SOPs).

Encouraging individuals to take reasonable care of their own and others' safety

Everyone in an organisation must play their part – to increase the safety of themselves and their colleagues. This starts with the need for individuals to be given the knowledge and information about how to keep safe.

Modelling good practice

Management must lead by example, such as washing hands and wearing appropriate PPE. This helps to create a culture of good practice.

This may not be enough in small organisations or where staff often work alone – they may not often be able to see good practice.

Following organisational policies and SOPs, including site-specific emergency procedures

As well as complying with regulations, following policies and SOPs should enhance safety. However, it does mean that these policies and/or SOPs need to be high quality, well designed and with health and safety addressed at every stage. Everyone has a part to play here. If you see any issues or weaknesses, you should raise these with your supervisor or line manager.

Ensuring there is clearly visible information and guidance

The HSE produces a health and safety law poster (Figure 3.4) and it is a legal requirement for any employer to display a copy where it can be easily read. As well as outlining health and safety laws, the poster lists clearly and simply what employers and employees must do to ensure safety in the workplace.

It is human nature that after a while we no longer notice the things we see every day. It can therefore be helpful to use a range of eye-catching and informative posters and other available materials that keep changing to continually promote good practice.

Following processes for recording and reporting issues and concerns

We can all learn from our mistakes – but it is better, where safety is concerned, if we learn not to make those mistakes. Employees must be free to raise issues and report their concerns. But that will be effective only if there are procedures in place to record and, most importantly, act on those concerns.

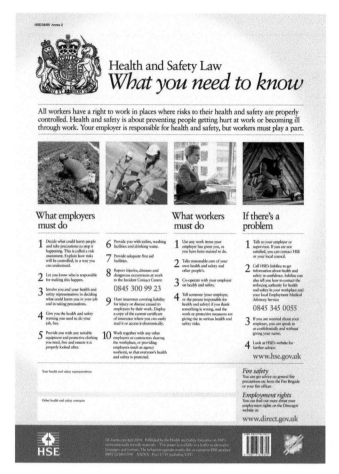

▲ Figure 3.4 The HSE safety law poster

Maintaining equipment and removing faulty equipment

Badly maintained equipment increases the likelihood of failure and can become a serious hazard. Faulty equipment can certainly represent a hazard and should be removed, or at least taken out of use, before it can cause harm.

Following correct manual handling techniques

Manual handling covers a wide variety of activities such as lifting, lowering, pushing, pulling and carrying – these are the cause of over a third of all workplace injuries. When these activities cannot be avoided, the risks of the task should be assessed and sensible measures should be put in place to prevent and avoid injury.

You should take account of:
▶ the strength and capability of the individual
▶ the type of load (box, crate, container for liquids, bulky item, etc.)

- environmental conditions, for example:
  - is the floor or the item being lifted wet?
  - could strong wind cause problems with light but bulky items?
- whether people have received adequate training
- how the work is organised – can it be reorganised to minimise handling or reduce the risk?
  - try to store materials in smaller quantities
  - try to store materials closer to where they are used.

Some points to remember when lifting by hand:
- Avoid, as much as possible, any twisting, stooping and reaching.
- Try not to lift from floor level or above shoulder height – particularly heavy loads.
- Arrange storage areas so as to minimise the need to lift and/or carry.
- Minimise carrying distances.
- Assess whether the load is too heavy – can it be broken down into smaller components, or can a colleague help?

If you have to use lifting equipment:
- use an aid such as a forklift or pallet truck, hoist (electric or hand-powered) or conveyor belt
- consider storage as part of the delivery process, i.e. heavy items could be delivered directly to the storage area.

Case study

Jack works as a technician in a hospital laboratory. Several times a day he collects items from the stores two floors below in a separate building. These include non-hazardous chemicals (such as 2.5, 10 and 25 litre bottles of solvent or 1–25 kg bottles of powder), large cartons of lightweight plasticware and heavy gas cylinders (compressed nitrogen and helium).
- What risks or hazards would Jack face in handling these items?
- What precautions should Jack take to minimise the risks?
- What changes could Jack's employer make to the way the work is organised?

Ensuring working environments are clean, tidy and hazard free

You may have seen signs in various workplaces saying, 'A tidy area is a safer area', and they are displayed for a good reason. Even when obvious hazards are removed, clutter can itself be a hazard:
- Items on the floor can be a trip hazard.
- Unnecessary items can conceal other hazards.

- The need to move items to get at other things can be a hazard.
- Dirty work areas can be a source of chemical or bacterial contamination.

Regular cleaning and tidying are important, and it may not be appropriate to leave the job to regular cleaning staff, for example, if there is specialist equipment or specific hazards. Making cleaning and tidying part of the regular laboratory routine will make for a much safer workplace.

Appropriately storing equipment and materials

The saying 'a place for everything and everything in its place' is an important way of ensuring safety in the workplace. It is the responsibility of the employer to ensure that appropriate storage facilities are provided – but it is everyone's responsibility to make sure that they are used properly.

Storage of hazardous substances is covered by regulations including COSHH Regulations 1994, subsequent amendments 2002, and the Hazardous Waste Regulations 2005.

We also need to think about moving equipment and materials in and out of storage and so the Manual Handling Operations Regulations 1992 (as amended) are also relevant. See pages 49, 51 and 52 for more on these three sets of regulations.

Completing statutory training

Question: who needs training in health and safety? Answer: everyone!

HSWA 1974 requires employers to provide all information, instruction, training and supervision needed to ensure (as far as reasonably practicable) the health and safety of employees.

The Management of Health and Safety at Work Regulations 1999 identify situations where training is particularly important, such as:
- when new people start work
- when there is exposure to new or increased risks
- when existing knowledge or skills have become rusty or out of date.

There are other regulations that include specific health and safety training requirements, for specific industries or for exposure to specific hazards, e.g. asbestos.

If you work with contractors or other self-employed people, they may still be classed as employees for health and safety purposes. This means that they need the same level of protection and appropriate training as regular employees – and they have the same responsibility to ensure their own health and safety and that of co-workers.

Test yourself

1   Identify three ways that management can promote health and safety at work.
2   Identify three ways that employees can promote health and safety at work.
3   Why is it important that equipment is properly maintained?
4   Why is it important that the workplace is kept clean and tidy?
5   A delivery of boxes has just arrived. You have been given the task of moving them to the storeroom and putting them onto shelves. Name three things you would have to consider to ensure safe handling.
6   Give three situations where the Management of Health and Safety at Work Regulations 1999 says that training is particularly important.

A3.4 How to deal with situations that can occur in a health or science environment that could cause harm to self or others

This is where we can put into practice what we have learned in the previous sections. Health and safety at work is governed by law and regulation (see section 3.1) that requires us to assess and minimise any potential hazards (section 3.2) and do all we can to ensure a safe working environment (section 3.3).

In any workplace, the response to a situation that could cause harm should follow a similar pattern.

Following organisational health and safety procedures

As well as helping to minimise the risk of harm, all organisations should have health and safety procedures that everyone can follow if something does go wrong. You need to be familiar with these and think about how they could prepare you to deal with any situation.

Keeping oneself and others safe, including evacuation as appropriate

In dealing with any situation, the priority is not to make things worse. For example, cleaning up a chemical spillage is important to prevent harm, but it must not be done in a way that exposes you or your colleagues to greater risk. Think about what actions and precautions you would need to take:

▶   The use of equipment such as a fire extinguisher or chemical spillage kit.
▶   The use of appropriate PPE.
▶   Do you have the training and capability to deal with the situation?
▶   Are you aware of procedures to be followed?

You should also realise that some situations are too hazardous for you to deal with yourself. In such cases, it might be necessary to evacuate the area. That could mean evacuating a room, a building or even a whole site. Are you familiar with the evacuation procedures?

Securing the area

It might be necessary to evacuate a room or building – but you do not want people wandering back in. Even if evacuation is not necessary, it is important to prevent unnecessary access while clean-up is taking place. Assuming that everyone is safe, the next step is to make sure that the situation does not get worse, for example, that a chemical spill is not continuing.

Reporting and/or escalating as appropriate

Even if the situation is relatively minor and fully controlled, you will still need to inform your supervisor, line manager, safety officer or other responsible person. If the situation is more serious than you can control by yourself, you need to know what action should be taken to escalate the response. This might involve bringing in more senior or experienced members of staff, a specialist response team or the emergency services, as appropriate.

Debriefing and reflecting on the root causes, to prevent the situation from recurring

Once the situation has been dealt with, it is important to learn lessons. This means that those involved need to review what happened and why. This will usually mean that management, safety officers or others will debrief those involved in the incident. The purpose is not to assign blame but to learn important safety lessons. It may be that procedures or working practices need to be changed to reduce the risk of future harm.

Test yourself

1 There is a chemical spillage in a school laboratory. Describe **three** actions that you would take to deal with it.

2 Under what circumstances should you evacuate an area?

3 Following a small fire in a chemical store, a debriefing is held for all employees involved. What is the main purpose of this?
   a To ensure there is no adverse publicity for the company.
   b To investigate the cause and assign blame.
   c To investigate the cause and learn safety lessons.
   d To remind employees that existing procedures must be followed without question.

Project practice

You have been recruited by a newly formed private physiotherapy company. The company has been formed by a group of qualified physiotherapists who have either worked for other private companies or in the NHS. They have formed a management team and recruited a manager with admin and finance experience. Neither the manager nor any of the physiotherapists has any experience of health and safety legislation.

You have been asked to prepare a report for the new company that achieves the following objectives:
– Makes the management aware of its responsibilities under current health and safety legislation and regulations.
– Makes recommendations for implementing a health and safety policy in the new company.

You need to complete the following steps:
1 Research a strategy.
   – Carry out a review of the relevant legislation and regulations.
   – Select the legislation and regulations that are applicable.
   – Justify why you have selected some legislation/regulations and not others.
2 Plan a project based on the legislation and/or regulations you have selected.
   – Summarise each piece of legislation and/or regulations.

– Describe the steps you would need to take to perform risk assessments, including identifying hazards.
– Identify the recording and reporting requirements.

3 Present your findings in a written report for the management team. You should cover the following areas:
   – obligations of the company and employees
   – roles and responsibilities
   – specific risk areas that need to be considered
   – how to promote the strategy within the company.

4 Discuss the following questions:
   – Does the company have the necessary information and expertise to prepare an adequate strategy for health and safety?
   – What further steps should be taken to draw up and implement the strategy within the company?
   – Who should be responsible for promoting the strategy within the company?
   – How should the roles and responsibilities be assigned? Think particularly about who should draw up the risk assessments and SOPs.

5 Reflection – write a reflective evaluation of your work.

1 Who does the Health and Safety at Work etc. Act, 1974 make responsible for the health of everyone at work?

2 To what extent does the Health and Safety at Work etc. Act 1974 compel employers to remove all risk from the workplace?

3 Which should come first, writing the SOPs or preparing the risk assessment?

4 Which of the regulations, **W** to **Z**, shown in the table, are relevant in each of the situations **A** and **B**? More than one of the regulations might apply to each situation.

Regulations		Situation in the workplace	
W	Management of Health and Safety at Work Regulations 1999	A	A company that does not handle hazardous materials needs to update its health and safety policies.
X	Control of Substances Hazardous to Health (COSHH) Regulations 2002		
Y	Environmental Protection Act (EPA) 1990	B	A technician in a school laboratory needs to dispose of old chemicals.
Z	Special Waste Regulations 1996		

5 A company is reviewing its training policy. All new employees undergo a half-day induction process that includes health and safety training. Half-day refresher courses are offered to all staff every five years. Evaluate this policy and suggest how it could be improved and why.

6 A new company has developed an approach to health and safety that includes the following:
 - The human resources department has the responsibility for carrying out all risk assessments.
 - The production department has the responsibility for preparing all SOPs.
 - Risk assessments and SOPs are made available on the company intranet.

 Assess what might be missing from the company's approach to risk assessment and SOPs. Your answer should include reasoned judgements.

7 Explain why the use of personal protective equipment should be considered only when all other steps have been taken to reduce risk.

8 You have been asked to dispose of large drums of solid and liquid chemical waste. Describe what the following legislation would require the process to include:
 - Environmental Protection Act (EPA) 1990
 - Control of Substances Hazardous to Health (COSHH) Regulations 2002
 - Manual Handling Operations Regulations 1992.

9 A company kept an accident book that was used to record all accidents that led to an employee being off work for more than seven days. Describe what the Reporting of Injuries, Diseases and Dangerous Occurrences Regulations 2013 (RIDDOR) requires in terms of recording and reporting accidents.

10 A technician has been given the task of producing SOPs for maintenance and disposal of scientific equipment. Outline the legislation and regulations that they would need to consider in producing the SOPs.

A4: Health and safety regulations applicable in the healthcare sector

Introduction

In the previous chapter, we covered the regulations that cover health, safety and the environment in the health and science sectors. We are now going to look in more detail at those that are particularly relevant in the healthcare sector.

Learning outcomes

The core knowledge outcomes that you must understand and learn:

A4.1 the purpose of workplace health and safety regulations in the health sector

A4.2 the purpose of specific health and safety regulations, guidance and regulatory bodies in relation to the health sector

A4.3 the overarching responsibilities of trained first aiders

A4.4 the purpose of guidelines produced by the Resuscitation Council (UK)

A4.5 the purpose of manual handling regulations and training, including why it's important to follow policy and guidance when moving, positioning people, equipment or other objects safely.

A4.1 The purpose of workplace health and safety regulations in the health sector

From what you learned in Chapter A3, you should now be aware of the purpose of workplace health and safety regulations in the health sector, namely:

▶ to maintain the safety and wellbeing of both the individual and healthcare workers
▶ to reduce risk to the individual and healthcare professionals
▶ to provide a duty of care to the individual and healthcare professionals.

In this context, the term 'individual' includes patients, care-receivers, members of the public, etc.

We covered the concept of a **duty of care** at the start of Chapter A3, and **safety** and **risk** were covered extensively. However, you will have seen a new term – **wellbeing**. This is a keyword in the World Health Organization (WHO) definition of health:

> 'A state of complete physical, mental and social wellbeing and not merely the absence of disease.'

It is not easy to define wellbeing – as we can see from the WHO definition, it is not simply the absence of disease. A dictionary definition will be something like 'being healthy, comfortable or happy'. Wellbeing is actually more complex than this. It is a combination of somebody's physical, mental, emotional and social health factors. It includes how well you get on with other people and how your surroundings affect you. It also includes how you feel about yourself and your life.

> Health and wellbeing is covered in more detail in Chapter A9 (page 147).

Research

The bullet points above identify the key purpose of workplace health and safety regulations. Use the information in Chapter A3 to identify the legislation and regulations that cover:

▶ Maintaining safety and wellbeing; this is covered mostly in section A3.1.
▶ Reducing risk; this is covered mostly in section A3.2.
▶ Providing a duty of care; this is also covered in section A3.1.

For each of these bullet points, identify the key features of the legislation and how it applies to your workplace.

A4.2 The purpose of specific health and safety regulations, guidance and regulatory bodies in relation to the health sector

You are highly likely to encounter all of these in the course of your work, so you need to be familiar with the purpose of each one and how it might affect you and your work.

Health and Safety (First Aid) Regulations (1981)

The regulations set legal guidelines for employers within the health sector to provide adequate and appropriate equipment, facilities and personnel to ensure their employees receive immediate attention if they are injured or taken ill at work. Notice the term 'adequate and appropriate' – what does that mean? It depends on the circumstances of your workplace.

An employer must carry out a **needs assessment** to decide on what is adequate and appropriate. This will cover aspects such as:

▶ the nature of the work done
▶ any workplace hazards and risks (this should have been covered as part of complying with HSWA 1974, see section A3.1)
▶ the characteristics and size of the workforce
▶ staff work patterns
▶ the history of accidents in the organisation.

On the basis of this needs assessment, the employer will then have to:

▶ ensure that there is an appointed person to take charge of first-aid arrangements, or that there are enough trained first aiders
▶ provide adequate facilities and a suitably stocked first-aid kit
▶ give all employees information about the first-aid arrangements.

Employees do not have any specific duties under these regulations. However, it is useful if you make your employer aware of any health issues that you have. This will allow them to take account of your needs and make appropriate provision. For example, if you have a serious allergy that might require you to use an adrenaline auto-injector (often known by the brand name EpiPen®), then (with your permission) first aiders can be made aware and, if necessary, receive extra training to help you should you be taken ill at work.

Care Act (2014)

The purpose of the Care Act (2014) is to improve people's independence and wellbeing.

Local authorities are required to provide or arrange services that make sure that people who live in their areas:

▶ are less likely to develop the need for care
▶ receive services that prevent their need for care and support becoming more serious
▶ get the information and advice they need to make good decisions about care and support
▶ have a range of provision of high-quality, appropriate services available to them.

Practice point

Central government often imposes new duties on local government but may not always provide extra financial resources for them to carry out those duties. This has been highlighted particularly since the start of the COVID-19 pandemic, during which local authorities gained extra responsibilities, for instance, around providing testing. Are you aware of any specific examples, either in the national or local news or through social media postings, where local authorities in your area have not been able to carry out their duties?

You may encounter situations in your professional life where budget constraints make it difficult or even impossible for you to provide what you believe to be the best level of care. This can lead to conflict with the ethical practice that you learned about in section A1.3.

Ionising Radiation Regulations (2017)

The IRR17 came into force on 1 January 2018, replacing the 1999 regulations. Ionising radiation includes:

▶ X-rays
▶ gamma rays
▶ radiation emitted by radioactive substances.

Ionising radiation carries more energy than other forms of radiation (known as **non-ionising radiation**) such as:

▶ visible light
▶ ultra-violet light
▶ infra-red radiation
▶ longer wavelength electromagnetic radiation (e.g. radio waves).

Just because radiation is non-ionising does not mean it cannot be harmful. For example, exposure to ultra-violet light in sunlight can cause skin cancer. For more information about ionising radiation, see sections B1.57–B1.61.

IRR17 forms part of the government's approach to radiation protection. This aims to protect people from exposure to the harmful effects of radiation.

The regulations make employers responsible for protecting employees and members of the public from exposure to:

▶ radiation arising from their work
▶ radioactive substances in the working environment
▶ any other forms of ionising radiation they encounter while at work or in the work area.

In the health sector, exposure to ionising radiation is likely to be from:

▶ X-rays and other forms of medical imaging (CT scans, PET scans, etc.)
▶ use of radioactive isotopes such as iodine-123 in diagnosis
▶ radiopharmaceuticals used in treatment, for example, to destroy or shrink tumours.

There is more information about the use of radiation in the health sector in section B1.61.

One important difference between IRR17 and the earlier regulations is that employees now have a greater obligation to co-operate with employers to ensure their own protection and the protection of others. This includes not knowingly exposing themselves or others to ionising radiation any more than is necessary to carry out their work. They must also exercise 'reasonable care'. However, employers have a duty to make sure that employees and outside workers understand how they can keep themselves safe.

Medicines and Healthcare products Regulatory Agency (MHRA)

One effect of the COVID-19 pandemic has been to increase the exposure or awareness of the public to the structures, organisations and procedures in healthcare. The **Medicines and Healthcare products Regulatory Agency** (**MHRA**) is one of those organisations. The MHRA is an executive agency of the Department of Health and Social Care and is responsible for ensuring that **medicines** and **medical devices** work and are acceptable and safe for use.

> **Key term**
>
> **Medicine:** any substance (or combination of substances) that is claimed to be able to prevent or treat human disease. Medicines are often referred to as (medical) drugs or pharmaceuticals. Medicines do not include food supplements, herbal products or cosmetics and so companies are not legally allowed to claim that these can be used to prevent or treat disease.
>
> **Medical device:** a healthcare product or piece of equipment that someone uses for a medical purpose. Medical devices can diagnose, monitor or treat disease and help people with physical impairments become more independent.

Medicines include a range of products, some of which can only be obtained with a doctor's prescription while others can be bought from pharmacies or even in supermarkets:

▶ drugs (pharmaceuticals) in the form of pills, capsules or liquids

▶ hormones such as insulin, glucagon, hydrocortisone ('cortisone')

▶ vaccines, such as those against flu or COVID-19.

The term medical device covers a wide range of items used in a healthcare environment – about 2 million different kinds worldwide, according to the WHO. These range from the quite simple to the highly complex, for example:

▶ tongue depressors used when examining the mouth and throat

▶ stethoscopes used for listening to heart and chest sounds

▶ hypodermic syringes used for giving injections or taking blood

▶ diagnostic test strips, e.g. for testing glucose concentrations in blood or urine

▶ ELISA tests used to test for the presence of HIV antibodies in blood samples

▶ RT-PCR instruments for use in diagnosing infection with SARS-CoV-2

▶ X-ray machines

▶ NMR whole body scanners.

Some types of medical device can be bought and used by the general public. For example:

▶ blood pressure monitors

▶ clinical thermometers

▶ condoms

▶ contact lenses and solutions

▶ pregnancy and other self-test kits (e.g. the lateral flow kits used in testing for COVID-19)

▶ wheelchairs.

Regulation of all of these is the responsibility of the MHRA. Approval of a medicine is given only once it has undergone strict and extensive testing for **safety** and **efficacy** (how effective it is at preventing or treating disease) through a series of **clinical trials**. Once approved, medicines are monitored for rare, harmful side-effects through the yellow card reporting system administered by the MHRA.

Testing and approval of medical products focuses more on making sure the product meets any applicable standards and is safe for use.

A4.3 The overarching responsibilities of trained first aiders

We saw in section A4.2 that employers have a duty to provide adequate first aid. This means that there must be a person appointed to take charge of first aid and that there are enough trained first aiders.

The role of a trained first aider includes several responsibilities:

▶ providing first-aid treatment for minor injuries and illness. These might include:
  – treating minor burns and scalds,
  – stopping bleeding using pressure or elevation,
  – keeping a fractured limb still and supported,
  – placing an unconscious casualty into the recovery position,
  – performing CPR or using an Automated External Defibrillator (AED); see section A4.4 for more information about this.

▶ ensuring, where necessary, that the casualty is referred for further treatment, appropriate to the circumstances of the injury/illness. This could be to their GP, an NHS walk-in centre or the Accident & Emergency department of the nearest hospital

▶ ensuring that the first-aid box/kit for which they have responsibility is kept clean, tidy and appropriately stocked. It is the responsibility of the employer to provide the contents, but the first aider must make them aware when items need to be reordered, or they need to order these themselves (e.g. from the central stores)

▶ any support provided, as far as possible, reflects an individual's needs and does not discriminate against them in any way. See section A1.3 for more information about ethical issues, particularly:

- Beneficence
- Non-maleficence
- Autonomy and informed consent
- Truthfulness and confidentiality.

When providing first aid, you must assess the situation quickly and calmly. This involves:

▶ Safety. Are you or the casualty in any danger? Is it safe to approach them (think about chemical spills or electrocution risk, for example)?

▶ Protecting yourself first, never putting yourself at risk. Only move the casualty if leaving them would cause them more harm.

▶ Preventing infection, either of you by the casualty or the casualty by you. This requires you to wear appropriate PPE.

▶ Comforting and reassuring the casualty. Introduce yourself to help gain their trust and explain the situation and any action you are going to take before you do it.

▶ Treating the casualty with respect at all times (consider the principles of ethical practice outlined in section A1.3).

▶ Assessing the casualty and giving first aid treatment as required.

A4.4 The purpose of guidelines produced by the Resuscitation Council (UK)

If someone stops breathing or suffers a cardiac arrest, there is very limited time available before they suffer permanent damage or even death. The Resuscitation Council UK states that for someone in cardiac arrest, every minute spent without receiving **cardiopulmonary resuscitation (CPR)** and having a **defibrillator** used on them reduces their chances of survival by 10 per cent. Therefore, if someone does not have a pulse (heartbeat – see section B2.11) or has stopped breathing, it is essential that they can receive CPR as quickly as possible. CPR involves chest compressions to maintain the flow of blood to the brain together with artificial ventilation (mouth-to-mouth resuscitation) to maintain an oxygen supply. A defibrillator (see below) uses a jolt of electrical energy to restart the heart.

Resuscitation Council

The Resuscitation Council UK helps to save lives in a number of ways, including by:

▶ promoting and publishing high-quality, scientifically informed resuscitation guidelines

▶ developing educational materials for learning resuscitation methods

▶ supporting research into resuscitation.

Resuscitation guidelines

The Resuscitation Council UK's guidelines help to ensure that healthcare professionals throughout the country share the same knowledge around teamwork and best practice for resuscitation. These guidelines include detailed information about basic and advanced life support for a range of individuals, including adults, paediatrics and newborns.

You can learn more about the guidelines and download the most recent version by visiting the website at **www.resus.org.uk**

Information for the use of external defibrillator

Section B2.6 describes how contraction of the heart is initiated by regular electrical signals produced by the SAN (the 'pacemaker' of the heart). In sudden cardiac arrest, these signals become disrupted and disorganised – this is described as fibrillation. Defibrillation uses a jolt of electrical energy to the heart to help restore the heart's rhythm so that it starts beating normally again.

Automated external defibrillators (AEDs) are becoming increasingly common in public spaces (on the outside of buildings or inside shopping centres, sports centres, entertainment venues), schools and colleges, as well as in many workplaces (see Figure 4.1). They are designed to be used by members of the public without any special training.

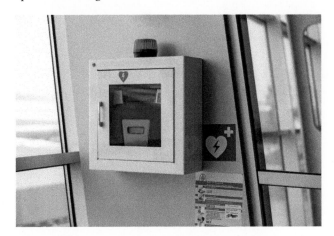

▲ Figure 4.1 An AED located in a public place

The location of an AED will be indicated with a sign (Figure 4.2) and there may also be a poster giving information about its use (Figure 4.3). Many are programmed to give verbal or audible instructions too.

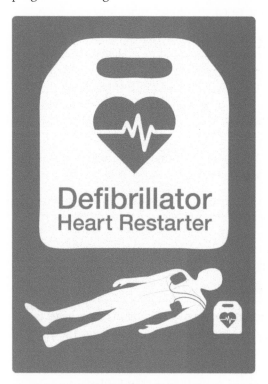

▲ Figure 4.2 Defibrillator sign

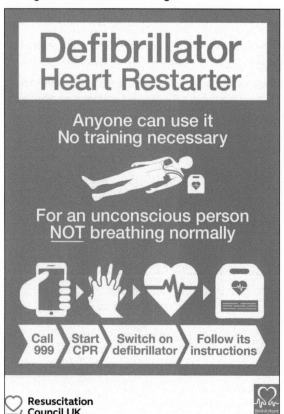

▲ Figure 4.3 Poster giving information about the use of a defibrillator

The first course of action, if someone suffers a cardiac arrest, will be to call 999 and ask for an ambulance (large organisations may have their own procedures as an alternative to calling 999). The call handler will be able to guide you through how to perform CPR and will also tell you the location of the nearest defibrillator.

AEDs or public access defibrillators are designed to be used by the public without any training. When you switch on the defibrillator it will give you clear instructions and guide you through what you need to do.

Employers are not obliged to provide AEDs to comply with the Health and Safety (First Aid) Regulations (1981) (see section A4.2) unless the needs assessment identifies a requirement for one. This might happen if:

▶ a large number of people pass through the site – the larger the number present, the greater the risk
▶ there are more older people present (employees and/or members of the public) as cardiac arrest is more common with increasing age
▶ risky procedures are undertaken, for example, the use of toxic chemicals.

If a need for an AED is identified, it is good practice to ensure that staff are familiar with its use. Grants are available from the government and charities such as the British Heart Foundation to increase the provision of AEDs in public spaces.

A4.5 The purpose of manual handling regulations and training

Section A3.3 in the previous chapter looked at manual handling throughout the science and healthcare sectors. It covered regulations, general guidelines for manual handling and why it is important to follow policy and guidance.

However, there are specific issues with manual handling in the healthcare sector because there is a frequent need to move and handle people (patients and care-receivers, for example). Poor practice can lead to:

▶ back pain and other musculoskeletal disorders that can make you unable to work, sometimes for a long time
▶ moving and handling accidents that can injure both the person being moved and the mover
▶ discomfort and a lack of dignity for the person being moved.

If your work requires you to move or position people, you must receive training on the general principles of safe handling, either on your own or with a colleague (as in Figure 4.4), as well as on any specialised equipment, such as slings or bath or bed hoists (Figure 4.5).

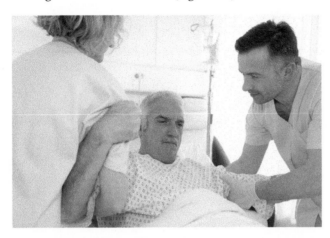

▲ Figure 4.4 Two healthcare workers help a patient out of bed

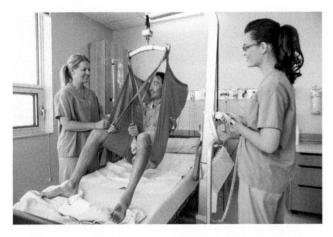

▲ Figure 4.5 Patients can be lifted from bed using a specialised bed hoist

The reasons for this are the need to:
▶ protect individuals (patients) and healthcare professionals from harm.
▶ comply with the requirements of health and safety law and regulations as well as the policy and guidance of the organisation.

Training should be given on a regular basis so that you maintain your skills and particularly when new lifting aids or equipment are introduced. Supervisors should also receive regular training so that they can monitor, identify and correct poor practice by their staff.

Research

The HSE publishes a useful information sheet 'Getting to grips with hoisting people' that has a lot of useful information about the problems associated with hoisting people as well as giving guidance on how to deal with those problems. This is available from **https://www.hse.gov.uk/pubns/hsis3.pdf**.

Does this provide sufficient information for your work situation? Do you need additional training on any specific equipment used in your workplace?

Manual handling regulations

We saw in section A3.3 that the main aim of the regulations is to prevent injury or harm. It is important to follow policy and guidance when moving or positioning people as well as moving equipment or other objects to protect the individuals and healthcare professional from harm.

Case study

A newly built hospital had carpeted areas that made it too difficult to manoeuvre the mobile patient hoists (such as that shown in Figure 4.5). As a result, healthcare staff had stopped using the hoists.

The staff identified the carpets as a risk factor. When a patient occupied the hoist, their weight caused the wheels to sink into the carpet, making it difficult to move the hoist. The wheels on the hoist were made of rubber, which is suitable for smooth and/or hard floors.

The supplier of the hoists offered a different type of wheel that was better suited for use on carpet. This reduced the amount of force required to move the hoist by about 40 per cent. As a result, the healthcare staff started to use the hoist again.
▶ What are the risks and possible consequences of healthcare staff not using the hoists?
▶ Two other possible solutions were to replace the carpet or to use larger wheels (these need less force to move but raise the hoist higher). Why do you think these solutions were discounted?

All employers must, by law, have **employer's liability insurance** to provide compensation to staff for injuries suffered in the workplace. It is normally a requirement of this insurance that staff are properly trained in manual handling procedures.

There are also legal requirements under health and safety legislation (see section A3.1) for employers to carry out risk assessment of manual handling techniques and for employees to co-operate by following the organisation's procedures.

Project practice

Think about your own workplace, or one that you are familiar with.

Prepare a report on the workplace health and safety regulations that would apply in your chosen workplace. This should include:
▶ a summary of the main points of the regulations that apply
▶ the risk assessments that should be undertaken
▶ any specific precautions that should be taken to ensure the safety of staff and members of the public
▶ ways in which you could increase awareness of the need for adherence to health and safety regulations and practices.

To what extent do you think your chosen workplace meets these regulations? Are there any areas for improvement?

You should present your report in the form of a Word document or PowerPoint presentation.

Write a reflective evaluation of your work.

Assessment practice

1   Outline the main purposes of:
    a   the Health and Safety (First Aid) Regulations (1981)
    b   the Care Act (2014).
2   Which **one** of the following statements about the Ionising Radiation Regulations (2017) (IRR17) is correct?
    a   Employers are solely responsible for protecting workers and the public from the harmful effects of ionising radiation.
    b   Employees have a duty to co-operate with their employer to protect themselves and others from the harmful effects of ionising radiation.
    c   IRR17 only applies to radiation from instruments such as x-ray machines and CT scanners.
    d   IRR17 only applies to radiation from radioactive isotopes used as medicines.

3   A friend says that they do not want to be vaccinated because 'vaccines aren't properly tested'. What arguments would you use to persuade them?
4   A colleague is a trained first aider. They are facing disciplinary action because there are several items missing from their first-aid box. In their defence, they say that other members of staff are taking them without their knowledge or consent, and they cannot afford to keep replacing the items that are taken. Evaluate your colleague's defence.
5   What is the purpose of the guidelines concerning the provision and use of external defibrillators?
6   You are working on a night shift in a care home and you are the only staff member on your wing. An alarm sounds and you discover that an elderly patient with dementia has fallen out of bed. How do the manual handling regulations determine the action that you should take?

A5: Managing information and data within the health and science sector

Introduction

Before we can think about managing information and data, we have to make sure we know what is meant by the terms **information** and **data**. We often use them interchangeably, as if they have the same meaning – but do they?

Data is a collection of values. These values can be characters or words, numbers or other data types. You may sometimes see the phrase 'units of information' as a description of data.

Information is data that has been processed in a way that we can read it, understand it and use it.

So, managing information and data allows us to use the data to generate useful information that can increase our understanding.

Learning outcomes

The core knowledge outcomes that you must understand and learn:

A5.1 a range of methods used to collect data

A5.2 the considerations to make when selecting a range of ways to collect and record information and data

A5.3 the importance of accuracy, attention to detail and legibility of any written information or data

A5.4 the strengths and limitations of a range of data sources when applied in a range of health and science environments

A5.5 how new technology is applied in the recording and reporting of information and data

A5.6 how personal information is protected by data protection legislation, regulations and local ways of working/organisational policies

A5.7 how to ensure confidentiality when using screens to input or retrieve information or data

A5.8 the positive use of, and restrictions on the use of, social media in health and science sectors

A5.9 the advantages and risks of using IT systems to record, retrieve and store information and data

A5.10 how security measures protect data stored by organisations

A5.11 what to do if information is not stored securely.

A5.1 A range of methods used to collect data

The methods that we use to collect data depend on the type of data. Data types will be discussed in a little more detail in section A5.2.

Focus groups

Focus groups are used widely in health research, as well as in parts of the science sector, as a way of discovering what individuals feel or believe. They can be very useful in understanding and explaining the factors that influence the feelings and attitudes of individuals as well as how they behave.

A focus group interview is usually highly structured. Participants are usually selected on the basis that they will have something to say on the topic – hence the term 'focus' – rather than being randomly selected. The focus group interview will have a facilitator or moderator whose job is to guide the discussion and manage the interactions between the participants. It is important that participants feel comfortable with expressing their views and opinions.

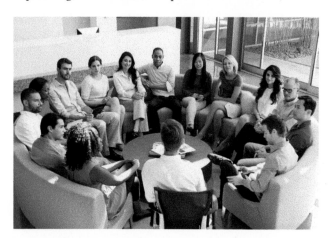

▲ Figure 5.1 Focus groups need a facilitator or moderator to lead the discussion

Focus groups can produce huge quantities of data that need to be processed and analysed to give useful information.

Surveys

A survey is a way of gathering factual information as well as views and opinions. They can be of two types: **closed-question** or **open-question**.

Closed-question surveys

Closed questions are questions that require a simple answer (see the table for examples). The advantage of closed-question surveys is that they can be quick and easy to carry out and produce a large amount of data that can be analysed quite easily. This can be made even more efficient when the survey is online or in some other electronic format so that the data is already available in electronic format for further analysis.

However, the questions must be carefully worded to obtain reliable data. This might involve giving people information and asking for their opinion, but there can still be ways in which the results might be influenced by the wording of the questions. Consider the following two questions:

1 People under the age of 40 are less likely to die of COVID-19. Do you think the risks of the COVID-19 vaccine outweigh the benefits in this age group?
2 People under the age of 40 are more likely to suffer with 'long Covid'. Do you think the benefits of the COVID-19 vaccine outweigh the risks in this age group?

Do you think you would have given different answers about the risks and benefits if you were asked these two questions?

Open-question surveys

Open questions are questions that require a longer answer or explanation (see the table). The advantage of open-question surveys is that they allow people to provide more information. This can be important when you are gathering information about complex issues or questions that do not have a simple yes/no answer. However, analysis of the data will take longer and be more complex.

Closed question	Open question
Have you been vaccinated against COVID-19?	What is your opinion of the COVID-19 vaccine?
Have you been admitted to hospital for an overnight stay?	What is your experience of staying in hospital overnight?
Who is your GP?	What is your opinion of the service provided by your GP?
When was the last time you were unwell?	How do you feel about your general state of health?

Interviews

An open-question survey can also be carried out face to face, in which case it can become an interview where the person asking the questions has the opportunity to follow up on answers to questions or adapt the interview to the individual. This can improve the quality of the data collected because it may not necessarily impose ideas or opinions on the individual responding to the survey. However, interviews can be even more complex to analyse and draw conclusions from.

Closed-question surveys are probably better at obtaining large amounts of data from a large number of people. Open-question surveys or interviews are probably better when the number of people being surveyed is relatively small.

Observation

This can be a good way of gathering data about behaviour, which explains its widespread use in healthcare and social science or animal behaviour studies (see case studies). It is an important part of the method known as **qualitative research** (see section A5.2).

In clinical and pharmaceutical research, randomised controlled trials are considered to be the most effective and reliable. In these, an experimental treatment or drug is compared either to a **placebo** (dummy treatment or drug) or to an existing treatment or drug. However, it is not always possible or desirable to carry out this type of trial. One example is where it is unethical to give a dummy treatment or drug.

In experimental studies, a researcher will usually have two groups: a test group and a control group. In observational studies, the researcher simply looks at (observes) groups of patients and compares the effectiveness of different types or treatment. An example is the **cohort** study, where a group of people (the cohort) is followed over a period of time. This can allow comparison of different treatment or care pathways to see which is the most effective. Cohort studies can be **prospective** or **retrospective**.

> ### Key terms
>
> **Prospective:** these studies take a group of people and observe them over a period of time. This could involve looking for correlations between factors such as diet or exercise and development of cardiovascular disease. The advantage is that the data collection methods can be tailored to the question being asked. The disadvantage is that these can take many years to complete.
>
> **Retrospective:** these studies look backwards at data from a group of people over many years. This often involves examining published data classifying people according to risk factors or medical outcomes. Although these can give results more quickly than prospective studies, the disadvantage of retrospective studies is that there is little control over data collection. This type of study typically looks at published data from many different sources that might involve different methods of data collection or analysis.

In clinical medicine, observation is very important in making diagnoses. However, the observational method used in qualitative research involves watching people to establish behaviours in a natural setting.

Public databases, journals and articles

You will notice, as you work through this book, that many of the Project practice items at the end of each chapter will start with asking you to research a topic. This is often to search published literature (see page 78), often for background information, but also to make sure that you are not just repeating work that has already been done.

Health Education England and the National Institute for Health and Care Excellence (NICE) provide access to a wide range of journals and other evidence-based resources for health and social care staff in England. Access to these requires an NHS OpenAthens account; you may be eligible for this if your course involves an NHS placement.

The Millennium Cohort Study (MCS)

The MCS is following the lives of about 19,000 young people born in the UK in 2000–2002. The study collects data on:

▶ Physical, social, emotional, cognitive and behavioural development (cognitive development is the ability to carry out conscious mental activities such as thinking, understanding, learning and remembering).

▶ Daily life, behaviour and experiences.

▶ Economic circumstances, parenting, relationships and family life.

▶ GCSE exam results.

The MCS has provided important evidence of how circumstances in the very early years of life can influence later health and development.

Research based on the MCS has shown that children born at or just before the weekend are less likely to be breastfed, because breastfeeding support services are less available in hospitals at weekends. Breastfeeding has been shown to have a strong influence on cognitive development.

The MCS has also contributed crucial evidence on two major health issues facing this generation – obesity and the high rates of poor mental health. There is more information about the MCS on the website: https://cls.ucl.ac.uk/cls-studies/millennium-cohort-study

1 How do prospective studies like the MCS differ from retrospective studies?

2 Do you think a prospective study can produce better quality data?

Observation of clinical practice

Observational research has been used to collect data on errors and potentially harmful events. A UK study on 10 wards in two hospitals showed that almost half of intravenous drug preparations and administrations had at least one error.

This research was an example of an ethnographic study – one where the researcher is immersed in the community being observed. In this case, the nursing staff were told that the observer was investigating common problems of preparing and administering intravenous drugs. The word 'error' was avoided so that the study did not appear to threaten the staff.

Source: K. Taxis & N. Barber (2003) BMJ 326, **684** (https://doi.org/10.1136/bmj.326.7391.684)

1 Do you think that observational research into patient care is important?

2 Is it always possible to build a complete and accurate picture of patient care by comparing outcomes in different hospitals or clinics?

The US National Library of Medicine has an online database, PubMed.gov, that has over 32 million biomedical research articles. Many of these have links to full text content, including free-to-access as well as paid-for content. PubMed is a free resource.

As well as literature databases (books, journals, articles, etc.) there are clinical databases that contain data rather than published research. These include:

▶ observational data on patients who meet certain criteria, such as disease type or population

▶ clinical trial data, such as **www.clinicaltrials.gov** (US based).

The World Health Organization (WHO) publishes databases in many health-related fields, including:

▶ life expectancy

▶ immunisation and vaccination data

▶ mortality.

From September 2021 NHS Digital (the part of the NHS that designs, develops and operates IT and data services in the NHS) began to collect patient data from GP medical records in England. This data includes information about symptoms, test results, diagnoses and medication as well as about physical, mental and sexual health. The intention is to use this data to improve health and care services through better planning, preventing spread of infectious diseases, help with research and monitoring the long-term safety and effectiveness of care. The data will not include people's names or where they live, but there are concerns that it will not be completely anonymous.

Another concern is that this data will be sold to private companies, such as pharmaceutical companies, as well as being made available to research organisations such as universities and charities.

Do you think that making this type of data available could help in the development of new treatments? NHS Digital plans to charge for access to this data. It says that this covers its costs in processing the data and delivering the service, but some people think that this amounts to selling patient data. Do you think this is ethical? Do you think the benefit of using the data to improve treatment outweighs the risk to patient privacy and confidentiality?

These databases are invaluable sources for health and healthcare researchers.

Carrying out practical investigations

When we think of data, we probably think first about the results of experiments in the lab rather than some of the methods just discussed. Practical investigations in the field of health and healthcare can include laboratory experiments, for example, in basic medical science, using knowledge and techniques that build on the subjects covered in Chapter B2: Further science concepts.

Practical investigations can form the basis of evidence-based practice, as discussed in section A2.9. These include:

▶ clinical trials of pharmaceuticals, usually run by pharmaceutical companies
▶ investigation of different types of care or treatment, such as comparison of drug treatment with talking therapies (talking to a therapist or counsellor) for treating mental illnesses
▶ investigation of different types of therapy, such as the RECOVERY trial into treatments for COVID-19.

Case study

The RECOVERY trial is the world's largest clinical trial into treatments for COVID-19. It was funded by the Medical Research Council and the National Institute for Health Research and led by the University of Oxford. The trial found one of the world's first effective drug treatments, dexamethasone. This cheap and widely available steroid medicine was shown to reduce deaths of patients in hospital with COVID-19 by one third.

Later the trial showed that tocilizumab, an anti-inflammatory drug used to treat rheumatoid arthritis, also reduces the risk of death in patients in hospital with severe COVID-19.

Do you think that low-cost treatments like dexamethasone would have been found if the investigations had been left to pharmaceutical companies that need to make profit for their shareholders?

Official statistics

Organisations such as Public Health England (PHE) and the WHO collect and publish statistics on disease, public health, health protection and health improvement. Official statistics available from PHE include those about:

▶ general public health
▶ alcohol, tobacco and drug use
▶ cancer
▶ cardiovascular disease
▶ child and maternal health
▶ chronic disease
▶ COVID-19
▶ diet and physical activity
▶ obesity
▶ end of life care
▶ immunisation and infectious diseases
▶ mental health
▶ sexual and reproductive health.

The WHO publishes statistics on an even wider range of health-related topics worldwide and by country.

Reflect

Collecting and publishing all these statistics is time consuming and can be expensive. So why do organisations publish official statistics? Think about how such statistics could be used.

Sometimes governments may be embarrassed if official statistics show that policies are not always working. For this reason, it is important that the collection and publication of official statistics is done in a transparent way so that we can have confidence in them.

Test yourself

1 State whether each of these questions is closed or open:
   a How often do you visit your dentist?
   b Have you found it difficult to find an NHS dentist in your area?
   c What type of extra services does your dentist offer?
2 What type of data collection would you use for the following?
   a To discover trends in the incidence of cardiovascular disease in the second half of the twentieth century.
   b To compare the amount of exercise taken by 18–24 year olds and 40–50 year olds in a local authority area.
   c To discover if vigorous exercise increases heart rate more in young people compared to middle-aged people.
   d To discover if young people are better than older people at using unfamiliar equipment.

A5.2 The considerations to make when selecting a range of ways to collect and record information and data

There are many ways we can collect data and turn it into useful information. If we choose the wrong way, we might discover that it is harder to analyse or present and so we cannot get and communicate the best information and understanding from our data.

Data type

Quantitative data includes measurements such as length, height, age, time or mass. Quantitative data can be either:

▶ **discrete** (or discontinuous), meaning something that you can count, such as number of patients, number of visits to the GP, number of cases of flu in a year. Discrete data is usually in whole numbers – you cannot have half a patient or visit your GP on 2.75 occasions in a year

▶ **continuous**, meaning something that can be measured, such as height, weight or blood glucose concentration. Continuous data can have any value within a range and so is usually not in whole numbers – you could have a weight of 94.7 kg or a blood glucose concentration of 5.2 mmol/litre.

Once you process data, for example, by taking an average, it is quite possible for discrete data to no longer be in whole numbers. For example, the average UK household size has been 2.4 for a number of years, but each household will have a whole number of members.

Source: www.ons.gov.uk/peoplepopulationandcommunity/ birthsdeathsandmarriages/families/bulletins/familiesandhouseholds/2020

Qualitative data is usually text-based, describing something in a way that may involve numbers (for instance, a rating of how good something is), but will also contain descriptive text. For example, a patient's medical history may contain their age, date of birth and blood pressure (all types of quantitative data) as well as qualitative data such as any diseases or other health conditions they have, operations or medical procedures they have undergone, and other information about their health and wellbeing.

Key terms

Quantitative data: is numerical, for example, the results from a laboratory experiment.

Discrete data: is numerical and can be **counted**. For example, number of patients (you cannot have half a patient). This is sometimes referred to as **integer** (only whole numbers).

Continuous data: is numerical and can be measured. It is possible to have any intermediate value, for example, height, mass, length.

Qualitative data: is descriptive, for example, a patient's medical history.

The most appropriate method of data collection

A laboratory notebook is the traditional method of collecting experimental data in the sciences and medicine, although paper notebooks are being replaced by electronic versions. These offer advantages in terms of security (e.g. backup of data) and data sharing (e.g. collaboration).

Quantitative data can be collected automatically. For example, a data logger can be connected to a piece of electronic equipment to capture the output (data) and transfer it to a computer. This offers several advantages:

▶ Data can be collected without the need for a human operator to be present.

▶ Data can be captured continuously, for long periods if necessary.

▶ Once captured by the computer, the data can be analysed and processed.

Qualitative data is usually based on observation and so cannot normally be collected automatically. However, qualitative data may be collected via questionnaires or surveys, and these can be set up in electronic format, either on computer, tablet or online. This means that much of the data collection can be automated. As with collection of quantitative data, this allows some (if not all) of the data processing and analysis to be automated.

Application of new technology to collection and analysis of data will be covered in more detail in section A5.5.

The most appropriate way to present the information or data

Before considering how to present information or data, we need to think about **dependent** and **independent variables**.

> ### Key terms
>
> **Dependent variable:** (often denoted by y) a variable whose value depends on that of another variable. In an experiment, we usually count or measure the dependent variable.
>
> **Independent variable:** (often denoted by x) a variable whose value does not depend on that of another variable. In an experiment, the independent variable is usually what we change.

Tables

When we collect data, we usually record it in a table, and this can often be a useful way to present the data.

There are rules to follow when presenting data in a table. This ensures uniformity so that anyone reading the table will be familiar with the layout of the data.

▶ Put the **independent** variable in the first column; the **dependent** variable should be in columns to the right.

▶ Put any processed data, such as means, rates or statistical calculations, in columns to the far right.

▶ Do not include calculations in the table, only **calculated values** (the results of your calculations).

▶ Head each column with the physical quantity and correct units and separate the units with brackets or a slash ('/'), for example, 'mass (g)' or 'body temperature/°C'.

▶ Do not include units in the body of the table, only in the column headings.

▶ Use consistent numbers of decimal places or significant figures throughout (see section B1.64 for more information about significant figures), even if it means writing 20.0 rather than 20.

▶ Calculated values, e.g. mean or other processed data, should be given to the same number of decimal places as the raw data, or one greater.

The table shows an example of how data should be presented. In this case, four 30-year-old men were asked to walk or run at a steady rate on a treadmill. The subject's heart rate (dependent variable) was measured in beats per minute (bpm) after 10 minutes. Following a period of recovery, the speed of the treadmill (independent variable) was increased and the experiment repeated. This was carried out at eight different speeds. The experiment was repeated for each of the four subjects and a mean value at each angle was calculated.

Speed of treadmill (km/hr)	Heart rate after 10 minutes (bpm)				
	Subject 1	Subject 2	Subject 3	Subject 4	Mean
2	75	78	80	76	77
4	80	82	85	88	84
6	88	89	92	90	90
8	95	98	101	105	100
10	110	105	115	112	111
12	125	100	128	130	128
14	155	158	160	165	160
16	170	175	178	185	177

> ### Reflect
>
> One reason for presenting data like this is that it can help identify anomalous results – ones that stand out as being 'different'. If you look at the highlighted cell in the table (subject 2 at 12 km/hr) you will see that the heart rate is lower than the same subject at 10 km/hr and is much lower than the other subjects at the same speed. Something is obviously wrong – maybe the heart rate monitor was not working properly – and so we discount this result as anomalous, and we have not included it in the calculation of the mean value (you can check that for yourself).
>
> As well as dependent and independent variables, there are **control** variables. These are things that we must keep constant (control) during the experiment. In this case, it means that anything that might affect heart rate, other than the speed of the treadmill, must be kept constant. One control variable would be the angle (steepness) of the treadmill as this makes walking or running more difficult.
>
> What other control variables can you think of?

Graphs and charts

The type of graph we use will depend on the nature of our data as well as what we hope to get from the graph.

Scatter graph

Scatter graphs are used when investigating the relationship between two variables that can be measured in pairs, for example, the age and height of children in a school. The graph can then be used to establish whether there is a relationship between the variables. This could be a **positive correlation** (as variable x increases, variable y increases, as in Figure 5.2), a **negative correlation** (as variable x increases, variable y decreases) or **no correlation** at all. To tell whether the correlation is significant or not you need to carry out a statistical test.

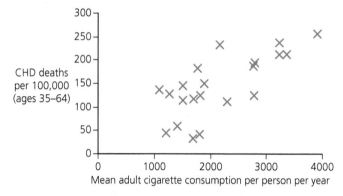

▲ Figure 5.2 Scatter graph showing the correlation between smoking and deaths from coronary heart disease (CHD)

Reflect

Does correlation imply causation?

This question means: just because there is a positive correlation between two variables, does that mean that one causes the other? For example, there is a strong positive correlation between ice-cream sales and deaths from drowning. Does that mean ice cream is a major cause of drowning? Should we ban ice-cream sales anywhere near open water? Or is there some other factor that is correlated with both? Hot weather, for example.

Line graph

Line graphs are used to show **continuous** data (see Figure 5.3). The independent variable, the one that we change, should be on the x-axis (the horizontal axis – think of it like changing a baby's nappy: the thing that is changed goes on the bottom). The dependent variable, the one that changes in response to changes in the independent variable, goes on the y-axis (the vertical axis). You would usually join the points with straight lines. You can draw a smooth curve or line of

best fit if you think that intermediate values will fall on the curve/line.

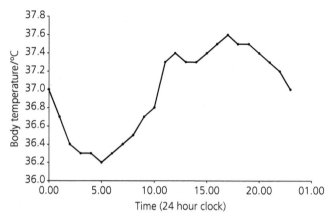

▲ Figure 5.3 Line graph showing how body temperature varies slightly during a 24-hour period

Bar charts and histograms

Bar charts are used to display **categorical data**. If you have an independent variable that is non-numerical (e.g. blood group, ethnic group of patient), then you should use a bar chart. These can be made up of lines, or blocks of equal width, that do not touch (Figure 5.4). The lines or blocks can be arranged in any order, although it can help make comparisons if they are arranged in order of increasing or decreasing size.

Bar charts can be turned through 90 degrees if it is easier to show or read horizontal rather than vertical bars.

Key term

Categorical data: is divided into groups or categories, such as male and female, ethnic group, city or country of residence.

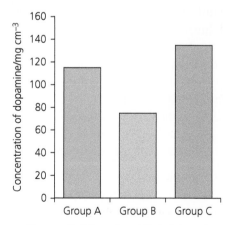

▲ Figure 5.4 Bar chart showing concentration of the neurotransmitter dopamine in three groups of patients

Histograms are sometimes called frequency diagrams. These can be used for either discrete data or continuous data grouped into classes, such as a range of heights or weights. The independent variable is usually on the *x*-axis and is grouped into classes. For example, the height of students in a class could be measured and grouped into 5 cm classes. Height is a continuous variable – students could be any height within a range – and so blocks are drawn touching. The axis is labelled with the class boundaries, e.g. 1600 mm, 1650 mm, 1700 mm, 1750 mm, 1800 mm, etc. and the *y*-axis would show the number or frequency within each class represented by the height of the bar (Figure 5.5).

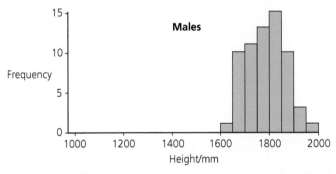

▲ Figure 5.5 Frequency distribution showing height of 18-year-old male students

Pie chart

Pie charts can be used when you need to show proportions or percentages (Figure 5.6). If you are drawing a pie chart by hand, you need to calculate the angle of each sector – divide the percentage by 100 and multiply by 360°, or just multiply the proportion by 360°. However, it is usually much easier to put your data into a spreadsheet and use the chart function to draw the pie chart!

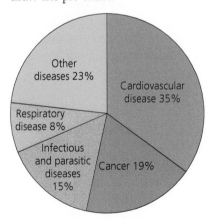

▲ Figure 5.6 Pie chart showing worldwide causes of death from disease, 2000–2019

Source: www.who.int/data/gho/data/themes/mortality-and-global-health-estimates/ghe-leading-causes-of-death

Case study

You have been asked to present data about the incidence (number of cases) of cardiovascular disease in the UK. You have been given the following data:

1 Total incidence of cardiovascular disease by age group (21–30, 31–40, 41–50, 51–60, 61–70, 71 and above).

2 Incidence of cardiovascular disease by the same age groups but separated into males and females.

3 Total incidence of cardiovascular disease (all ages) broken down by ethnic group.

You decide to use a histogram for the first data set. For the second data set, you have two options. You could draw two separate histograms, one for males and one for females. Alternatively, you could use a single histogram and draw two columns for each age group, one for males and one for females.

▶ Which do you think would be better?

▶ Are there advantages and disadvantages of each?

For the third data set you know that you cannot use a histogram. You could use a bar chart or you could use a pie chart.

▶ Think about the two ways of presenting the data. What advantages and disadvantages of each can you see?

Depth of analysis required

Collecting data is the start of the process. To convert raw data into useful information we usually need to carry out some form of analysis. Using graphs and charts can help in analysing the data or they can be the end point, i.e. how we present the data.

The depth of analysis required can determine how we record and present the data. Spreadsheet programs, such as Microsoft Excel or Apple Numbers, are convenient ways of recording data. We could enter the data manually, or even download data collected by a data logger directly into a spreadsheet. Once in a spreadsheet we can use a range of tools to analyse the data:

▶ simple analysis such as calculating the mean (average)

▶ more complex analysis such as statistical tests.

Another advantage of using a spreadsheet to record data is that we can use the graphing tools to present our data in different ways, such as the types of graphs and charts described on pages 73–75.

Qualitative or text-based data, e.g. from observations, surveys or focus groups, would normally be recorded and stored in a database, such as Microsoft Access or Apple FileMaker. Databases can contain huge quantities of data. They can also be used to analyse qualitative data as well as to organise it in ways that helps gain insight into connections, trends or groupings within the data.

Databases also allow others, such as collaborators or the general public, to access the data (if permitted), so this can be a way of presenting and sharing information as well as collecting, storing and analysing data.

The intended audience

This is a consideration largely when deciding how to present our data. Simple graphs and charts can make data and information more accessible to a non-specialist audience. This might be the case with an information leaflet or poster aimed at patients or the general public. Meanwhile, a more specialist audience might require more complex graphs that may give greater insight into the finer detail of the data. This would be the case if we wrote a research paper aimed at fellow health professionals for publication in a scientific or healthcare journal.

Collecting and storing data in electronic format (spreadsheet or database) also allows collaborators to get easy access to the data so that they can use it in their own work.

Storage method

How we store data depends in part on how it is collected and how it is used. Paper-based surveys, questionnaires or records of interviews or observations can, of course, simply be kept on paper. The same is true of results of experiments in a lab notebook. However, if they can be converted to digital format, then we can analyse them in the ways described. Data that has been collected in digital form would usually be stored in that form.

A5.3 The importance of accuracy, attention to detail and legibility of any written information or data

There are a few rules we must always follow in keeping written records of our work:
▶ We must be able to understand the record.
▶ It should be legible and contain enough detail for someone else to understand it and be able to repeat the work.
▶ It should be a faithful, honest and accurate record of what we did.

Always write up your work as you go along; do not make notes on scraps of paper and write it all up later – even if you do not lose the scraps of paper, you may not remember all the details. It is always good practice to date all your notes. In some organisations there may even be a legal requirement to do so.

There are numerous reasons why we must pay attention to detail and accuracy in written information or data.
▶ It may be necessary to comply with legal requirements, for example, the General Data Protection Regulation (GDPR) – see section A5.6.

- We may need to limit liability, either our own or that of the organisation – for example, by ensuring anonymity and to record informed consent.
- We should be able to provide an accurate account of events. That might be obvious when recording the details of an experiment, but it is also important in a healthcare situation. Knowing exactly what happened in the lead-up to a patient's condition improving or deteriorating can be essential in learning from experience. It might also be needed if there is an investigation into the patient's care.
- It will help collaboration in integrated working and data sharing. You may be able to remember the details of an experiment, treatment or patient's observations. However, unless you record those details clearly and accurately, colleagues may not have sufficient information without asking you for more detail. Sharing of data is essential in multidisciplinary teams, where healthcare professionals with different specialisms must work together.
- It helps to ensure accurate analysis of findings. Accurate analysis begins with good quality data. If the data is poor, then the processed or analysed data will also be poor, and the conclusions may be invalid. Recording a patient's **clinical observations** (see section B2.10 and B2.11 for more detail about this topic) is an important aspect of monitoring a patient. If these observations are not correctly and accurately recorded, it may not be possible to identify whether they are within the normal range.
- It can provide evidence needed in support of audit trails. This could include things as diverse as:
  - keeping a record of a patient's clinical observations
  - providing evidence that a medication or treatment has been given and when.
- To help ensure reproducibility of results. Our work can be reproduced only if it is clear what we did, how we did it and what our results were.

Results are **repeatable** when we carry out an investigation several times in the same place, using the same method under the same conditions, and get the same result.

Results are **reproducible** when investigations are carried out by different people, in different places using different methods or equipment, and get the same result. This means that our findings can be replicated by others.

Case study

A study at a large hospital in England found that nurses sometimes completed documentation retrospectively (after the event) without full knowledge that the recorded care had been completed. One nurse described how a patient had collapsed, but their notes did not contain any information about why they had been admitted. In another case, nurses completed the documentation before they carried out procedures because they were worried about forgetting to complete the paperwork. Accurate record keeping was particularly important for older patients because of the complexity of care that they require and also the problems they may have with communication. However, nurses working with older patients found completing the documentation was very time consuming and took them away from patient care.

The authors of the study recommended that electronic methods of documenting patient care could be used to reduce the amount of unnecessary paperwork as well as to make sharing of information more effective.
- Can you see lessons for your own practice?
- Do you feel that there is sometimes a conflict between accurate record keeping and providing care?
- Should that be the case?

A5.4 The strengths and limitations of a range of data sources when applied in a range of health and science environments

If we are going to be able to draw valid and useful conclusions from data – get good quality information – we need to have an appreciation of the strengths and limitations of the type of data source. Otherwise we risk producing poor quality information based on invalid conclusions.

Results of investigations

Scientific or medical experiments ('investigations') should, if properly designed, give consistent and reliable results. This is because they should be well designed. This includes:
- formulating a clear hypothesis to be tested
- designing an experiment to test that hypothesis
- controlling all variables

- repeating measurements, excluding anomalous results (these are outliers, or results that lie outside of the range of the others) and calculating mean values
- performing a statistical analysis to test the significance of the results.

However, there can be limitations. For example, we might be tempted to apply the results of an investigation done under highly controlled conditions to the more complex situation of the 'real world'. A potential new drug might show promise when tested in test-tube experiments, for instance. However, complex interactions in living systems might mean that the drug does not work as hoped when tested in humans, or it might have unexpected and even harmful side-effects.

Patient history

At its simplest level, this approach involves taking medical histories of patients. This is a skill that many healthcare professionals need to develop. Done well, a medical history will provide detailed information about a patient over a long period. However, the data may be incomplete, particularly if it relies on the patient's memory.

If you consult some of the databases described in section A5.1 you might come across many studies looking at patient histories over time. Some of these will look backwards at patient data – these are known as **retrospective** studies. Others will follow a group of normal subjects (a selection of the general population, perhaps of a particular age) or patients over a long period to look for development or progress of disease over a period of time – these are known as **prospective** studies.

In either case, the studies are likely to involve a **cohort**, which is a group of individuals that have something in common. It could be age, sex, state of health or disease, occupation, etc. Examples of this are the two Whitehall studies. Each of these followed a large group of British civil servants over many years and looked at factors that affected the health of the cohort, in particular cardiovascular disease and mortality rates. One finding was that there was a correlation between employment grade and reduced risk of cardiovascular disease – more senior civil servants enjoyed better health.

The strength of this type of study is that it can provide detailed information over time. However, there are cases where the data may not be accurate or complete, particularly with retrospective studies.

Patient test results

Patient test results usually mean the results of biochemical and other laboratory analysis. These should offer a high level of accuracy. Also, testing laboratories and the tests themselves must usually go through an accreditation process to ensure that they operate to approved standards and give reliable results. This means that test results this week should be comparable with results of tests taken weeks or months ago. It should also be possible to compare test results performed in different laboratories.

However, as humans are complex, a patient's test results will often need careful interpretation. This can introduce an element of subjectivity. Two healthcare professionals might look at the same set of patient test results and make different interpretations or draw different conclusions.

Published literature

The medical and scientific literature is a huge and invaluable resource in the health and science sector. This is the reason why most research projects will start with a literature review, to see what work has already been done and how that can inform and influence the research you plan to undertake. It is also an important tool for learning and diagnosis.

As well as the sheer volume available, another strength of published literature is that it goes through a process of **peer review**. This is where, before it can be published, a research paper is examined by other experts in the field. They might find flaws in the experiments or the logic or interpretation of the results and request that any deficiencies are put right before publication. This process improves the validity of the published research.

This process is not perfect. Professional rivalry means that reviewers are not always impartial. Also, the process can be slow and cumbersome, taking weeks, months or even years. This has led to a trend for **preprints**. These are papers that are published rapidly before peer review. This has the advantage of putting information into the scientific community very quickly. This is important during an event such as the COVID-19 pandemic, because information about new treatments can be made available rapidly in order to save lives.

However, not all published literature is of equal high quality. Some research might be based on studies with very small sample sizes, for example, clinical trials with only a few patients. The methods used in the experiment or study might be biased in a way that produces the results the investigators hoped for. The work might even be based on fraudulent data.

Andrew Wakefield and the MMR autism fraud

Andrew Wakefield was an academic physician who published a paper in the medical journal *The Lancet* in 1998. In this paper, Wakefield claimed that there was a link between the measles-mumps-rubella (MMR) vaccine and autism, based on a study involving 12 children. The publication, and particularly news conferences given by Wakefield, led to a loss of confidence in the MMR vaccine.

After the original publication, other researchers were unable to reproduce Wakefield's findings and it was found that Wakefield had a number of undeclared financial conflicts of interest. As a result, he was charged with gross professional misconduct and in 2010 the General Medical Council's Fitness to Practise Panel judged that Wakefield should be struck off the UK medical register, meaning he would no longer be allowed to practise as a doctor. Following this judgement, The Lancet retracted the paper, stating:

'It has become clear that several elements of the 1998 paper by Wakefield et al are incorrect, contrary to the findings of an earlier investigation. In particular, the claims in the original paper that children were "consecutively referred" and that investigations were "approved" by the local ethics committee have been proven to be false.'

Source: www.thelancet.com/journals/lancet/article/PIIS0140-6736(10)60175-4/fulltext

As a result of the original publication and the publicity it received, many parents chose not to have their children vaccinated and by 2012/13, cases of measles, mumps and rubella had reached the highest level for 18 years.

Source: www.gov.uk/government/publications/measles-confirmed-cases/confirmed-cases-of-measles-mumps-and-rubella-in-england-and-wales-2012-to-2013

Real-time observation

Some prospective observational studies can last for many years. However, observation does not need to be carried out over such a long period. We can get a great deal of information observing patients or test subjects for a relatively short time. The advantage of this is that we get the data immediately.

Of course, the disadvantage is that our observations might become subjective. **Objective** observations are things that can be measured, such as pulse, temperature or respiration rate. **Subjective** observations are signs that cannot be measured, such as how a person or patient feels. These can be very important, particularly when we observe someone over time and can tell when there is a change in their condition or behaviour. However, we have to take care that we do not misinterpret or over-interpret such observations.

1 Give two advantages and one disadvantage of using results of experiments or investigations in healthcare.
2 Give one advantage of using data or information from published research.
3 What is the difference between **objective** and **subjective** observations?

A5.5 How new technology is applied in the recording and reporting of information and data

In section A5.2 we saw the advantages of automated data collection. New technologies are being used to improve both the quality and quantity of data that can be collected, even allowing us to collect new kinds of data. New technology has also transformed the way we can analyse the data collected.

This is particularly true when applied to **longitudinal** research, where measurements or observations are made over a long period. By allowing passive measurement of health-related factors, we can avoid the bias that can occur when we rely on people self-reporting. The widespread use and acceptance of fitness trackers and smartwatches means that these can also be used for monitoring physiological data in subjects that are part of a cohort study or clinical trial.

AI/machine learning

Big data is a term that you hear more often these days, usually to describe the massive amounts of data collected by companies such as Amazon, Facebook and

Google. However, there are many areas of science and healthcare that now generate very large data sets, for example:

▶ DNA sequences, such as from the Human Genome Project
▶ proteomics – the study of the proteins produced by the body and how the presence or absence of some proteins is correlated with various diseases
▶ high content imaging – the automated collection and analysis of microscope images to provide information about processes within cells and tissues
▶ results from clinical trials
▶ epidemiology data looking at the spread of diseases (see sections B2.18 and B2.19).

Machine learning is a branch of **AI** (artificial intelligence) that uses computers to imitate the ways in which humans learn. The **algorithm** (a list of rules that a computer follows to solve a problem) can be trained to interpret a sample set of data and then automatically improve the algorithm. This can go through many rounds so that, eventually, the computer is able to interpret very large data sets.

This approach has been used to develop algorithms that can help to interpret medical images, such as those from CT scans or radiography for use in diagnostics, particularly of cancer.

Case study

Research carried out by Moorfields Eye Hospital, DeepMind (part of Google) and UCL uses AI to help identify diseases that can lead to blindness. AI and machine learning technology was trained on thousands of historic eye scans, previously used by specialists to diagnose the disease, to identify features of eye disease and recommend how patients should be referred for care. The AI system can recommend the correct referral decision for more than 50 eye diseases with 94 per cent accuracy. This is the level of accuracy achieved by world-leading eye experts.

Some of these applications come under the general heading of **bioinformatics**. This describes the use of tools and software methods to analyse and process large data sets, such as DNA and protein sequences, genetics, cellular organisation and the mutations that lead to cancer. A related area is **systems biology**, which looks at the chemical and enzyme interactions and pathways within the cell.

Mobile technology and applications

Smartphones and high-speed mobile data networks such as 4G and 5G mean that devices can be connected to the internet almost anywhere in countries with more developed economies – and in many other parts of the world as well. Smartphones and tablets can also be used within a hospital, care home or other healthcare facility to connect to Wi-Fi. This opens up many opportunities for using mobile devices to collect and transfer data.

Health informatics is the use of computer science and AI/machine learning to assist in the management of healthcare information.

Case study

Nottingham University Hospitals NHS trust (NUH) has issued 6500 mobile devices to its clinical staff to allow implementation of electronic observations. Alongside this, NUH developed an app called 'Safer Staffing'. This allows the trust to see the nurse staffing position in real time across more than 85 wards and departments. The nurse in charge of each ward is asked to declare whether they judge that the ward is safe to deliver the required level of care to its current group of patients with the staff on duty. This allows the trust to see where support might be required.

Smartphones also have GPS (global positioning system) receivers built in, which means that they can be used for physical tracking of individuals. This, together with Bluetooth® wireless technology, was used in the NHS COVID-19 app that was the basis of 'track and trace' during the pandemic. If you had been in close contact with someone who tested positive for COVID-19, the app would 'ping' you and you would be told to self-isolate for 10 days. Unfortunately, in the summer of 2021, as lockdown restrictions were eased, the number of people who had to self-isolate grew to such high levels that there were severe staff shortages in areas such as hospitality, transport, retail and healthcare. As a result, there were reports of people deleting the app to avoid being contacted. This was a good example of how technology does not always offer an ideal solution, particularly if it is not properly implemented.

Cloud-based systems

Cloud computing means the availability of computers and computer resources, especially data storage, without active management by the user. Cloud-based systems usually have functions distributed over multiple locations or data centres connected via the internet. This distribution can make cloud-based systems more robust, because they will usually recover quickly if a single server fails. However, it can also make them more susceptible to malicious attacks, as described in section A5.9.

An important application of cloud-based systems in healthcare is the use of **electronic health records (EHRs)**. Because cloud-based systems are accessible to anyone with the appropriate permission, patient data can be available to anyone who needs it across the whole healthcare system. NHS Digital is implementing systems like this – see section A5.1 for an example.

As well as making patient data available to all appropriate healthcare professionals, cloud-based systems mean easier data sharing for further analysis, for example, by AI/machine learning systems that can be used in diagnosis or to gain insight into treatment and prevention of disease.

Digital information management systems

In 2018, the Department of Health and Social Care published a policy paper entitled 'The future of healthcare: our vision for digital, data and technology in health and care'. This addressed many of the areas that we have covered here, such as the use of cloud-based systems, AI/machine learning and mobile technology.

Digital information management systems also offer the advantage of a digital audit trail. This can show, for example, who accessed a patient's records and when, which can help ensure patient confidentiality and protect their personal information (see section A5.6).

Data-visualisation tools

One problem associated with the vast amount of healthcare data that is now available is the difficulty in understanding the complexity of numerical and text-based data. The simplest data visualisation tool is the graph (see section A5.2). Modern technology makes it possible to take multiple data sources, often from cloud-based systems such as patient databases, and present them in a way that makes it easier to understand and interpret them.

Every modern hospital will use data-visualisation tools to manage its in-house processes, such as:

▶ maintaining electronic medical records to track and monitor patient health
▶ avoiding diagnosing errors by eliminating human error
▶ accessing information about patients' demographics (factors such as age or ethnic background) and lifestyles (diet, exercise, smoking, alcohol consumption, etc.) in order to improve care and treatment of the patient.

Test yourself

1 Explain what is meant by the following terms:
   a Artificial intelligence (machine learning).
   b Cloud-based systems.
2 Give one advantage of the use of mobile technology in healthcare data capture.
3 Give one advantage of using digital information management systems.
4 Give one advantage of using data visualisation tools in healthcare.

A5.6 How personal information is protected by data protection legislation, regulations and local ways of working/organisational policies

We have covered the various applications of modern technology in the health sector. We all know that electronic systems are not always secure from all the hacking incidents that have happened over the years. To maintain faith in these different uses of modern technology, patients and staff must feel confident that their personal information will be protected.

This applies equally to personal information stored on paper or in electronic format. In this section we will look at the ways in which personal information is protected. These issues are covered by legislation as well as local policies that most organisations have in place.

Data Protection Act 2018

The DPA 2018 revised earlier data protection law passed in 1998, but its main purpose was to implement the GDPR of the European Union (EU). Although the UK has now left the EU, the legislation remains in force at the time of writing.

The DPA 2018 controls the use of personal information by organisations, businesses or the government. The Act is enforced by the Information Commissioner's Office (ICO), which is funded by a charge on **data controllers**, who must register with the ICO. A data controller is a person or organisation that stores or processes personal information, either on paper or electronically. Personal information is defined quite widely, so it includes aspects such as:

▶ your name and telephone number
▶ your National Insurance or passport number
▶ your location data, such as home address or smartphone GPS data – i.e. your smartphone tracking you
▶ online identifiers such as email or IP address.

However, there are other types of personal data that are also covered by the Act and GDPR, including:

▶ biometric data such as facial images or fingerprints that can be used to identify you
▶ health data that can reveal information about your physical or mental health status
▶ genetic data that can also give information about your health or physiology
▶ ethnic origin
▶ political opinions and religious or philosophical beliefs
▶ sexual orientation.

GDPR 2018

The GDPR came into force within the EU in 2018. It provides a set of principles with which any individual or organisation processing sensitive personal data must comply. There are six legitimate reasons why an organisation may process your personal data:

▶ You have given your consent for them to process your data for a specific purpose. This must be explicit (for example, you tick a box on an online form saying 'I wish to receive emails from you') rather than default – where you must untick a box to opt out of receiving emails.
▶ The processing is necessary to fulfil a contract you have entered into. For example, if you place an online order with a company, it has the right to process your personal data so that it can deliver the goods or inform you if there are any delays.
▶ There is a legal obligation for them to process your data. For example, an employer is obliged to pass employee salary details to HMRC for tax purposes.
▶ The data processing is necessary to protect you or someone else. For example, if you are admitted to A&E with life-threatening injuries following a road traffic accident, disclosure to the hospital of your medical history is necessary to help save your life.
▶ Processing is necessary to perform a task in the public interest or for an official function. This applies to any organisation that exercises an official authority that has a clear basis in law. Examples include local authorities, courts and the criminal justice system, and other agencies carrying out duties that are laid down in law. For example, a government agency has statutory powers to research the online shopping habits of consumers. The agency can ask retailers to share the personal data of a random sample of their customers so that it can carry out this function.
▶ Processing is necessary so that the organisation can pursue its legitimate interests. For example, companies and other organisations need to maintain personnel records.

GDPR includes a number of rights of individuals, for example:

▶ the right to be informed about the collection and use of their personal data
▶ the right to have access to their personal data
▶ the right to have incorrect personal data corrected or completed if it is incomplete
▶ the right to have personal data erased – but only in certain circumstances
▶ the right to restrict the processing of their personal data – again, only in certain circumstances
▶ the right to data portability, so that they can copy or transfer their personal data between different systems, for example, if you have accounts with different banks you may be able to view the details of all of them in a single app
▶ the right to object to processing of personal data, for example, you can refuse to have your personal data used for direct marketing (sometimes called 'spam' or 'junk mail').

GDPR also regulates the processing by organisations outside the EU of personal data of people within the EU. It prevents transfer of data from within the EU to countries outside the EU (such as the UK) unless those countries have appropriate safeguards in place. If you think about the widespread use of cloud computing described in section A5.5, you can see how easily personal data might be transferred across national borders. Partly as a result of this, the GDPR has become the model for many national data protection laws around the world.

Local ways of working/organisational policies

The DPA 2018 and GDPR are not the only things that regulate and protect personal information. Many organisations have their own ways of working, rules and policies that ensure compliance with legislation and regulations, as well as to protect the organisation (for example, from reputational damage if personal information is misused). The ICO expects organisations to have their own policies in place to ensure that they and their staff will comply with GDPR.

Examples of this include:

▶ ensuring that data is stored securely (electronically or paper-based) so that there will not be any loss of data or loss of confidentiality

▶ restricting the use of mobile devices as ways in which personal information may be misused or divulged. This helps to ensure confidentiality

▶ preventing potential conflicts of interest. For example, organisations must appoint a Data Protection Officer (DPO) who should be relatively senior in the organisation. However, there are some senior jobs (such as Chief Executive, Chief Medical Officer or Head of Human Resources) that would be in conflict with the job of DPO, so the roles should not be combined.

Reflect

Clearly it is essential to protect personal information and ensure patient confidentiality is maintained, but can that be taken too far? A patient's medical history must be kept secure when sharing it with another provider involved in their care, but is there a risk that vital information could be missed if the medical history is kept confidential? Could keeping data confidential from those who need to know put effective care at risk?

Test yourself

1 Name the legislation and regulation that protect personal information.
2 Which of the following are examples of the acceptable processing of personal information?
   a Collecting contact details from social media so that you can advertise a new patient support group.
   b Providing a patient's medical history to a life assurance company without the patient's permission.
   c Providing a patient's medical history to an intensive care doctor when the patient is in a coma.
   d Transferring a database of patient data to a computer located in an unknown country for analysis.

A5.7 How to ensure confidentiality when using screens to input or retrieve information or data

Having considered the legal framework around the protection of personal data, we should also consider ways in which confidentiality could be lost or compromised through carelessness or poor practice.

Computer systems should always have password-protected access. This helps to protect sensitive personal information from being accessed by anyone without authorisation. It also means that it is possible to see who accessed what information – it provides an audit trail if there is a data breach.

That means that we should always protect login details and passwords. Unfortunately, many organisations insist on the use of passwords that are difficult to remember (although not always difficult for computer hackers to guess). It should be obvious that 'Password1234' is not a secure choice. Nor is it good practice to write your login details on a sticky note on your computer screen. Sadly, both of these – and other – poor practices are widespread.

We should always log out of a system when leaving the screen (PC, laptop, tablet, etc.) so that someone else cannot come along and access sensitive personal information. Alternatively, if you have a password-protected lock screen (which is a basic computer security feature), you should lock the screen when you leave it, even if it is just for a minute.

You should also be aware of your surroundings when dealing with personal information. When you get money out of a cash machine, you should be cautious of 'shoulder surfers' trying to see your PIN as you enter it. The same can be true in the workplace where it might be possible for unauthorised people (colleagues, patients, visitors) to overlook you and your screen. For this reason, privacy screen filters can be useful as they make it difficult to read information on screen unless you are directly in front of it.

Another area that is important is the use of secure internet connections. We should all be aware that regular email is not secure – it passes through so many different systems, any one of which could be compromised. Another potential insecurity is the use of public Wi-Fi, such as in coffee shops. Any information shared over a public Wi-Fi network can be intercepted easily. Your home Wi-Fi may not be completely secure either. For this reason, many organisations now use VPN (virtual private network) to access the internet or exchange information safely and privately.

A5.8 The positive use of, and restrictions on the use of, social media in health and science sectors

It is becoming more common for employers to look at the social media of prospective employees. So think carefully before you post pictures of wild nights out on your social media! Of course, social media can offer many advantages as well.

Positive uses

Section B2.20 covers the ways in which health promotion helps control of disease and disorder and refers to a number of health promotion initiatives, particularly by Public Health England (PHE). Section A9.5 also covers some ways of promoting health and wellbeing.

Social media can play an important part, particularly in:
▶ awareness campaigns and disseminating information – this could be as simple as reminding social media followers to follow common-sense health practices, but it is also possible to target relevant population groups with specific health messages
▶ correcting misinformation – there is a lot of health misinformation on social media. This might be simply untrue statements. There can also be misinformation in the form of facts presented without context, or in the wrong context. Unfortunately, people are often more inclined to believe information that supports their existing prejudices
▶ crisis communication and monitoring, for example, during an epidemic or pandemic (such as COVID-19). More people now get their news from social media than from newspapers.

PHE uses a wide range of social media to share news and information about its work as well as public health incidents – the COVID-19 pandemic, for example.

Other uses of social media in the health and science sectors include:
▶ monitoring public health. People post about everything online, including their health. Hashtags such as #flu can show when diseases are spreading in new locations. Health data from social media has improved prediction of infectious diseases such as flu
▶ data gathering
▶ establishing patient support networks. This can be particularly effective among younger people
▶ recruitment – both of new employees or of subjects for clinical trials and other health research
▶ marketing by commercial and healthcare organisations.

Restrictions

We have already seen how social media can be a useful tool but can also have disadvantages. To try to minimise the disadvantages, we need to follow some basic rules when using social media in the health and science sectors.
▶ Do not post sensitive or personal information about yourself or others on social media. This should be common sense, but it is also likely to be covered by an organisation's code of conduct.
▶ Maintain professional boundaries when interacting with individuals outside the organisation. Again, it should be common sense, but it can sometimes be easy, in the context of social media, to be less professional than you would be face to face.

▶ Do not share inaccurate or non-evidence-based information. In fact, it is a criminal offence under the Care Act 2014 (see section A4.2) for care providers who 'supply, publish or otherwise make available certain types of information that is false or misleading'.

More employers in the health and science sectors are implementing social media policies to avoid risks associated with misuse of social media by their employees. These risks can include:
▶ reputational damage
▶ infringement of the intellectual property rights of others, e.g. by posting copyright material such as images, videos or music
▶ liability for any discriminatory or **defamatory** (reputation-damaging) comments posted by employees
▶ possible unauthorised sharing of confidential information.

A5.9 The advantages and risks of using IT systems to record, retrieve and store information and data

Compared with paper-based systems, IT systems have huge advantages – some of which were discussed in section A5.5. However, while being aware of the advantages, we must also guard against the risk associated with IT systems.

Advantages

The advantages of IT systems in the health and science sectors include:
▶ ease of access, sharing and transferring data – particularly with greater use of cloud-based systems
▶ the speed of data analysis as well as the ability to use AI/machine learning (see section A5.5)
▶ greater data security, for example, when it is password-protected
▶ standardisation of data. This can be a barrier to be overcome when transferring information and data from old, particularly paper-based, systems to modern IT systems because the older data is likely to be in a variety of non-standard formats. However, moving forward, standardisation can be a great advantage
▶ the ability to have continuous and/or real-time monitoring of data. This can be particularly

important during disease outbreaks such as epidemics and pandemics
▶ cost and space saving. This is another reason why cloud-based solutions are becoming more widespread
▶ integrated working, making for greater collaboration between colleagues. It also supports safeguarding practices.

Risks

We have covered some of the risk factors, particularly security breaches – accidental or malicious – that can compromise patient confidentiality. However, there are other risk factors to consider.

There is the potential for corruption of data, making databases unusable. This is one reason why all IT systems need robust procedures for backup of data – although making a backup of corrupted data can just mean that you have a corrupted (and so useless) backup. Organisations need to be aware of the risks of data corruption as a result of ransomware attacks. This is where malicious software is installed on a system (usually by someone in the organisation clicking on a link in an email or on a website) which then corrupts or encrypts all the data held on the system. Some organisations have paid millions of dollars in Bitcoin to ransomware criminals so that they can retrieve their data.

Have you ever called a company, only to be told 'I'm sorry, but our system is down'? That might be annoying when you are trying to find out when you will get the item of clothing you ordered. But when you are trying to access critical patient information, it can be much more serious. This is why many healthcare systems have built-in redundancy – there may be multiple computers handling access to data so that a single failure does not bring the whole system down.

> **Reflect**
>
> It is hard to think about how we managed without modern IT systems. But, do we always appreciate the risks as well as the benefits? We have seen the importance of following policies and procedures, but do we always think about whether that is enough? Are the systems that we use sufficiently secure? Are there procedures to monitor and enforce the policies that are in place? These are questions for management, rather than individual health professionals. However, it is good to ask ourselves these questions, if only to reinforce the need to comply fully with required procedures and policies.

A5.10 How security measures protect data stored by organisations

We have already looked at how security measures can help to preserve patient confidentiality and keep personal information secure. However, that is not the only reason that data must be protected by appropriate security measures. Loss of data can be catastrophic in a modern healthcare setting.

Malicious operators (hackers) may try to access sensitive patient information, or they might have some other criminal intent, such as installation of ransomware. State-sponsored groups have been implicated in various attacks on computer systems in recent years – this has been given the name 'cyber warfare' – and healthcare systems have been targeted. In May 2020, the International Committee of the Red Cross called for governments to take immediate and decisive action to prevent and stop cyber attacks on hospitals, healthcare facilities and organisations, research organisations and international authorities that provide critical care and support for healthcare. This followed cyber attacks against medical facilities in the Czech Republic, France, Spain, Thailand and the United States as well as international organisations such as the WHO.

There are various ways in which an organisation's data can be protected:

▶ Controlling access to information, for example, through levels of authorised logins and passwords. This can also mean that some staff can access information but not change it ('read only' access). This helps protect against inadvertent change to or deletion of data by inexperienced staff.

▶ Allowing only authorised staff into specific work areas so that they cannot physically access sensitive computer equipment. In some organisations, the USB ports on computers are disabled so that data cannot be transferred onto USB memory devices.

▶ Requiring regular and up-to-date staff training in complying with data security. Technology and the methods used by cyber criminals change rapidly, so staff need to keep up to date.

▶ Making regular backups of files. Often there will be multiple backups so that there is no risk of replacing 'good' backup data with corrupted or encrypted data.

▶ Using up-to-date cyber security strategies to protect against unintended or unauthorised access. Organisations need to employ good cyber security staff or consultants and make sure that their recommendations are taken seriously.

▶ Ensuring that backup data is stored externally, for example, cloud-based or on (ideally multiple) servers elsewhere. If there is a fire in the IT suite, you need to be able to get up and running again quickly and this will not be possible if all the backups are stored in a cupboard in the IT suite.

A5.11 What to do if information is not stored securely

Sometimes things go wrong, often due to human error or carelessness. If you discover sensitive information that is not stored securely, you need to take action. This could apply equally to paper-based and electronic patient data.

The first step must be to secure the information where possible. This is mostly likely to be the case with paper records left lying around. However, a colleague might have gone home and left their screen running or still be logged into a sensitive system. In such cases you should log them out and shut the screen down.

Having taken immediate action to secure the information, you must then record and report the incident to the designated person. This will depend on your organisation's policies and procedures, but it might be your line manager or a specialist computer security person or department.

Research

In 2016 the Care Quality Commission (CQC) published a report into whether personal health and care information is being used safely and is appropriately protected in the NHS. The review is available from the CQC website at **https://www.cqc.org.uk/publications/themed-work/safe-data-safe-care** (or search online for 'safe data safe care').

Think about what the CQC found. Can you see any lessons for your own workplace or professional practice?

There were six recommendations made. Can you see evidence of them being applied in your own organisation?

Project practice

You have been asked to prepare a report on data collection, recording and handling in your organisation.

You should research:
▶ The methods used to collect data.
▶ The types of data that are collected.
▶ The way(s) in which data is stored, analysed and presented.

You should also consider how your organisation addresses:
▶ the use of technology to assist in recording and reporting of data
▶ the ways in which data is shared amongst those who need to have access to it
▶ how personal data is protected
▶ procedures and policies that apply to ensuring confidentiality and security of personal data.

Prepare an evaluation of the methods used, covering:
▶ ways in which procedures ensure accurate collection and recording of data
▶ how information sharing is helped or hindered by the procedures in place
▶ areas that might be improved, such as:
  – reducing the time needed to document activities
  – improving sharing of information
  – increasing security of data and personal information (concentrate on how the systems are used, rather than on the detail of the systems themselves).

Present your report as a written document or slide presentation, infographic or scientific poster.

Discuss your findings with the group.

Write a reflective evaluation of your work.

Assessment practice

1 For each of the following, state whether it is qualitative or quantitative data:
   a Blood pressure readings.
   b Responses to a questionnaire about patient perception of the quality of their care.
   c Height.
   d Hair colour.

2 For each of the following, state whether it is continuous or discrete data:
   a Number of weeks that a pregnancy lasts.
   b Number of children in a family.
   c Average number of children in families.
   d Size of the UK population.
   e Blood glucose concentration.

3 Suggest **two** security measures that can be used to protect personal data stored on a computer network.

4 Give **two** advantages of using automated data collection.

5 Discuss the advantages and disadvantages of using surveys to collect healthcare data.

6 Discuss the impact of machine learning on the role of healthcare practitioners.

7 Discuss the importance of having policies to prevent unauthorised access to patient data.

8 Discuss the ways in which security measures can protect stored data.

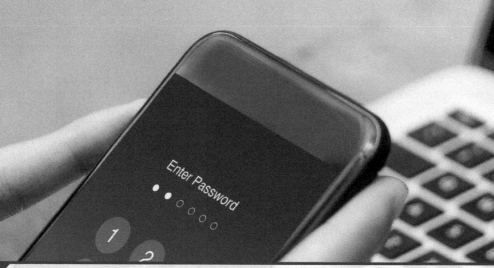

A6: Managing personal information

Introduction

Collecting and recording information is an essential part of the role for anyone working in healthcare. Much of the information recorded is personal and sensitive, and must therefore be kept private. Being able to implement good practice when managing patient information is extremely important and a legal requirement.

Breaches of security and confidentiality are serious and result in upset and anxiety for service users and possibly, in the worst-case scenario, prosecution for the care provider. This chapter will help you to understand your responsibilities and the requirements for collecting, recording and handling information through knowledge of the law and regulations that govern and protect individuals whose information is being held. You will develop an understanding of the need for secure systems for recording, storing and sharing information.

Considering the reasons why personal information is collected when obtaining a client history and how it can be stored appropriately are very important in healthcare. It is also essential to understand when and how it is appropriate to share information and the procedures that need to be followed when this is done.

Learning outcomes

The core knowledge outcomes that you must understand and learn:

A6.1 your role in relation to record keeping and audits

A6.2 why personal information is collected, stored and protected

A6.3 the types of information needed when obtaining a client history

A6.4 the purpose of common abbreviations used in the healthcare sector

A6.5 the advantages of reporting systems for managing information with regards to incidents, events and conditions

A6.6 when it may be appropriate to share information and the considerations that need to be made when sharing data

A6.7 the different formats for the sharing of information

A6.8 the reasons for record keeping and how this contributes to the overall care of the individual

A6.9 the responsibilities of employees and employers in relation to record keeping and when to escalate issues.

A6.1 Your role in relation to record keeping and audits

Your role in relation to record keeping

A 'record' is any information about an individual (a patient or service user) that is collected by being written down or recorded electronically. An employee in a healthcare setting has personal responsibility for any record keeping they are expected to complete as part of their job role.

NICE guidelines state that record keeping is an integral part of health professionals' practice and is essential to their provision of safe, effective care (see www.evidence.nhs.uk/document?id=2162183 &returnUrl=search%3fq%3drecord %2bkeeping%2bmidwifery).

Ensuring timely, accurate records for every interaction and how you have provided care for the individual

It is important to record information in a timely way, and this means as soon as possible. The longer recording is left, the less likely it is that the record will be fully accurate. Completing records too long after an event can result in gaps in the information due to not remembering exactly what happened. The information may also be time-sensitive and needed urgently in order to continue providing appropriate care.

It is also essential that records are accurate. Incomplete or muddled record keeping can have serious consequences for patients if something is misunderstood because a record is incomplete or misleading.

Every interaction and type of care you provide must be recorded. If there is no record, how does anyone know that they happened? For example, if medication is provided for a patient but not recorded on the medicine administration record (**MAR**), another member of staff may think it has not been given. They may then administer the medication again and this double dose could have serious consequences, primarily for the patient but also for the member of staff who had not completed the record.

If a patient's actual words are being recorded, which is preferable, it is important that this is indicated by using quotation marks.

> **Key terms**
>
> **NICE:** the National Institute for Health and Care Excellence. This organisation provides guidelines and information on standards and effectiveness of care.
>
> **MAR:** a medicine administration record that is updated every time any medication is given to a patient in a healthcare setting, i.e. a hospital, nursing or care home, etc. It contains a list of what has been administered and when, and can be an electronic or paper-based record.

Ensure you are competent in using systems to record data where applicable

If your role involves record keeping, you should always use the agreed ways of working that you should have been informed about in your induction or training. You should ask to be trained in this if this has not happened. You must always ask your supervisor if you are not sure about how or whether to record information – it is better to check than to guess and potentially cause problems by getting it wrong.

Ensure confidentiality/security is not compromised by leaving records in public places or data unprotected

Maintaining confidentiality limits access or places restrictions on sharing certain types of sensitive information, so that it is kept private to only those who need to be aware of it and only certain personnel can access it.

Records of individuals using care services and staff records are confidential and so must be kept safe and secure. When working in a care setting you should never leave folders or reports lying around – they should always be put away appropriately in the correct place as soon as they are finished with, and stored securely when unattended. You must always log out of electronic records, and never move away from the computer leaving documents open, as anyone could read private information that they are not authorised to access. Electronic records are usually password protected – you must never share the password with anyone. In order to maintain proper security, those who need to access electronic records will have been given a password.

Ensure the information recorded is factual and recorded in line with legislative requirements

Information that is recorded should be factual, i.e. a record of what has actually happened. It is not an opinion of what you think might have happened, or speculation about reasons why, it is a statement of the facts reflecting what did happen.

The records kept in a care setting are in fact legal documents as they form a record of the care provided, how it was decided on, who provided it and the results of the care. They can be referred to at a later date and would be used as evidence if complaints were made, including in court.

Key aspects of legislation that guide the recording, storing and sharing of information include the following:

▶ The Data Protection Act (2018), including the provisions of the GDPR (General Data Protection Regulation (2018)) described in sections A6.2 and A5.3, places an emphasis on 'consent'. This means that information should be shared only if the individual has given permission; it also limits how long information should be kept, stating that information should be kept 'no longer than necessary' and should be deleted or shredded when it is no longer needed. These regulations state that all staff have the responsibility for ensuring that confidential information is kept securely and not disclosed inappropriately.

▶ The Care Act (2014) gives local authorities the responsibility to ensure that appropriate information is shared to assist in multidisciplinary team working.

▶ The Human Rights Act (1998) provides individuals with the right to 'respect, privacy and family life'. This supports the maintaining of confidentiality of information in care settings to ensure an individual's privacy.

▶ The Equality Act (2010) identifies nine 'protected characteristics' against which it is illegal to discriminate. This means, for example, you should not share information about someone's sexuality without their consent, so that they are not treated differently because of it.

▶ The Freedom of Information Act (2000) gives individuals the right to view any information kept about them by public bodies, such as the UK government, the NHS and local authorities. This includes documents, reports and emails between co-workers.

Healthcare organisations' procedures and policies for handling information are designed to help staff ensure they are complying with the relevant legislation. They should also support individuals' rights to have their information kept confidential, only shared with consent and destroyed if no longer needed.

Avoid abbreviations where possible

While using abbreviations can save time when record keeping, they are open to misunderstanding and may mean different things in different care settings. For example:

Abbreviation	Possible meaning
CCU	critical care unit OR coronary care unit
DNR	do not resuscitate OR district nurse referral
CNS	clinical nurse specialist OR central nervous system

You should never use your own abbreviations as this could cause confusion. You should only use abbreviations that you have been told to use by your supervisor which are appropriate for the setting and/or records in question. If you use your own abbreviations, it is likely that other people using the records will not understand what they mean.

Your role in relation to audits

An **audit** is when a review or inspection is carried out to ensure compliance with regulations, policies or legislation. For example, financial accounts are subject to regular audits to ensure they are accurate. In a healthcare setting an audit could be carried out to check if staff are following record-keeping policies and procedures. This helps to identify good practice and also to indicate whether any improvements are required.

Accurate record keeping also helps to provide an 'audit trail', i.e. a clear path of evidence showing what actions have been taken, when and by whom, which would be especially useful in any investigation about misconduct, abuse or an accident.

When record keeping, it is your responsibility to:

▶ ensure information is legible where records have been recorded by hand, using black ballpoint pen

▶ all information must be legible – i.e. if writing records by hand, others must be able to read your handwriting. Be honest with yourself – if your handwriting is difficult to read, it is much better to print rather than use joined-up writing. A black ballpoint pen is more easily read than pale blue or green, for example, and can be photocopied more clearly if necessary

▶ ensure all records have a date, time and signature Do not guess the time – get used to noticing the time you do something that needs recording, taking someone's blood pressure, for example. Note this down as soon as you can

▶ use a signature rather than initials, as more than one person may have the same initials. It is good practice to sign and then print your name to ensure it can be clearly understood

▶ ensure care is taken to enter the data record accurately if using electronic systems.

Your main responsibility is to ensure that any record keeping that you carry out is done accurately, so for digital records, enter information carefully. Do not type too fast as errors are more likely to occur. Always read through quickly to check electronic records when you have finished entering the information. Remember to save the file regularly where necessary.

> See also section **A5.3** for more on accuracy of data and written information.

Reflect

Consider any record keeping that you have done in your placement organisation.
▶ Identify any good practice in this area which you have used or observed.
▶ Are there any areas for improvement?

Test yourself

1 Describe four main features of accurate records.
2 Choose one piece of legislation relevant to personal information and describe the guidelines each one provides for record keeping.
3 Explain why it is recommended *not* to use abbreviations when record keeping.
4 What should you do if you are unsure whether something needs to be recorded on a patient's record?
5 Describe your role in record keeping and audits in your placement organisation.

A6.2 Why personal information is collected, stored and protected

Why personal information is collected

Obtaining personal information about an individual's current state of physical and mental health is essential to inform their diagnosis and the type of treatment that may be required (see Figure 6.1). Anything that has affected their health previously may have an impact on their present health and wellbeing. So, it is important to get a full picture of the individual's overall health and any other factors, such as work, family or housing issues, that affect their wellbeing.

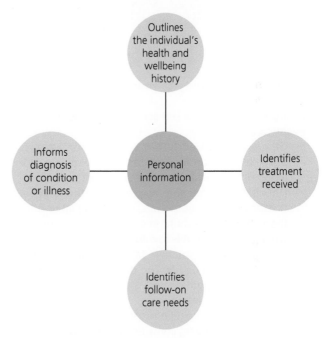

▲ Figure 6.1 Why personal information is collected

Why personal information is stored

Information is stored so that it can be shared, as appropriate, within the wider network of multidisciplinary teams. This is an important aspect of person-centred care. Often an individual receives care from several different practitioners or services, like George in the case study below.

It is important that all practitioners involved in his care have access to information about George, such as problems he is having, the treatment he is receiving and the success, or otherwise, of any support provided. This gives everyone involved a full picture of his health and wellbeing. Keeping detailed records means the information can be shared quickly and efficiently.

Case study

George

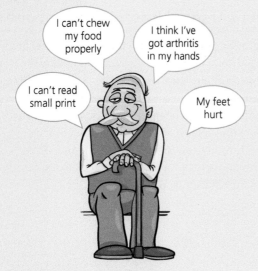

I can't chew my food properly

I think I've got arthritis in my hands

I can't read small print

My feet hurt

▲ Figure 6.2 George – 86 years old

George is 86 years old and accesses a range of healthcare services:

▶ GP – examines George and writes a prescription for painkillers and refers George to the hospital to see a doctor specialising in bones and joints.

▶ Hospital – George sees a specialist orthopaedic doctor who arranges x-rays, examines him and then diagnoses arthritis in George's finger and wrist joints. George is told to keep taking the painkillers and to return to his GP if they are not sufficient for his needs. The doctor refers George to a podiatrist (foot doctor), a physiotherapist and an occupational therapist.

▶ Podiatrist – this practitioner provides foot care for George by removing corns and hard skin and trims his toenails. This should help to stop his feet hurting.

▶ Physiotherapy – the physiotherapist teaches George some simple exercises to help him to strengthen his muscles and keep mobile to make grasping objects and moving around easier. The physiotherapist refers George to an occupational therapist.

▶ Occupational therapy – the occupational therapist carries out an assessment of the problems

George is having with using his hands. The occupational therapist visits George at home and arranges to supply him with some specialist aids to help with everyday tasks. These include a 'tap turner' and 'kettle pourer' to help him make a cup of tea more easily.

▶ Optician – George makes himself an appointment with his optician. The optician thoroughly checks George's eyesight and tells him there are no serious problems. He is prescribed a stronger pair of glasses so that he can read his newspaper once again.

▶ Dentist – George makes an appointment to see his dentist. His teeth and gums are checked and his teeth are cleaned. George is advised he needs to have two teeth removed and a dental bridge fitted to replace them. The dentist tells George he will be able to chew properly again when this dental work is done.

▶ Social worker – the social worker visits him at home for a review as George told the occupational therapist he was finding it difficult to prepare his food because of his arthritis. The social worker arranges for a home care assistant to visit George for half an hour twice a day to help him prepare meals.

Each member of the team needs to know what treatment or support George is receiving. At each stage the practitioners will record information about the treatment or support they have provided for George and it will be available to the whole team. This enables everyone to be fully informed to monitor George's progress. They can assess his needs holistically, changing his ongoing care package when necessary and keep the whole team up to date.

Read the case study information about George and the treatment he has received.

1 Describe four examples of information about George that is shared by the practitioners – these could be problems he has, treatment or support provided.

2 For each example you gave in Question 1, explain the benefits for George of the information being shared between the practitioners.

Another reason information is stored is for future use. Records of someone's previous illness and treatment could have an influence on future needs. They may have fully recovered at the time, but sometime in the future their previous illness may have relevance to a current condition.

Individuals have a right to access data records and so this is a further reason for storing information. The GDPR regulations, Caldicott Principles (see page 94) and the Freedom of Information Act are just some examples of legislation and guidelines that require personal information to be made available to individuals if they request to see it.

How personal information is protected

Data protection regulations

General Data Protection Regulation (GDPR) 2018

The GDPR is a set of data protection rules for the European Union that were brought into UK law as the Data Protection Act 2018. This law applies to the processing of data by care organisations and settings. Processing data is the act of obtaining, recording or using an individual's personal information.

The GDPR sets out seven key principles:

▶ **Lawfulness, fairness and transparency.** This means that people have a right to know and view any information that is being held about them, to know how their information is being used, to have any errors corrected, and to prevent any data being used for advertising or marketing.

▶ **Purpose limitation.** Information should only be collected for a specific purpose. Organisations such as the NHS and health and social care settings can hold information about staff and clients for a clear purpose and must only use it for that purpose.

▶ **Data minimisation.** Data collection should be limited to that which is necessary and relevant to the purpose. This means that organisations and care settings must not collect information that is not relevant.

▶ **Accuracy.** Data found to be inaccurate should be destroyed or corrected. Staff have a responsibility to ensure information they collect and use is correct and up to date.

▶ **Storage limitation.** This means that information should be kept for no longer than necessary. Data should be deleted or destroyed when it is no longer needed, for example, staff should delete or securely shred sensitive or personal data.

▶ **Integrity and confidentiality** (i.e. security). Information must be held and processed securely. So, in care settings access should be restricted. For example, non-authorised staff/people should not be allowed to access the information – it should be kept in secure conditions and stored safely, for example, in a locked filing cabinet, and electronic records should be password protected to limit access.

▶ **Accountability.** Care organisations must have appropriate systems and records in place to demonstrate that they are complying with the data protection regulations. They have to be able to show how they gained an individual's consent for processing their information (see Figure 6.3). If there is a serious breach of an individual's data, there is a duty to inform the individual straight away.

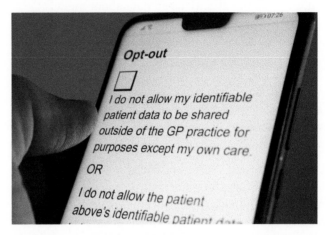

▲ **Figure 6.3 Withdrawing consent to share data**

The GDPR provides the rights outlined in the table for individuals.

Rights	Meaning for individuals
Right to be informed	Must be told data is being collected
Right of access	Must be allowed to see the data held
Right to rectification	Inaccurate information must be corrected
Right to erasure	Can request the deletion of data
Right to restrict processing	Can request data is not used
Right to data portability	Can request their data (usually digital) is transferred between organisations
Right to object	Can stop their data from being used
Rights related to automated decision-making, including profiling	There are controls about the automated collection and use of data

Source: Adams, J, *L2 Technical Award in Health & Social Care*, Hodder Education, 2019, pp. 69–70

Information governance (IG)

Various laws govern the use of personal confidential data in healthcare, including the NHS Act 2006, the Health and Social Care Act 2012, the Data Protection Act, GDPR and the Human Rights Act.

These laws allow personal data to be shared between those providing care for patients but also protect patients' confidentiality when data about them is used for other purposes. These 'other purposes' are referred to as **secondary uses**. The permitted secondary uses include:

▶ reviewing and improving the quality of care provided
▶ researching what treatments work best
▶ commissioning clinical services
▶ planning public health services.

People working in health and social care who use data for secondary purposes must only use data that does not identify individual patients unless they have the consent of the patient themselves. Names and other identifying features must be removed.

Further detail about NHS information governance can be found at **www.england.nhs.uk/ig/about**

See also section A5.6.

Research

Watch the NHS Information Governance Training Film:

https://youtu.be/9FflMuJaxBs

This is an Information Governance Training Film from the Leeds Teaching Hospitals NHS Trust.

Using information from the clip, create a guidance sheet for NHS staff explaining the correct way to securely manage the following types of information:
▶ paper records
▶ digital records
▶ sharing information.

The Caldicott Principles

The Caldicott Principles were developed in 1997 as a result of a review of how patient information was handled across the NHS. The review was named after the chairperson, Dame Fiona Caldicott. The principles have become widely used across health and social care to help ensure that confidential information is protected and used appropriately. The most recent review was in December 2020 and an eighth principle was added.

The eight Caldicott Principles are:

1 Justify the purpose for using confidential information.
2 Use confidential information only when it is necessary.
3 Use the minimum necessary confidential information.
4 Access to personal confidential data should be on a strictly **need-to-know basis**.
5 Everyone with access to confidential information should be aware of their responsibilities.
6 Comply with the law.
7 The duty to share information for individual care is as important as the duty to protect patient confidentiality.
8 Inform patients and service users about how their personal confidential information is used.

Source: www.gov.uk/government/publications/the-caldicott-principles

The Caldicott Principles cover all personal data collected that is necessary for the provision of health and social care services. This includes health history, diagnosis, treatment, symptoms and personal details, such as address and family circumstances information.

Key term

Need-to-know basis: information is only shared with those directly involved with the care and support of an individual. They need the information to enable them to provide appropriate care.

Practice points

Consider how the Caldicott Principles are applied in your placement organisation.

Give an example of practice at your placement organisation for each of the eight principles in action.

A6.3 The types of information needed when obtaining a client history

A client history consists of factual information about the person; it establishes relevant background information about their life. It also gathers information about their lifestyle that can contribute to developing an understanding of their illness or condition.

Some information is required to confirm who the person is and their age:

▶ name
▶ date of birth
▶ individual NHS or hospital number.

Access to NHS health records may be required.

Further details are needed to gain an insight into the person's state of health and their circumstances. These details include:

▶ presenting complaint – a description of any symptoms that they are experiencing and that are concerning the individual
▶ drug history – this includes details of any prescribed or over-the-counter medicines they are taking. Information about recreational drug use is also relevant
▶ family history:
  – are they a parent? do they have any dependants, that is family members, or others, relying on them for financial or other support?
  – do they work and if so, what type of employment?
  – type of housing.

These aspects of the individual's family, work responsibilities and type or standard of housing could have an influence, either positive or negative, on their state of health. Poor (or lack of) housing, stress and pressure at work or with family responsibilities could be having a negative impact. Equally, the individual may have extended family and friends who are available for support if required.

▶ Social history:
  – culture
  – beliefs
  – religion.

These aspects of the individual's social history may have an impact on the care that can be provided, for example, many women strongly prefer to be treated by a female doctor or nurse, including but not exclusively for cultural or religious reasons. If a female practitioner is not available, this could impact the individual's willingness to seek help for an illness. Another example is that Jehovah's Witnesses, a Christian faith group, will not accept blood transfusions. Religious beliefs and cultural views must be taken into account when planning and providing care for an individual in order to prevent discrimination.

Test yourself

1   Make a list of the different types of information collected about service users in your placement organisation.
2   Choose three and explain why each type of information is needed.

A6.4 The purpose of common abbreviations used in the healthcare sector

To facilitate and shorten written narratives

Using common abbreviations enables patient records to be produced more quickly as whole words will not have to be written out repeatedly. Also, the records will be shorter due to fewer words being used, which means they take less time to create and to read.

Standardisation

Having a set of common abbreviations that is agreed and used by everyone in the care setting will ensure a consistent standard across all departments, regardless of who has completed the record. If a common set of abbreviations is used, all staff and practitioners can be trained and made aware of them so will be familiar with them and there should not be any misunderstanding when the records are referred to.

See also section A6.1 (page 90) for guidelines on the use of abbreviations in official records.

Common abbreviations used

Abbreviations	Meaning
PRN	pro re nata (meaning 'given as needed', would refer to, for example, medication)
BP	blood pressure (usually taken regularly over a period of time and recorded by a health practitioner)
MAR	medication administration record (consists of the dates, times, types and quantity of medication given to an individual patient each day)
DNR	do not resuscitate (see below)
MUST	Malnutrition Universal Screening Tool (see below)
NEWS	National Early Warning Score (see below)
PEWS	Pediatrics Early Warning Score (see below)

DNR

This stands for 'do not resuscitate' and means that the person has requested that they should be allowed a natural death without any attempt at CPR (cardiopulmonary resuscitation) if their heart stops beating.

MUST

This is a five-step screening tool to identify adults who are malnourished, at risk of malnutrition, those who are undernourished, and obese individuals who are lacking certain nutrients. It includes management guidelines which can be used to develop a care plan. It is for use in hospitals, community and other care settings and can be used by all care workers

NEWS (National Early Warning Score)

The purpose of NEWS is to help early identification of patients who are in danger of developing a sudden, serious, severe illness, such as sepsis. It is a system for scoring the regular measurements that are routinely recorded at a patient's bedside. Measurements taken include breathing rate, oxygen saturation, pulse rate and level of consciousness. Each of the results is scored from 0 to 3 and then they are totalled up. The higher the total, the more serious the illness – a score over 7 usually results in the patient being moved to intensive care.

PEWS (Pediatrics Early Warning Score)

This is a similar system to NEWS but specifically for children aged up to 16 years. Monitoring of heart rate, quality and rate of breathing and blood pressure results are scored regularly so any deterioration is noticed as soon as possible. By calculating the PEWS score, action can be taken straight away.

A6.5 The advantages of reporting systems for managing information with regards to incidents, events and conditions

The advantages of reporting systems

Figure 6.4 outlines the advantages of having a reporting system.

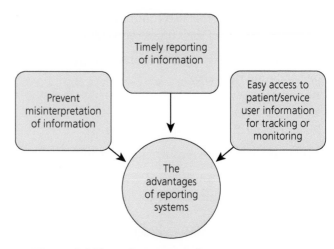

▲ Figure 6.4 The advantages of reporting systems

All care organisations have their own policies and procedures to guide staff when handling information. The reporting systems in place should result in a consistent approach from all staff and ensure controlled access to patient records, for example, when needed for test results, monitoring their condition or response to treatment.

A reporting system prevents misinterpretation of information as all staff should be recording the information required in the correct format. For example, as explained above, to avoid errors in understanding the information, staff will use only agreed, standard abbreviations.

Having a reporting system makes it quicker and more convenient for staff to update records regularly and ensures that they record only the necessary information. Use of a standard form, either electronic or paper based, helps to ensure that only the relevant and necessary data is obtained and recorded.

In addition to patient care reporting, healthcare settings will have specific reporting systems for certain incidents or events, including:

▶ accidents/injuries
▶ complaints
▶ fire safety
▶ outbreaks of certain diseases
▶ risk assessments
▶ safeguarding.

Research

▶ Find out about reporting systems at your placement organisation for specific incidents and/or events (examples listed above).
▶ Explain the benefits of two of these reporting systems.

A6.6 When it may be appropriate to share information and the considerations that need to be made when sharing data

When it is appropriate to share information

In some situations, such as those in the table, it is essential that information is shared.

Essential to share information
For the purpose of ensuring effective diagnosis, treatment and care of individuals – such as a handover briefing at the shift change on a hospital ward.
When there is risk of harm to individuals, for example, in a serious situation regarding someone's mental health or in an emergency healthcare event such as a seriously injured child.
A crime has been committed or there is risk of it being committed, for example, the misuse of medication.
Safeguarding issues, for example, suspected harm or abuse of a child or older adult.
Legislative requirements, for example: ▶ Care Act 2014 ▶ GDPR and Caldicott Principles

In some situations, however, it is helpful and beneficial to share information with colleagues. These could involve successful projects or initiatives, or successful everyday care practice that care workers can share with their colleagues.

Examples of when it is beneficial to share information include:

▶ for the purpose of sharing improvements to practice – such as sharing a successful therapy method for a particular sports injury, as a result of research

▶ for the purpose of sharing good practice – such as dressing wounds

▶ for the purpose of introducing new ways of working and innovations in practice to colleagues, for example, a project using new ways of involving patients in decision-making about their care.

Before sharing information/data you should always consider whether it is appropriate and necessary. Consider why you are sharing.

Considerations when sharing data

▶ The reason why information is being shared, for example, to support the individual's care or to present outcomes of a project. Is it essential or desirable to share the information?

▶ The need to inform the individual that the information needs to be shared and why. The individual must be asked for consent unless it is required by law to share or the benefit in sharing information outweighs keeping it confidential (for example, safeguarding risks).

▶ The individual's information and confidentiality requirements, as set out in relevant regulations: GDPR, Caldicott Principles and Freedom of Information Act (see section A6.2). This includes principles for protecting the individual's identification – for instance, using the individual's NHS number as an identifier rather than their name is more appropriate because they cannot be as easily identified. The NHS identifier would be used in research and on patient records, but not in person to the individual.

▶ Where the age or mental capacity of the individual is of concern, in which case there may be a need to inform an **appropriate adult** or **advocate** if sharing an individual's information.

▶ The intended audience for the information, for example, the individual or health professionals. The depth and level of detail, use of terminology and amount of information will depend on the audience: patients may not understand healthcare acronyms or terms or the precise implications of more formal medical notes, and consideration should be given to tone and whether reassurance or explanation might be helpful. Method of presentation should be considered, such as handouts, slide presentations, leaflets or posters.

> **Key terms**
>
> ***Appropriate adult:*** their role is to protect the wellbeing and best interests of a young person aged 17 or younger, or someone of any age with a learning disability, when they are interviewed or attend a meeting. Usually this will be a parent or guardian, or alternatively a social worker or someone who has been trained as an appropriate adult.
>
> ***Advocate:*** someone who speaks on behalf of an individual who is unable to speak up for themselves.

A6.7 The different formats for the sharing of information

The format used for sharing information will differ depending on the type of information that is being shared and who it is being shared with.

Oral reports

Spoken information is useful and efficient when information needs to be summarised and passed on quickly.

An example is the shift changeover on a hospital ward. This is called the 'handover'. The nurse in charge will speak to the new team, giving an overview of patients on the ward so that the new staff taking over have all the key information to start looking after the patients straight away. Any issues or problems will be flagged and a brief review of the condition of each patient will be given.

Written reports

Written information could be on paper or in an electronic format. The information can be brief or very detailed depending on the type of information being recorded. For example, the report could be a family's record of interactions with a social worker or details of test results sent from the hospital to a GP. Written information is usually more detailed than oral reports and can provide a permanent record of information over time.

A transfer report is a document that would be provided, for example, when a patient leaves hospital and moves into the care of social services. The report would detail treatments received, success of recovery and any specific requirements for continued recovery at home, such as physiotherapy. The social worker would use this report as a starting point for developing a care package with the patient.

Forms and documents

These are for a specific purpose such as a complaint form, a risk assessment document or an accident report. They will usually consist of sections, sometimes with questions, that have to be filled in with the specific information required. Often this type of form has a series of **mandatory fields**. Mandatory means compulsory and these fields (spaces for information)

have to be filled in – they cannot be left blank. This is because they gather necessary specific information.

Presentations

These are usually delivered with the aid of slide shows, presented on a screen to a group of people, but could also involve video or audio. The presenter talks through the slides, giving a commentary. The slides can include pictures, diagrams, charts and written information. They are useful for the delivery of training or providing information for a group of people. Quite a lot of information can be given, with the benefit that it can be revisited easily at a later date if delegates are sent a copy. Presentations can be used for sharing good practice in a team meeting or reporting the results of a research project.

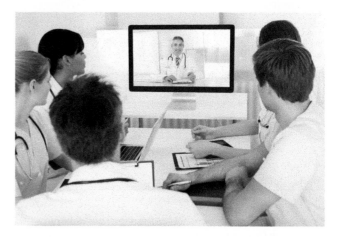

▲ Figure 6.5 A presentation

Graphs and tables

Graphs provide a visual display of data – they can contain a lot of information gathered over time in a way that is easy to understand at a glance (see Figure 6.6). They are particularly useful for numerical and statistical data.

A graph could be used to show the results of research, for example, average waiting times at an A+E department and the trends in the numbers of people attending at particular times.

Tables are useful for organising information in columns and rows. They can contain just numbers or just words or a combination of both as required. They could be used for recording staff on duty at times through the day or as a food or exercise diary.

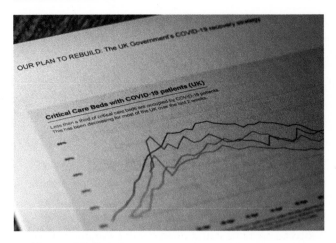

▲ Figure 6.6 Graph

Leaflets or posters

These are useful for providing 'chunks' of information, for instance about topics such as heart health, healthy eating, exercise and other health-related information for individuals. Leaflets provide more information than a poster and have the benefit of individuals being able to read it through at their own pace at a later date. They could provide information about treatment options for a condition that has been newly diagnosed, for example.

The government has used posters extensively from the beginning of the COVID-19 pandemic to publicise public health guidance and legislation.

Web pages and social media

Websites can provide access to a vast amount of information (see also section A5.8). It is important to use reliable sites to ensure the information is trustworthy and correct. For example, the NHS website (www.nhs.uk) has comprehensive information about health, illness and services provided.

Social media reaches a large number of people very quickly. This is the reason why, for example, the NHS used tweets about getting vaccinated against COVID-19 in 2021 in an attempt to increase the numbers of younger people in particular getting vaccinated.

Test yourself

1 Suggest suitable formats for delivering an induction training session about data protection to a group of new nurses on their first day. Give reasons for your choice.
2 State one format you would *not* use in this situation and explain why.

A6.8 The reasons for record keeping and how this contributes to the overall care of the individual

Reasons for record keeping

▶ It is important to provide an overall view and history of the individual's medical history and care needs. A record that includes all services accessed by the individual ensures each new service or practitioner will be informed about the effectiveness the treatment or support provided previously.
▶ Individuals should be at the centre of the care provided and should be treated as a whole person, not, for example, just someone who has diabetes. Everyone involved in an individual's care needs access to an individual's information.
▶ Most people are treated and supported by a multidisciplinary team of practitioners, like George (see page 92), and so multidisciplinary team members must have access to records to get the whole picture of an individual and their holistic care needs.
▶ **Continuity of care** is supported by good record keeping. For example, it is not always possible to see the same practitioner at each hospital visit, but if the individual's records are of a good standard and continuous over time, they will support the provision of good quality care.

As stated in section A6.1, in the event of any issues, the records can be used as evidence. The care practitioner should have recorded details of care provided, stated reasons for any decisions made, and dated and signed the record.

How it contributes to the overall care of the individual

Record keeping ensures uniform care is provided regardless of the service accessed.

It ensures there is a record of what has been discussed (for example, next steps) and what took place within each interaction.

A6.9 The responsibilities of employees and employers in relation to record keeping and when to escalate issues

Responsibilities

Legal requirements and inspections

The Care Quality Commission carries out inspections of health and social care services for England to ensure essential standards of quality and safety are met. The quality and effectiveness of record keeping is one of the aspects inspected. Procedures and practices must be of the correct standard to pass the inspection. Actions such as fines or closure can result if standards are not met.

Duty of care

Healthcare providers have a **duty of care** for individuals who use their services. This means that all organisations and practitioners must put the best interests of the individuals using the service first. They also have to ensure the safety of staff and service users.

Duty of candour

This means care workers must be open and honest with individuals and their families when something goes wrong. They should give a transparent explanation of what has happened, apologise and explain fully what occurred. They should also inform the individual of any potential consequences of the incident. This includes what steps will be taken to avoid or prevent it from happening again.

Further reading about the duty of candour, from the Nursing and Midwifery Council, can be found at **www.nmc.org.uk/standards/guidance/the-professional-duty-of-candour/read-theprofessional-duty-of-candour/**

Investigation and tracking incidents and accidents

If a patient safety incident occurs, NHS investigation procedures must be followed. Full details and procedures used can be found at **www.england.nhs.uk/patient-safety/patient-safety-investigation/**

All care providers have a responsibility to have procedures in place, so that in the event of an accident or incident an investigation can take place and any necessary changes can be made to avoid similar incidents in future.

Accountability

Record keeping provides an audit trail that can evidence what actually happened if there is an investigation into an incident. This may help to determine who was responsible or accountable for what happened.

However, the point is not about finding who to blame but rather about preventing and fixing issues in the interests of good practice. Thus, accountability also means being honest and open if you have made a mistake – you are responsible for the care you provide and the consequences of that care. You should always follow your organisation's policies, practice and agreed ways of working in order to prevent any harm.

When to escalate

'Escalate' means to take an issue very seriously and to take further action, usually by involving more senior members of staff or management.

Often just taking someone aside and speaking with them and explaining the issue, possibly also giving a verbal warning if necessary, will be enough for them to improve their practice. However, in some cases the issue is very serious and could lead to (or may already have led to) consequences such as abuse or harm. If this is the case, you have a duty to escalate the situation to a senior manager.

Safeguarding concerns

Safeguarding refers to the measures taken to protect people's health, wellbeing and rights, enabling them to be kept safe from harm, abuse and neglect. All practitioners in health and social care organisations must be aware of the need for safeguarding.

Some individuals may be more at risk of abuse, maltreatment or neglect than others. Examples include individuals who have a learning or physical disability, those with a sensory impairment (visually or hearing impaired) or those who lack mental capacity due to dementia or being unresponsive, in a coma, for example.

For many reasons these individuals may not want to, or be able to, report poor care or abuse. They are dependent on carers and may not want to upset them as their treatment might get worse. They may not know or understand their rights and not realise they are being abused. They may not see or hear who is abusing them. Staff have a duty of care to report concerns of suspected abuse or poor care to the organisation's safeguarding lead.

See Chapter A11 for more on safeguarding.

Whistleblowing

If you become aware of someone neglecting their duties, resulting in causing harm to others, you have a duty to report this to the senior manager or other person designated to be responsible for whistleblowing reports. Whistleblowing is the procedure used when you have really serious concerns about behaviour that may be illegal. Unsafe medical practice or suspecting someone is under the influence of alcohol at work are examples of when whistleblowing would be appropriate. Healthcare settings must have a whistleblowing policy, and employees are protected from losing their job as a result of raising these concerns.

See section A11.7 for details of this and more on whistleblowing in general.

Radicalisation concerns

Radicalisation is a process by which 'an individual or group adopts increasingly extreme political, social, or religious ideals and aspirations that reject or undermine the status quo or undermines contemporary ideas and expressions of freedom of choice'.

Source: http://lhp.leedsth.nhs.uk/LeedsPathways/files/adultsafeguarding/event_training_competencies_framework.pdf

The Prevent duty requires all NHS trusts to ensure that all healthcare staff can identify any early signs of radicalisation and know to refer them either to their safeguarding lead or to the police.

See section A11.9 for more on Prevent.

Research

Visit the Let's Talk About It website to find out about the signs of radicalisation: **www.ltai.info/spotting-the-signs/**

Project practice

1   View the Skills for Care presentation for Standard 14 Handling Information – Care Certificate presentation (**https://skillsforhealth. org.uk/wp-content/uploads/2021/01/Care-Certificate-Standard-14.pptx**).

    Make notes of key points. You may wish to refer to the Skills for Care workbook for Standard 14, 'Handling Information': **www.skillsforcare. org.uk/Document-library/Standards/Care-Certificate/Standard%2014%20CC%20 Workbook.pdf**

2   You have been asked to assist a midwife by gathering information from Amaya, who is pregnant for the first time and is attending her first appointment. You will have 30 minutes to speak with Amaya.

    (a) You need to create a plan for the session. Consider the following:
    ▶ What types of information will you need from Amaya?
    ▶ What methods will you use to gather the information?
    ▶ How will you record the information?
    ▶ How will you provide the information you have gathered to the midwife?

    (b) As part of your plan, reference how your information gathering meets the requirements of three pieces of legislation.

    (c) Carry out a role play of the session and then write a personal review:
    ▶ stating how successful the interview was in gathering the information required
    ▶ giving examples of good practice that you used.

Assessment practice

1 Explain why it is so important that a healthcare worker ensures that their records about a service user are timely and accurate.

2 What should you do if you are not sure:

(a) whether to record some information about a patient

(b) where to record some information?

3 Describe how you can ensure confidentiality when using electronic records.

4 Outline **one** piece of legislation that relates to the recording, storing and sharing of information. Include the people responsible for data management and their duties under this legislation.

5 Discuss the purpose of using abbreviations when record keeping. Your response should demonstrate:

▶ examples of abbreviations used in record keeping

▶ a reasoned conclusion about the use of abbreviations.

6 Describe the responsibility of healthcare professionals in relation to audits.

7 Describe **three** different formats that would be appropriate for sharing information with patients.

8 (a) List **three** of the seven key principles of the GDPR.

(b) Briefly state how each influences practice.

9 Explain the types of information needed when obtaining a client history and why each is necessary.

10 Discuss when it is appropriate and permitted for a care assistant to share an elderly person's health information with their family members. Your response should demonstrate:

▶ examples of different types of information that might be shared

▶ a reasoned conclusion about when sharing information is appropriate.

A7: Good scientific and clinical practice

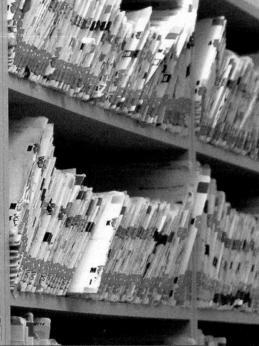
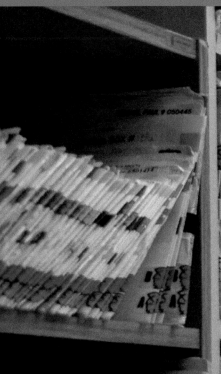
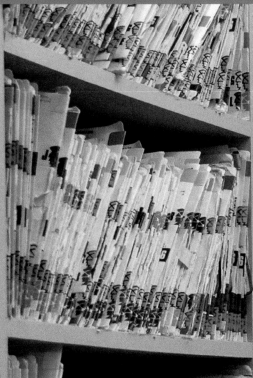

Introduction

If you bake a cake, you follow a recipe. If you strip down and rebuild an engine, you follow a workshop manual. If you have done either of these many times before, then you may not have to keep looking at the recipe or the manual. But if you are new to baking, then failure to follow the recipe carefully is likely to give disappointing results – something that looks and tastes more like a pancake than a light, fluffy sponge. Not paying attention to the workshop manual might result in a few parts left over and a reassembled engine that may never work again.

The same principles apply to our work in science and healthcare. Therefore, we have to follow proper procedures and do our best at all times – particularly when the consequences of getting things wrong can be disastrous. This is why we must always adhere to the standards and procedures that we call good scientific and clinical practice.

Learning outcomes

The core knowledge outcomes that you must understand and learn:

A7.1 the principles of good practice in scientific and clinical settings

A7.2 what an SOP is

A7.3 why it is important for everyone to follow SOPs

A7.4 how to access SOPs for a given activity

A7.5 the potential impacts of not regularly cleaning and preparing work areas for use

A7.6 the potential impacts of not maintaining, cleaning and servicing equipment

A7.7 why it is important to calibrate and test equipment to ensure it is fit for use

A7.8 how to escalate concerns if equipment is not correctly calibrated/unsuitable for intended use

A7.9 why it is important to order and manage stock

A7.10 the potential consequences of incorrectly storing products, materials and equipment.

A7.1 The principles of good practice in scientific and clinical settings

Whatever our work environment, whatever branch of science or healthcare, we must aim to achieve:

▶ consistency
▶ predictability
▶ reproducibility
▶ reliability.

On top of all this, we must ensure the health, safety and wellbeing of ourselves and others.

We can achieve these objectives in several ways, as described in this chapter, but they all share these common principles:

▶ using standard operating procedures (SOPs)
▶ effectively managing calibration and maintenance of equipment and work areas
▶ effectively managing stock
▶ appropriately storing products, materials and equipment.

The following sections will look at how all of these contribute to good scientific and clinical practice.

A7.2 What an SOP is

A **standard operating procedure** or **SOP** is simply a set of steps or instructions in a sequence that are designed to standardise the approach to a process or action, so that everyone learns to do it the same way. SOPs can be used for everything we do in the workplace, including:

▶ receiving goods, booking them into stock and informing the accounts department that the invoice can be paid
▶ cleaning a room in a healthcare facility or a microbiology lab
▶ producing a batch of a pharmaceutical ingredient
▶ analysing that batch to make sure it meets standards of purity, activity and safety.

Some SOPs may be just a few lines of instruction, others will be long and complex. They will always aim to ensure that the process or activity is done correctly and consistently.

Research

Find one or more examples of an SOP. Ideally these should be from your workplace, but if none is available, an internet search for 'SOP in healthcare' should provide numerous examples.

Review the SOPs. Are there any common features? Would they allow you to carry out the task without further information? Do some of them require prior knowledge or training, or refer to other SOPs?

A7.3 Why it is important for everyone to follow SOPs

SOPs are created for a reason – to ensure that processes can be followed consistently, which can be crucial in health and science facilities. Ultimately, if you do not follow an SOP, you might get fired from your job, or at least disciplined. Of course, this is not the main reason we must all follow SOPs – failure to follow SOPs might have legal consequences in some organisations, or someone may be injured as a result – but it does illustrate why doing so is so important.

Maintaining health and safety

In Chapter A3 we looked at various health, safety and environmental regulations. You will have learned the importance of following proper procedures, especially in areas that are tightly regulated. Part of this is to perform a proper risk assessment. Every SOP should include a risk assessment of the process being carried out and the steps taken to minimise harm. Following the SOP is essential to reduce harm to employees, the public or the environment.

Enabling consistency of approach

The key word is 'standard'. An SOP should ensure that a process or procedure is always carried out in the same way. The outcome should be predictable. An SOP helps ensure that everything is done in the same way each time, producing consistent outcomes.

Of course, it is important that quality is also built into SOPs. Consistency is no good if all it means is that the product is always consistently poor. Consistency without quality is not enough.

Meeting any legal or organisational requirements

The science and healthcare sectors are highly regulated – for good reason. Companies and other organisations can see the importance of good-quality SOPs that are strictly followed, but some SOPs will ensure that any applicable laws are followed.

Here is a range of examples of how SOPs might be required for organisational or legal reasons:

▶ cleaning staff writing their initials on a chart to show that regular scheduled cleaning has been carried out

▶ following government (specifically, Home Office) requirements for storing and issuing controlled drugs in hospitals or care homes

▶ storing and disposing of hazardous waste (see COSHH Regulations in Chapter A3, page 49)

▶ carrying out clinical trials of new medicines or therapies

▶ obtaining regulatory approval for new medicines, medical devices or treatments.

Upholding professional standards

Membership of all sorts of professional bodies from the Royal Society of Chemistry to the various medical colleges (Royal Colleges of Nursing, Midwives, Physicians, Surgeons, etc.) requires adherence to certain professional standards. By following appropriate SOPs, you can show that you are upholding those standards.

Some regulated activities, such as production of pharmaceuticals, have to be supervised by a **qualified person (QP)**. European Union regulations state that a medicinal product cannot be supplied for sale without a QP certifying that it meets the relevant requirements or standards. A QP is typically a pharmacist (MRPharmS), chartered chemist (CChem) or chartered biologist (CBiol). These roles are administered by the Royal Pharmaceutical Society, Royal Society of Chemistry and the Royal Society of Biology.

Demonstrating compliance for audit purposes

It is not enough to do something properly – you need to be able to show that you did it properly. Having an experienced person watch over you might be useful, but it will not be enough to show that the job was done correctly when your organisation is audited or inspected months or even years later. Having robust SOPs, following them carefully and recording how they were followed provides documentary evidence that will satisfy inspection bodies such as the Medicines Agency, Home Office or Care Quality Commission when they review this at a later date.

Test yourself

1   What is a standard operating procedure (SOP)?
2   Explain two reasons why it is important for everyone to follow SOPs.
3   Give two consequences of not following an SOP.
4   Explain why SOPs often require you to complete a log or record your actions.

A7.4 How to access SOPs for a given activity

Most organisations should have SOPs for all the procedures and processes that are carried out in the workplace. These should be kept in either hard copy or electronic format and be readily available for use. However, if SOPs are not available, you might need to look elsewhere.

Carrying out detailed index searches (for example, via intranet/manual)

If the SOP is available in your organisation, you might need to search for it. This might involve searching an electronic or paper-based index. SOPs may be held centrally or located in the departments to which they relate. SOPs that are used infrequently might require some tracking down.

Finding SOPs in electronic format via your organisation's intranet or computer network should be quite straightforward – particularly if it has good search facilities, ideally based on one of the online search engines such as Google or Bing.

Completing detailed staff induction and ongoing training

If you wrote an SOP for how to run an efficient organisation, staff induction (processes for getting new employees set up and informed about their new role) and regular training would certainly be very prominent. New staff must be aware of SOPs that affect their area of work – it is not good enough to expect them to learn, sometimes the hard way, 'the way we do things round here'. As well as being part of the induction process for new employees, staff need to be kept up to date with the new SOPs or modifications to SOPs. This should be part of a regular training programme for all staff.

Ensuring the SOP is the most up-to-date version

Using a version of an SOP that was written 20 years ago and has been updated once since then can be worse than useless. Much could have happened in the meantime:

▶ Methods may have changed.
▶ Equipment or processes may have been updated.
▶ Regulations may have changed.
▶ Roles and responsibilities may have evolved.

It should be obvious that some form of **version control** is needed (for instance, giving each new updated version a new number – e.g. v2, v3, etc.). But it is not enough to know which version you are using – you need to know that you have the latest version. This can be achieved in a number of different ways:

▶ Controlling the production and distribution of SOPs so that old versions are returned or destroyed when new versions are introduced.
▶ Maintaining a central deposit (electronic or paper-based) that can be accessed but not removed or downloaded.
▶ Maintaining a central index or database so that version numbers of SOPs in use can be checked to ensure they are the most up to date.

Research

It is unlikely that you will have responsibility for production of SOPs, at least in the early years of your career. However, you will almost certainly have to use them. You should always know where and how to access the SOPs that cover your work. Find out how your organisation stores, makes available and maintains its SOPs. Think about the tasks you undertake (or are likely to undertake) in your role and obtain copies of the relevant SOPs. Do they provide sufficient information and guidance for you to carry out the task adequately? If not, do you know where to go to get additional help or support?

Ensuring all relevant documentation has been completed and signed

Although people sometimes complain about 'box-ticking exercises', 'mountains of red tape' or

'bureaucracy', good documentation is essential to keep track of:

▶ what is done
▶ when it is done
▶ it being done correctly
▶ who does it.

These are all essential to make sure not just that things are done correctly but that we can show they have been done correctly. 'Signing off' the records helps to emphasise the importance of following procedures and taking responsibility. It encourages taking ownership of a process.

If something goes wrong and a product does not meet specification, or someone is injured, there is likely to be an investigation. It is important to have good records and an **audit trail** to ensure that lessons can be learned for the future. Learning lessons, in the spirit of continual improvement, is more important than assigning blame. There are examples of this in sections A3.3 and A3.4.

Test yourself

1. Describe the ways in which an organisation may:
   – keep or store its SOPs
   – make them available to staff.
2. Give two reasons why it is important to use up-to-date SOPs.
3. Describe one way in which organisations ensure that the most up-to-date version of an SOP is the one that is used.
4. Explain why it is necessary to ensure all relevant documentation is completed.

A7.5 The potential impacts of not regularly cleaning and preparing work areas for use

Risks to health and safety

Some of the more general risks in this area are covered in section A3.3 ('Ensuring working environments are clean, tidy and hazard free', page 55). Other risks can be specific to certain environments or workplaces.

Spread of infection

The COVID-19 pandemic has made us all aware of the importance of hygiene in reducing the spread of infection. Different micro-organisms can spread in different ways, but regular cleaning and preparation can reduce routes of transmission:

▶ Contaminated surfaces, known as **fomites**, can transmit bacteria and viruses when touched. These can include:
  – hard surfaces (door handles, handrails, light switches, mobile phones)
  – fabrics such as clothing, towels and furnishings.
▶ Aerosols, produced by breathing, coughing or sneezing, can transmit infected droplets directly between people. This is why good ventilation is so important. Aerosols can also transfer infectious agents to fomites.
▶ Accumulations of waste, rubbish, dirt, etc. can provide a breeding ground for infectious micro-organisms or for vermin that can be **vectors** for disease (see section B1.26, page 253).

Production of toxic/dangerous by-products

Aseptic technique is used in microbiology to prevent contamination of bacterial cultures as this can have serious consequences. For example, if a pathogen contaminates the culture, this could lead to disease or even death of anyone who comes into contact with the culture.

In some chemical processes, failure to clean equipment properly can lead to contamination of the product and could also lead to production of hazardous by-products that are toxic, explosive or harmful to the environment.

Health and safety

Think about the risks we have covered. Do any of these apply in your workplace? Do you need to get more information about precautions to take and procedures to follow? Are there any ways that you could modify your work practices that will help to reduce risks to health and safety?

Invalid results

Contamination can introduce other micro-organisms (bacteria and fungi) that can compete with the one being cultured. This can obviously ruin an experiment. However, there are many other situations in laboratory or clinical settings where contamination, or cross-contamination, can invalidate results.

Here are some examples:
▶ Environmental samples for water analysis can be contaminated during the sampling process or during transport or storage.
▶ Analytical reagents can be contaminated. This is likely to invalidate any analysis performed using them.
▶ DNA samples are at particular risk from contamination – especially cross-contamination. See the case study for more information.

Case study

The polymerase chain reaction (PCR) is an enormously powerful technique for 'amplifying' DNA or RNA. It uses the enzymes involved in DNA replication to take a few hundred copies of DNA or RNA and create billions of copies. PCR is used in many applications in research (genetic engineering), forensics (DNA samples from crime scenes) and diagnosis (the PCR test for SARS-CoV-2 virus). However, it is also highly susceptible to contamination and so precautions must be taken to prevent this. Use of DNA in evidence in a criminal trial could be invalidated if there were any possibility of 'foreign' DNA being introduced.
▶ What precautions should be taken to minimise risk of contamination when working with PCR? Think about use of SOPs and staff training.

Reflect

Have you had a COVID-19 PCR test? Did you notice any signs of an SOP being followed, or precautions being taken to avoid contamination during collecting the samples?

If you have taken a COVID-19 lateral flow test, think about the instructions provided. Do they have the characteristics of an SOP? Is the information provided sufficient for you to carry out the test correctly?

Inefficient working practices

'Time is money' is a saying you are likely to encounter many times in your working life, largely because it is true. Lack of efficiency means that the job takes longer – and that means it is not just your time that is being wasted but other people may be waiting on your work, so they are wasting time as well. This means higher staff costs as they have to be paid for more hours. And inefficiency is not just about waste of time – it could mean a waste of valuable materials or resources, some of which could be incredibly difficult to obtain.

Damage to equipment

Not following an SOP can have many consequences, including breaking essential and/or expensive equipment. Once again, it is likely to cause your organisation extra costs – such as repair or replacement – as well as increasing the time it takes to get the job done.

A7.6 The potential impacts of not maintaining, cleaning and servicing equipment

All of the factors that we considered in section A7.5 about not cleaning and preparing work areas apply just as much to not maintaining, cleaning and servicing equipment properly:

▶ Risks to health and safety:
  – increased risk of injury
  – spread of infection.
▶ Invalid results:
  – contamination or cross-contamination.

Reduced function of equipment

Lack of proper maintenance can lead to decreased lifespan of equipment. That is why second-hand cars sold with a 'full service history' are considered better buys. As well as this, equipment being out of service for repair or because it has not been properly maintained is likely to increase costs and cause delays in getting the job done.

For all these reasons, it is quite common for regular maintenance (sometimes called **preventative maintenance**) to be included in various SOPs.

Similarly, there might be SOPs for regular maintenance of some or all key equipment. These could include:

▶ regular checking that all connections are secure to make sure there are no leaks
▶ regular lubrication of moving parts
▶ replacement of batteries to ensure they do not cause damage if they leak
▶ regular calibration of equipment, as described in the next section.

A7.7 Why it is important to calibrate and test equipment to ensure it is fit for use

The **true value** of a measurement is the ideal or perfect value. Except for some of the physical constants used as the basis of SI units (see section B1.62, page 295), we can never determine the true value because of the inherent **uncertainty** in any measurement.

The uncertainty in any measurement reflects the difference between the actual measurement and the true value as a result of the level of **accuracy** of the measuring equipment or apparatus.

> ### Key terms
>
> *Accuracy*: measurements that are close to the **true value**.
>
> *Precise*: measurements that are close to each other, but they may be inaccurate.
>
> *Calibration*: the process of comparing measurements, usually against a **reference standard**.
>
> *Reference standard*: something of known size, mass, concentration, etc. that we can use to calibrate equipment or methods.

Ensuring accuracy of measurements

Accuracy and **precision** are terms that are not always used correctly. Figure 7.1 illustrates this using the analogy of shooting at a target.

High accuracy   Low accuracy   High accuracy   Low accuracy
High precision   High precision Low precision   Low precision

▲ Figure 7.1 The target analogy of accuracy and precision

Accuracy in measurement depends on the quality of the apparatus used for measurement, the skill of the person using it and how well the apparatus has been **calibrated**. The degree of precision of a piece of equipment is related to the number and size of **random errors** that it generates. The accuracy will depend on whether and how well it has been calibrated.

Calibration methods will depend on the equipment being used, but they usually involve use of a standard. Calibration is essentially the process of comparing measurements. One measurement is of a known size or correctness, e.g. a **reference standard**. The other is on the device or instrument being calibrated.

Calibration is required for:

▶ any instrument that has moving parts, such as an analogue ammeter or voltmeter, because movement can upset the balance of the instrument
▶ anything that can be affected by temperature change
▶ electronic equipment, as the performance of various electronic components can change over time, for example, the glass membrane in a pH electrode can be affected by deposits (dirt, oils and grease, protein, inorganic materials) and should be calibrated before each use.

However, calibration is only as good as the reference standard used, so it is important to take care of standards, for example, by preventing cross-contamination of standard solutions, corrosion of standard masses, etc.

Prolonging the life of equipment

As well as ensuring the accuracy of measurements, calibration and testing equipment will form an important part of any programme of preventative maintenance. This will help to extend the useful life of the equipment.

Meeting legal requirements

It is not so common to buy loose produce in a grocery store these days. It takes a lot longer to weigh out 1 kg of rice than it does to simply pick a packet off the shelf. However, you also have to consider the time and expense in maintaining and calibrating the scales used. There is a legal requirement for all measuring equipment used in trade to be certified to meet certain standards. This ensures that consumers are not cheated and that they can be confident in their purchases.

Now imagine you are not simply buying 1 kg of rice in the supermarket. If you buy a medicine, you need to have confidence that the dosage shown on the packaging is correct. For this reason, all equipment used in every stage in the manufacture of the raw materials and finished products has to be certified so that it meets the necessary standards of accuracy.

Test yourself

1 Give two consequences of not keeping up with a regular cleaning programme of both work areas and equipment.
2 What is meant by an **accurate** measurement?
3 Explain how proper calibration reduces the risk of error.

A7.8 How to escalate concerns if equipment is not correctly calibrated/unsuitable for intended use

The details of the procedures to follow will vary according to the workplace. However, the principles to follow if any equipment is not fit for purpose remain the same. For some critical pieces of equipment, the course of action might be covered in the SOP.

Taking the equipment out of action

This should be obvious, for the reasons discussed in the previous sections. If a pH meter or thermometer is found to be out of calibration or specification, it should be simple to stop using it and find another one. However, it is not always possible to simply throw a switch. Whenever you encounter new equipment or a new task, give some thought to what you would need to do if that equipment had to be taken out of action.

Labelling the equipment as being out of use, if appropriate

It is not enough to simply stop using the equipment yourself, you need to let other people know that the equipment should not be used. Ideally, there should be signs or stickers available that can be used – if not, perhaps you should suggest some. It is important that any sign or label is prominent so it cannot be overlooked. Also, make sure that it cannot simply fall off or be removed too easily.

Reporting concerns to the relevant person, in line with organisational policies and procedures

You might have to report any concerns to your line manager. Alternatively, there may be someone, such as a safety officer, who should be informed of any issues that could have an impact on safety.

You need to make sure that some action is taken, even if you do not need the equipment right away. Repairs or re-calibration may take time. It may not be your responsibility to actually do that, or arrange for it to be done. However, you should certainly take responsibility for informing the appropriate person so that they can take the necessary action.

Recording concerns according to organisational procedures

Reporting concerns is important, but so is making a record of those concerns. We saw in section A7.3 that you need to be able to demonstrate that an SOP has been followed for audit purposes. The same is true about documenting concerns about equipment being fit for purpose. This might look like 'covering your back' in case there are any repercussions. That may be a benefit, of course, but it is not the real reason that you need to document everything related to equipment – particularly if it has a safety implication.

Key equipment will often have an associated log, either on paper or electronically. This might cover:
▶ who used the equipment
▶ when it was used
▶ what it was used for
▶ any routine calibration or maintenance carried out.

A log of this sort might be the appropriate place to record concerns about the equipment so that everyone using the equipment is aware of any issues, either current or historical.

Research

Think about any pieces of equipment that are used in your workplace. Which of these require regular calibration? How often are the different pieces of equipment calibrated? Some types of equipment might require calibration before each use (do you know which these are in your workplace?) whilst others might need calibration at regular intervals, such as weekly, monthly, quarterly or annually. Are there SOPs covering this? Is there a record or log of what was calibrated, when it was calibrated and what the outcome was? Do you know whether each piece of equipment that you use will be fit for purpose?

If you feel that any equipment is not fit for purpose, what are the procedures for escalating your concerns? For example, should you report it to your supervisor or line manager? Is there an individual or department that is responsible for maintenance and/or calibration of equipment? Is there a procedure for reporting issues with equipment? Do you feel confident that you could handle this? If not, what steps can you take, such as asking for training or other form of support?

Case study

In August 2021, Becton Dickinson, a company that makes consumables for the NHS, announced that there was a global shortage of blood collection tubes. This was due to record demand for these tubes, partly because of the increased need for tests for COVID-19 patients. An additional factor affecting the UK was transport and import issues related to Brexit.

As a result of this, the NHS in England and Wales told GP surgeries and hospitals to temporarily stop some blood testing. Patients would only be able to get tests if they were urgent. The tests that were suspended included those for fertility, allergy, and pre-diabetes.

Doctors and nurses in GP surgeries were asked to:
▶ only request blood tests where they were clinically urgent, or time-critical (such as in pregnancy)
▶ when taking blood samples, not send an extra tube 'just in case'
▶ not duplicate tests that may have already been carried out in hospital.

Source: www.hey.nhs.uk/wp/wp-content/uploads/2021/08/bloodTubeShortageCCGs.pdf

In addition, practice managers in GP surgeries were asked to:
▶ review their local stocks to ensure they had a maximum of 3–7 days' supply
▶ not over-order tubes so that the central Pathology stores teams could manage stocks based on expiry dates and availability
▶ return any short-dated blood tubes that would not be used before the expiry date to the central stores.

Source: NHS blood test tube shortage: Doctors 'facing difficult choices' - BBC News www.bbc.co.uk/news/health-58374553

This was an exceptional situation, based on the combination of worldwide and local factors. Nonetheless, can you see aspects of how normal stock control was managed?

What are the lessons for proper ordering and managing of stock?

A7.9 Why it is important to order and manage stock

Ensuring sufficient supply of required consumables and materials

Clearly, it is important that you have access to sufficient stocks of all the items you need to carry out your work. You may not be responsible for the purchase or ordering of **consumables** or **materials**, but you will almost certainly be responsible for ensuring that you have access to everything you need. That may mean knowing how to get them from stores or ensuring you have your own stock in your work area.

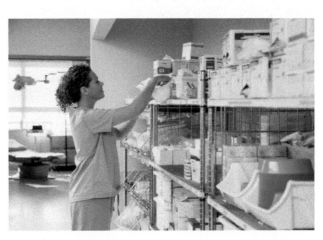

▲ Figure 7.2 Make sure you always have the right amount of stock

Key terms

Consumables: items that are used and then disposed of. They are mostly single-use but might be re-used in some circumstances.

Materials: include items such as ingredients or components used in the manufacture of a product.

Ensuring that materials are used before their expiry date

We are used to seeing 'use by' or 'best before' dates on most of the items we buy in the supermarket. Do you know what they mean? In general, they mean what they say. Some products might become harmful if kept beyond the 'use by' date. On the other hand, something eaten after the 'best before' date may not be as tasty but it is unlikely to cause you harm.

In a science or healthcare environment you are more likely to come across products with expiry dates. Some of these will be more important than others.

If the expiry date on a pack of self-adhesive envelopes has passed, the adhesive may not be fully effective and you might have to resort to sticky tape to seal the envelope. That is inconvenient but is not dangerous and is therefore minor in the overall scheme of things.

However, most of the items that you encounter in a healthcare or clinical setting are likely to have expiry dates that must be respected, including:

▶ medicines that may no longer be sufficiently effective, meaning the patient does not receive the effect of a full dose
▶ packs of fluids, swabs, dressings, etc. that may no longer be sterile and could cause harm to the patient if used.

Reducing the costs of excess stock

Sometimes it is necessary to maintain high levels of stock, such as:

▶ items for which there is a long lead time, meaning we need to order them well in advance
▶ items that are critical to patient care, where running out might harm the patient.

However, in your working environment it is possible that excess stock will be wasted for no good reason. That puts a drain on resources and means there will be less budget available for essentials. Implementing robust stock control procedures can save huge amounts of money.

Improving efficiency and productivity

Efficiency and productivity are linked. Whether you measure productivity in the amount of work you get done in a given time or how much product goes out of the door every day, if you can work more efficiently, you will be more productive. However, being productive does not necessarily mean being quick. If you rush things and make a mistake, you may find that everything takes longer and costs more than if you had worked at a more steady, methodical pace. Efficiency and productivity also mean being careful.

Ensure safety of stock

We have considered the importance of good stock control. It should be obvious that stocks need to be looked after, which we will cover in the next section.

Ensuring stock is safely looked after might mean keeping it under the correct conditions, for example, in a fridge or freezer. It might also mean ensuring the security of stock. That might be to prevent unauthorised use or to prevent access to hazardous or controlled substances. For example, the Misuse of Drugs Act 1971 and Misuse of Drugs Regulations 2001 apply strict procedures to storage of **controlled drugs**, including:

▶ ensuring safe and secure storage, including restricting personnel access (for example, by use of locked storage cabinets, keycard access, etc.)
▶ undertaking inventory record-keeping
▶ following sign-in/sign-out protocols.

A7.10 The potential consequences of incorrectly storing products, materials and equipment

Are you the sort of person who reads the small print on jars of jam or bottles of tomato sauce? If so, you may notice that they nearly always have the instruction 'refrigerate after opening'. This is increasingly common, as food manufacturers reduce the amount of artificial preservatives added to foodstuffs. The consequence is that something that may have been kept in a cupboard many years ago should now be stored in the fridge. It probably explains why large fridges are becoming more popular, but it also illustrates the importance of proper storage.

Cross-contamination

Keeping with the domestic theme, we are told that cooked foods should never be stored in the fridge on a shelf below raw meat. Raw meat may be contaminated with harmful bacteria. Although these are destroyed by cooking, fluids from the raw meat may drip down onto the cooked food. The benefits of cooking are lost if cooked foods become contaminated. You will encounter many similar situations in your workplace, so pay attention to procedures for safe storage of any items that might be at risk of cross-contamination.

Breakdown of limited stability products

Many products that you will encounter in a healthcare setting are sensitive to heat or light and need to be stored accordingly.

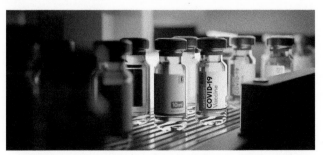

▲ Figure 7.3 COVID-19 vaccine vials in refrigerated storage

Consider the recent example of two COVID-19 vaccines (see Figure 7.3):

▶ The Pfizer vaccine needs to be stored and transported at –70 °C.
▶ The Oxford/AstraZeneca vaccine can be stored at up to +4 °C.

It is clear from this that the Oxford/AstraZeneca vaccine is easier to handle, particularly outside of hospitals or in developing countries that may not have access to ultra-cold storage.

Light-sensitive products are often stored in brown glass bottles (see Figure 7.4), so take care if you need to transfer such liquids to other containers.

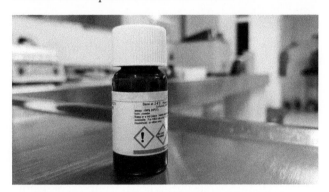

▲ Figure 7.4 A light-sensitive laboratory reagent packed in a brown glass bottle

Products exceeding expiry dates

Stock rotation is a term you are likely to encounter. It means always using the oldest batch first, providing the oldest has not passed its expiry date. Stock should always be kept in a way that makes proper stock rotation possible, rather than in such a way that items are left for months or years at the back of a cupboard. Physically arranging stocks of materials with the oldest batches at the front of a shelf can help, for example.

Loss of samples or degradation of reagents not stored at the correct temperature (–20 °C, –4 °C, 4 °C or room temperature)

NHS guidance to GP surgeries is that blood samples and urine samples should be sent to the lab the same day (see Figure 7.5). If this is not possible, they must be stored refrigerated at 4–8 °C and analysed within 24 hours. Cells in the blood can start to break down and release substances that mean the results may not be valid. It is not just high temperatures that can be damaging.

In general, blood samples should not be frozen before analysis as this can also lead to damage to cells.

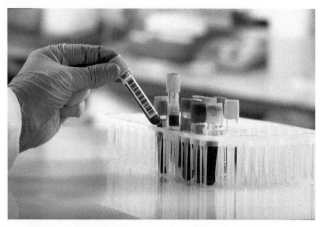

▲ Figure 7.5 Blood samples ready for analysis

The World Health Organization (WHO) has strict guidelines for transport and storage of water samples. Microbiological analysis should ideally be performed within 6 hours or no later than 24 hours after sample collection. Failure to do this means that the results may not be valid.

Correct storage of reagents is equally important. Here are some examples:

▶ Antibodies and proteins usually need to be stored at −20 °C or −80 °C, but conjugated antibodies (antibodies with enzymes attached) must not be frozen and so should be stored at 4 °C.

▶ Antibodies and other reagents that have a fluorescent dye attached must be kept dark to prevent photobleaching of the fluorescent dye, which will make it useless.

▶ Many solids are **hygroscopic**, meaning that they will absorb moisture from the air. When they do so, they are more likely to degrade by **hydrolysis**. This is when a compound is broken down by water – see section B1.7 or B2.5 for examples of hydrolysis. Also, if the solid has absorbed moisture, you cannot weigh it accurately.

So far, we have described the need for low-temperature storage. What about storage at room temperature? Obviously, it can be expensive to maintain large fridges or freezers, particularly ultra-cold freezers at −80 °C. Therefore, it makes sense to store materials at room temperature where possible. However, there is another reason why it can be better to store at room temperature. Whenever a bottle of solid is removed from a fridge or particularly a freezer, there is a risk of condensation forming on the powder when the bottle

is opened. This can also cause damage to the material by hydrolysis. For that reason, it is important that you leave a bottle to reach room temperature before opening. This could take several hours, so if there is no need to store the product at low temperature, it would be better to keep it at room temperature.

Practice point

One useful tip when handling products that require storage at low temperature is to **aliquot**. This means sub-dividing a larger amount into single-use quantities. This will avoid many freeze–thaw cycles that can be damaging to temperature-sensitive materials.

If you do this, you need to make sure that the process of aliquoting does not introduce contamination.

Risks to health and safety

Incorrect storage can have serious, sometimes life-threatening, consequences.

▶ Cultures or samples containing pathogens could be released and that could lead to spread of infection.

▶ Toxic, corrosive or other dangerous chemicals could be released into the lab or into the environment.

▶ Heavy items stored above a safe height could fall and cause injury or could injure someone trying to reach or lift them.

Stock is difficult to locate

What happens when one member of staff goes on holiday and they are the only person who knows that the spare toner cartridges are kept in a particular cupboard in an obscure location? Storage of stocks of consumables and materials should follow a logical pattern so that things can be found easily (see Figure 7.6).

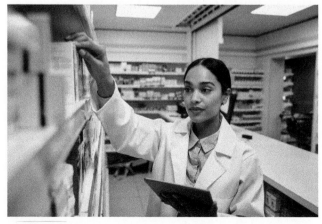

▲ Figure 7.6 Computerised stock control has many advantages

Financial loss

We have focused mainly on the health and safety consequences, but incorrect storage that leads to loss of or writing off stock has a financial implication as well. Think about the high cost of medicines and other clinical supplies and consider how much money could be saved if you reduced losses from incorrect storage.

Research

Think about your workplace and the materials, products or samples that are stored. Do they require any special storage conditions? Is it always clear what these conditions are? For example, are the containers marked or is there information about correct storage conditions in any relevant SOPs?

What would be the consequence of incorrect storage of any of these items?

Project practice

You have been asked to review the way in which SOPs are used in your organisation (you can base this on your own workplace or an organisation you are familiar with). The results of the review will be considered by the management and used as the basis for future action.

You need to complete the following steps:

1 Research a strategy.
  a Carry out a review of the legislation and regulations that affect your organisation.
  b Gather information about clients, customers, stakeholders of different types and how they are affected by your organisation's performance.
2 Plan a project based on the information that you have gathered.
  a Identify who is responsible for production and maintenance of SOPs.
  b How and where are SOPs kept, issued or referred to and by whom?

c What procedures are in place for documenting and auditing adherence to SOPs?
d How are SOPs incorporated into induction and training?
3 Present your findings in the form of a written report or PowerPoint presentation. You should include the following:
  a What weaknesses are there in the existing SOPs?
  b Who is responsible for maintaining SOPs and do they have the relevant training and experience?
  c Are all members of staff familiar with the SOPs that affect them?
  d Recommendations for improved systems.
4 Discuss the following questions:
  a How should members of staff be made aware of the importance of following SOPs?
  b Is the culture of the organisation to impose or to encourage the following of SOPs?
  c What are the risk factors if SOPs are not followed correctly?
5 Write a reflective evaluation of your work.

Assessment practice

1 What are the main principles of good practice in scientific and clinical settings?
2 Give **two** advantages and **one** disadvantage of keeping all SOPs on an organisation's intranet/computer network.
3 You notice that an SOP does not include a procedure for calibrating an important piece of measuring equipment. Justify why it should be included in a revised SOP.

4 Which of the following is the correct course of action if you find a piece of equipment is not performing correctly?
  a Put a note on the door of the room containing the equipment.
  b Unplug the equipment, stick a label on the front saying 'Do not use' and inform your line manager.
  c Inform the safety officer when you next meet them.
  d Put a note in the equipment log to say that it is not working correctly.

5   Amir and Sofia are arguing about the terms 'precision' and 'accuracy'. Amir says that calibrating a piece of equipment makes the results more **precise**, but Sofia says this makes the results more **accurate**. Who is correct? Explain why.

6   A package arrives by next-day courier containing several bottles of a therapeutic enzyme. Explain what should happen to the package.

7   A healthcare practitioner is supporting a patient with reduced immunity during chemotherapy. The patient has complained of feeling unwell and the practitioner is taking the patient's temperature and blood pressure. Give **two** reasons why it is important to ensure that the information is accurate, and for each, explain a possible impact of not doing so.

8   What precautions would you take when preparing blood samples for transfer to an analytical laboratory?

9   You have been asked to review the way in which stocks of consumables are handled in a large care home. Each floor has a supervisor who is responsible for ordering and maintaining stocks of cleaning materials, hygiene products and some patient medications such as insulin. Identify **two** weaknesses in the current approach.

10 Explain the importance of proper stock control.

A8: Providing person-centred care

Introduction

An understanding of person-centred care is essential for anyone working in the healthcare sector. This unit provides an introduction to the purpose and key features of person-centred care and planning, and considers how it can be achieved.

Relevant legislation such as the Mental Capacity Act and its impact on the provision of person-centred care are considered. The ways that healthcare is regulated to ensure high standards of care are examined by looking at the roles of a range of regulatory bodies within the health sector, such as the Care Quality Commission and the Health & Safety Executive.

We also discuss how an individual's stage of development and long-term conditions and diseases impact care needs and types of service provision required throughout the lifespan and relating to death and bereavement.

Promoting independence and self-care can have positive effects on the care and service provision. These are considered with reference to the 6Cs, linked with understanding the need for safeguarding and the importance of managing relationships and boundaries when providing person-centred care.

Learning outcomes

The core knowledge outcomes that you must understand and learn:

A8.1 the purpose of the Mental Capacity (Amendment) Act 2019 in relation to healthcare

A8.2 the key principles of the Care Act 2014

A8.3 the role of a range of regulatory bodies within the health sector

A8.4 how the stages of human development impact on physical and mental function and the support provided in relation to person-centred care

A8.5 the key values of the healthcare sector when providing care and support

A8.6 the purpose of the Personalisation Agenda 2012 and the importance of using holistic approaches in order to place individuals, their carers and significant others at the centre of their care and support

A8.7 a range of verbal and nonverbal communication techniques, potential communication barriers and how to overcome them to support an individual's condition

A8.8 the application of relevant legislation, including Mental Capacity Act (2005) plus Amendment (2019) and Liberty Protection Safeguards (LPS) on the provision of person-centred care

A8.9 the considerations when providing person-centred care to people with pre-existing conditions or living with illness

A8.10 how mental health conditions, dementia and learning disabilities can influence a person's needs in relation to overall care

A8.11 how to promote independence and self-care and the positive impact on the healthcare sector

A8.12 the range of terms used in the healthcare sector in relation to death and bereavement, including their meaning

A8.13 the role of healthcare professionals in providing person-centred care for the individual during the active dying phase

A8.14 how to support people with bereavement and how to communicate with families

A8.15 what the 6Cs are in relation to person-centred care

A8.16 the importance of practising and promoting the 6Cs in relation to demonstrating person-centred care skills, through own actions and promoting the approach with others

A8.17 the concept of safeguarding in relation to providing person-centred care

A8.18 the importance of managing relationships and boundaries when providing person-centred care.

A8.1 The purpose of the Mental Capacity (Amendment) Act 2019 in relation to healthcare

This Act is designed to help safeguard and support individuals over the age of 16 who may lack the **mental capacity** to make choices about their own treatment or care.

> **Key term**
>
> **Mental capacity:** the ability to make a decision. It involves being able to understand information and remember it for long enough to make a decision and to be able to communicate it to others.

The Mental Capacity (Amendment) Act (2019) protects and supports the rights of individuals, aged 16 or older, who lack the mental capacity to make their own decisions. An individual who has dementia, someone with certain learning difficulties or an individual who has a serious head injury are all examples of people who may lack mental capacity and who would be protected by this Act.

The 2019 Amendment to the Act replaced the 'Deprivation of Liberty Safeguards' (DoLS) with the 'Liberty Protection Safeguards' (LPS). This amendment aims to improve and simplify the process of assessing mental capacity and the care that is required. It also clarifies the Act's provisions, aiming to ensure that individuals are only deprived of their liberty, or freedom, in order to protect them and keep them safe.

The Liberty Protection Safeguards seek to:
▶ introduce a simpler process that involves families more and gives swifter access to assessments
▶ support carers, families and local authorities
▶ allow the NHS, rather than local authorities, to make decisions about patients, allowing a more efficient and clearly accountable process
▶ consider restrictions of people's liberties as part of their overall care package
▶ remove repeat assessments and authorisations when someone moves between a care home, hospital and ambulance as part of their treatment.

Source: www.gov.uk/government/news/new-law-introduced-to-protect-vulnerable-people-in-care

A8.2 The key principles of the Care Act 2014

The six key principles of the Care Act 2014 are as follows.

Empowerment

Individuals should be supported to make their own decisions based on the best possible information. They should be encouraged to take control of their lives, be confident and make their own independent decisions.

Protection

This Act gives safeguarding adults a legal framework for the first time and stipulates that service users who are in greatest need of support and protection should be provided with representation. This could be an independent advocate, whose job is to facilitate the involvement of a vulnerable person who is the subject of an assessment or review of a care package.

Prevention

Since it is better to take action to prevent harm before it occurs, all staff should be trained in safeguarding procedures (see Chapter A11) and how to recognise signs of neglect or abuse. The Act states that local authorities must put in place preventative services that can help reduce or delay the development of care and support needs, including those of carers.

Proportionality

Actions should be proportionate to the risk: being overprotective can disadvantage service users by preventing them from being able to make their own decisions.

Partnership

This involves working with a range of professionals, groups and communities to prevent, detect and report neglect or abuse. This includes information sharing, when appropriate and always in line with data protection regulations.

Accountability

Healthcare professionals are accountable for any activities in relation to safeguarding. They need to be able to justify their actions and decisions. The organisation's policies, practices and agreed ways of working should be followed.

Research

Watch this video (or read the transcript) about the Care Act from the Social Care Institute of Excellence (SCIE): www.scie.org.uk/care-act-2014/video.asp

Make notes of any additional information you find in addition to the key principles listed above.

Produce a factsheet for yourself about the Care Act for future reference.

A8.3 The role of a range of regulatory bodies within the health sector

Regulatory bodies and their role

Healthcare services are regulated by official government organisations. The regulations (rules) are set by law and state the standards that have to be met by healthcare settings. **Inspections** are carried out by the **regulators**, for example, the CQC and Ofsted, to see whether services are safe, effective and well managed, and whether they meet the needs of their service users. Reports are published as a result of an inspection and healthcare settings may have to make improvements to their services in order to continue providing care.

Regulations and inspections enable service users to be informed about the quality and standard of care that is being provided and to have trust in the services they use.

Some regulatory bodies are responsible for registering care professionals as '**fit to practise**', for example, the Nursing and Midwifery Council. A midwife may be '**struck off**' the register if there are fitness to practise concerns. (See also section A2.11.)

Key terms

Inspection: the process of observing and carrying out checks to see whether services provided meet the required standards.

Regulator: independent organisation that carries out inspections to monitor and rate the quality of services provided.

Care Quality Commission (CQC)

The CQC is the regulator of health and social care for England. It carries out inspections of care services such as hospitals, GP surgeries, care homes, community care services, mental health services and social service departments to ensure that care standards are being met.

The CQC sets out 13 fundamental standards of care. Care should not fall below these standards. You can find the standards using this link: www.cqc.org.uk/-what-we-do/how-we-do-our-job/fundamental-standards

The role of the CQC includes:

▶ registering and licensing care services to ensure essential standards of quality and safety are met

▶ carrying out inspections of health and social care settings to monitor that the care provided continues to meet the standards required

▶ publishing inspection reports which rate care settings (see Figure 8.1)

▶ issuing cautions, warning notices and fines if standards are not met

▶ providing recommendations of how the service can improve

▶ putting a care provider into special measures – this means informing them of improvements which have to be made within a specified time limit and with re-inspection within six months

▶ closing down a service to protect service users if it does not improve and continues to provide inadequate care.

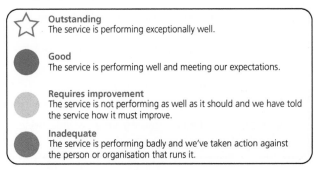

Outstanding
The service is performing exceptionally well.

Good
The service is performing well and meeting our expectations.

Requires improvement
The service is not performing as well as it should and we have told the service how it must improve.

Inadequate
The service is performing badly and we've taken action against the person or organisation that runs it.

▲ Figure 8.1 Care Quality Commission inspection grades

Source: Care Quality Commission, www.cqc.org.uk

The CQC aims to ensure health and care services provide people with safe, effective, compassionate, high-quality care. The organisation focuses on how services can improve.

There are various impacts of regulatory inspections:
- There is **transparency** about the standard of services being provided.
- The public know that independent checks are carried out.
- They give people confidence in the quality of health and care services.
- The inspection grade may help individuals to choose whether or not to use that service.
- The grades enable individuals to compare services and care settings.
- The strengths of the quality of care provided are identified.
- They help practitioners do their job effectively, they know what needs to improve.

Key term

Transparency: nothing is concealed, hidden or covered up, the inspections show things exactly as they are, whether good or not.

Research

Go to the CQC website using the link: **www.cqc.org.uk/search/services/**

Refine your search by selecting, from the 'All information' drop-down menu at the top left, a type of service, e.g. care home, GPs, hospitals, mental health services. Then click on 'search' on the right.

Scroll down and choose a care setting – try to find one with 'requires improvement' or 'inadequate' grading. Click on the care setting's inspection grade, download and read the report.

What features of the care setting gained good or outstanding grades?

What features of the care setting were considered to require improvement or were inadequate?

Health and Safety Executive (HSE)

The HSE is the national independent regulator for health and safety in the workplace. This includes public and private healthcare services. The HSE was created by the Health & Safety at Work Act 1974.

The HSE's role is to:
- enforce health and safety law in the workplace by ensuring health and safety standards and regulations are followed
- inspect health and care workplaces following health and safety incidents of a non-clinical nature
- provide advice on health and safety in the workplace
- improve health and safety in workplaces.

The HSE has the right to enter premises to carry out investigations of incidents and accidents, and to check on safety compliance. If there has been an accident it might, for example, collect samples, take photographs and ask questions about safety procedures and risk control as part of the investigation.

Following an investigation, the HSE may give advice on how to minimise risk in future and issue instructions that must be carried out by law. It may also issue 'improvement' and 'prohibition' notices which would detail action that must be taken and the timescale.

Health and safety

Read the following questions. Do you know the answers to these already? What are they?
1 The health and safety concerns in healthcare settings are different from those in other industries or organisations. List three examples of the special needs in healthcare settings.
2 Why are there extra risks for fire evacuations in some healthcare settings?
3 Consider the health and safety policies in your placement organisation. Choose three examples and explain how each addresses risks in your workplace.

Then watch this video on YouTube about health and safety in healthcare and compare your answers: **www.youtube.com/watch?v=nqf08O7WS-4**

The table shows the main health and safety legislation that applies to healthcare services. In the event of a serious incident or accident, the HSE investigation would involve checking evidence that the relevant legislation was being followed by the care service.

Regulations	What they mean for care settings
Manual Handling Operations Regulations 2002 **Lifting Operations and Lifting Equipment Regulations (LOLER) 1998**	These regulations relate to ensuring staff are trained in moving and handling activities, including lifting, lowering, pushing, pulling and carrying, so that they are carried out safely. This would include using moving and handling equipment such as hoists or slide boards to assist with transferring individuals in care settings in and out of bed, for example. See A3.1, page 52 for details of the Manual Handling Operations Regulations.
Reporting of Injuries, Diseases and Dangerous Occurrences Regulations (RIDDOR) 2013	See A3.1, page 50.
Management of Health and Safety at Work Regulations 1999	**Risk assessments** (see A3.2) have to be carried out and **control measures** put in place. Care settings must appoint a manager of health safety and security. See A3.1, page 48.
Food Safety (General Food Hygiene) Regulations 1995	Requires care settings to identify food safety hazards and put procedures in place to ensure the safe storage, preparation and serving of food.
Control of Substances Hazardous to Health Regulations (COSHH) 2012	See A3.1, page 49.

Key terms

Risk assessment: the process of evaluating the likelihood of a hazard causing harm.

Control measures: actions that can be taken to reduce the risks posed by a hazard or to remove the hazard altogether.

General Dental Council (GDC)

The GDC is the UK statutory independent regulator for dental care professionals. The GDC was created in 1956 with the role of setting and maintaining standards of dental care practice and so protecting people from unqualified dental practitioners.

The GDC maintains a register of qualified dentists and other dental professionals such as dental nurses and hygienists.

The GDC ensures the quality of dental education and training. It sets the standards of training required for students, for continuing professional development (CPD) and for providers of dental education and training. It monitors whether dental professionals have completed the minimum CPD required to maintain their registration. This ensures knowledge and skills are kept up to date and that practitioners know how to meet and maintain high professional standards.

The GDC website provides information for the general public including guidance and advice about topics such as teeth whitening, home aligners and braces.

To protect individuals' safety and maintain public confidence in dental services, the GDC also provides information about how to raise a serious concern about the ability, health or behaviour of a dental professional. The GDC will investigate complaints regarding dental professionals' fitness to practice, such as:

▶ serious or repeated mistakes in patient care
▶ failure to respond reasonably to a patient's needs, including referring for further investigations where necessary
▶ violence, discrimination, serious breaches of confidentiality and other inappropriate behaviour.

Nursing and Midwifery Council (NMC)

The NMC is the professional regulator of nurses and midwives in the UK and nursing associates in England. Anyone practising as a registered nurse or midwife or a nursing associate in England has to be registered with the NMC.

The registration has to be revalidated every three years to demonstrate that skills and knowledge are kept up to date and that the practitioner is maintaining safe and effective practice. To revalidate, some of the evidence that is required includes at least 35 hours of CPD and five written reflective accounts.

The NMC establishes the expectation that registered professionals will uphold the standards and behaviours set out in the NMC code.

Research

Research

Use this link to find the NMC code of professional standards of practice and behaviour for nurses, midwives and nursing associates: **www.nmc.org. uk/globalassets/sitedocuments/nmc-publications/ nmc-code.pdf**

Use information from the NMC code to make notes about the key aspects of each of the four standards. The standards are:
▶ Prioritise people.
▶ Practise effectively.
▶ Preserve safety.
▶ Promote professionalism and trust.

The NMC sets the education standards professionals must achieve to practise in the UK, it promotes self-reflection and evaluation of practice to improve services, and it encourages lifelong learning of professionals. It supports professionals to have the knowledge and skills to deliver consistent, quality care that keeps people safe, for example, 'Caring with Confidence: The Code in Action' (**www.nmc.org.uk/ standards/code/code-in-action/person-centred-care/**). This gives a series of animated examples of how to follow the standards when providing care.

The NMC can investigate reported incidents and take action ranging from providing additional training, allowing time off work, suspension or deregistration, depending on the seriousness of the incident. The NMC website gives examples of different situations, such as theft of medication or concerns about clinical competence, with explanations of how they were investigated and resolved.

Health and Care Professions Council (HCPC)

This organisation regulates 15 health-related professionals including paramedics, physiotherapists, dieticians, occupational therapists, radiographers, **prosthetists**, **orthotists** and speech and language therapists.

Key terms

Prosthetist: specialist in prosthetics, which are artificial replacements for a missing limb such as a leg, foot, hand or arm.

Orthotist: someone who makes splints or braces for weakened limbs for patients who require support due to an accident, injury or disease.

This organisation sets standards for professionals' education, training and practice, providing information about how to ensure training programmes meet the standards required by the HCPC. Some examples of the standards training programmes must meet include:
▶ practice-based learning must be integral to the programme
▶ the course must be relevant to current practice
▶ the delivery of the programme must support and develop evidence-based practice.

For in-depth details of the standards visit: **www.hcpc-uk.org/standards/standards-relevant-to-education-and-training/set/**

The HCPC registers qualified professionals who meet the required standards. It publishes **standards of proficiency** for each of the 15 specialisms, which all registrants must meet in order to become registered and to remain on the register.

The HCPC can take action if professionals on the register do not meet the required standards or if there are concerns about a professional's conduct, such as:
▶ bringing the profession into disrepute, e.g. inappropriate comments on social media
▶ failure to maintain adequate records.

The HCPC website has a series of case studies that demonstrate the action that can be taken when professional standards are not met.

Ofsted

This government organisation inspects and regulates social care services that care for children and young people. It has responsibility for regulating children's homes under the Child Standards Act (CSA) 2000 where regulated activities take place, for example, providing personal care. These organisations must register with the CQC.

Ofsted is also responsible for inspecting any services providing education and skills training for learners of all ages.

Following an inspection, the setting is given one of the following ratings: 'Outstanding', 'Good', 'Requires improvement' or 'Inadequate'. The inspection report will identify good practice that the inspectors observed and also indicate what needs to be improved. These areas for improvement will be checked again at the next inspection with the expectation that the issues will have been dealt with and improvements made. Ofsted will put failing settings, rated 'Inadequate', into 'Special measures', which means they will be re-inspected and checked to monitor progress and improvements to the aspects of service that have been identified as unsatisfactory.

Information Commissioners Office (ICO)

The ICO is an independent body whose role is to uphold and promote information rights in the public interest, encouraging transparency in terms of data usage and data privacy for individuals.

The ICO provides guidance for maintaining data protection in care settings and explanations of data protection legislation, such as GDPR regulations. Its website has 'At a glance' summaries, for example, data protection involving children, and checklists organisations can use to review their data protection policies and procedures.

The ICO carries out audits and advisory visits across health organisations in relation to personal data. It then produces reports indicating areas of concern, good practice and recommendations for future practice. To see an example of a report on NHS Trusts, visit: **https://ico.org.uk/media/action-weve-taken/audits-and-advisory-visits/2618960/health-sector-outcomes-report.pdf**

Practice points

Do you know which regulatory body is responsible for your placement organisation? If not, find out.

Using the regulatory body's website and any information you are given from your placement, find:
▶ the standards set for practitioners
▶ what the requirements are to become a registered practitioner
▶ what action could be taken if a practitioner does not meet the standards.

Describe the benefits of a regulatory body for your placement organisation.

Test yourself

1 a State one benefit of regulatory inspections for individuals using a service.
  b State another benefit of regulatory inspections in terms of public trust.
2 Figure 8.2 shows nurses being trained to use equipment to lift a patient from a hospital bed.
  a Which piece of legislation requires that this training should take place?
  b Which regulatory body would investigate a care setting if a serious accident occurred when lifting a patient?

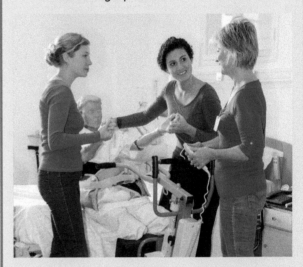

▲ Figure 8.2 Nurses learning to use equipment for lifting a patient from a hospital bed

3 Give four examples of how the Information Commissioners Office (ICO) provides support for care settings when handling information.

A8.4 How the stages of human development impact on physical and mental function and the support provided in relation to person-centred care

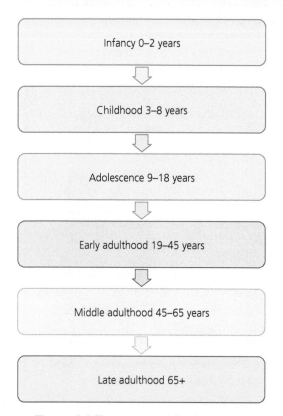

Infancy 0–2 years

⬇

Childhood 3–8 years

⬇

Adolescence 9–18 years

⬇

Early adulthood 19–45 years

⬇

Middle adulthood 45–65 years

⬇

Late adulthood 65+

▲ Figure 8.3 Key stages of the human lifespan

Development happens throughout life – it does not stop when you reach adulthood (Figure 8.3). There is a generally accepted pattern of development known as 'norms' and while not everyone achieves these norms at the same time, they will do so at their own pace; however, the general progression through the stages is similar.

Most growth and development occur during infancy, childhood and adolescence; an individual's skills and abilities become more sophisticated and complex as they progress towards adulthood. But learning and development continue throughout every life stage.

Transitions and significant life events occur across the life stages. Transitions mean changes and are a natural part of maturing through life. Some are expected or planned, such as starting school, while others are unexpected, such as illness.

Each life stage of human development

Birth and infancy 0 to 2 years

A baby relies totally on their carers to provide support with hydration, nutrition and personal care needs. A possible significant transition is moving from being home all day to starting at nursery, which means leaving the primary carer for the first time and may cause separation anxiety.

Care needs in infancy:
▶ food, clothing, shelter
▶ love, safety, a carer they can trust
▶ activity and sleep
▶ immunisations, protection from injury and illness
▶ stimulation to learn new skills.

Early childhood 3 to 8 years

There is an impact on physical and mental function, for example, a child may well need support with self-esteem and independence when starting primary school. Other transitions requiring physical and mental support may include the birth of a sibling or moving house, for example.

High self-esteem	Low self-esteem
Motivated to do something because you have often been successful	Lacking motivation because when you have tried new things before, you often did not do very well
Confident in social situations because you usually get on well with people	Lacking confidence, especially when meeting new people; new people make you feel anxious as you fear you will have nothing to say
Generally happy with your life	Unhappy a lot of the time
Enough self-confidence to cope with new challenges and to view them positively	Often find life difficult and do not enjoy new challenges as you are afraid of failure

Care needs in early childhood:
▶ health – immunisations, personal hygiene, nutrition and balanced diet
▶ exercise
▶ rest and sleep
▶ opportunities to play and learn
▶ opportunities to develop social skills.

Adolescence 9 to 18 years

Children and adolescents will need support with a wide range of expected and unexpected transitions, such as:

▶ transferring to secondary school
▶ taking exams
▶ puberty
▶ navigating learning about sex and relationships
▶ driving test
▶ further education and/or going to university
▶ leaving home
▶ first job.

Adolescents who feel confident, who accept they have strengths and weaknesses and who feel loved and wanted, tend not to undervalue themselves and usually have higher self-esteem.

Possible care needs for adolescents:

▶ health – problems relating to menstruation, skin problems such as acne or issues such as eating disorders and self-harm, drugs and alcohol abuse
▶ social and emotional needs – relating to relationships, feelings and the physical changes of adolescence or peer pressure and exam stress.

Early adulthood 19 to 45 years

At this time there may be a need for support with general health and wellbeing as this is a life stage that can present many demands, such as changing jobs, promotion or unemployment, causing stress and upheaval. Getting married, having children and going through the menopause are other stages. Divorce and family break-up may occur during this life stage, resulting in physical and mental support needs.

Possible care needs in early adulthood:

▶ pregnancy/contraception/fertility
▶ emotional needs – relating to relationships, work, personal social problems
▶ possible injury such as broken bones
▶ drug and alcohol problems
▶ dietary intolerances, e.g. coeliac disease, IBS
▶ unexpected illnesses or accidents affecting physical or mental health.

Middle adulthood 46 to 65 years

Needs at this life stage could include, for example, support with diagnosis and treatment of conditions and possible loss of parents. Retirement may be a positive or negative transition depending on the physical and mental health of the individual.

Possible care needs in middle adulthood:

▶ menopause (a woman's ovaries stop producing eggs) may cause symptoms such as hot flushes, night sweats, mood swings
▶ coping with stress due to work, redundancy, unemployment, family responsibilities
▶ emotional needs due to, for example, relationship breakdowns or family responsibilities, or bereavement
▶ illness may develop – Type 2 diabetes, heart disease, arthritis, cancer.

Part of the body affected	Ageing effects
Eyesight	Cataracts and glaucoma may develop, if untreated may cause blindness
Hair	Starts to thin, growth slows, men may go bald. Hair turns grey or white
Hearing	Can deteriorate, losing quiet and high-pitched sounds, and a hearing aid may become necessary
Heart	Heart becomes less efficient; blood pressure may increase Blood vessels become less elastic and this can lead to strokes, heart attacks, etc.
Lungs and respiratory system	Lungs become less elastic and the respiratory muscles weaken. Less able to take exercise due to reduced lung function Need to be vaccinated against flu and pneumonia as more susceptible to developing these
Reproductive system	Menopause means the end of menstruation. This may cause unpleasant side effects such as hot flushes and disturbed sleep
Skeleton and muscles	Shrink in height, bone mass reduces, women in particular can develop osteoporosis. This increases the risk of fractures. Knee and hip joints can cause mobility problems. Muscles become less flexible and balance can be affected
Skin	Loss of elasticity, wrinkles develop
Urinary system	Kidneys become less efficient at filtering waste products; may need to pass urine more frequently

Later adulthood 65 years onwards

The effects of aging (outlined in the previous table) may begin to have an impact.

Care needs due to illness, for example, support with hydration, nutrition, personal and mobility care, may become necessary.

A range of major transitions occurs at this life stage – some may be welcomed, but others may not be wanted or expected. Freedom from work may bring time for hobbies and travel. However, downsizing to a smaller house, moving into a retirement home, bereavement, family illness or disability are all life events that may result in the need for mental health or physical health support.

Care needs in late adulthood:

▶ **chronic** health problems may develop, such as heart disease, arthritis, **osteoporosis**, Alzheimer's disease, cancer

▶ sensory problems – vision and hearing may start to decline

▶ loss of mobility – needing care and support in the home

▶ emotional needs as a result of social isolation due to loneliness or feeling they are a nuisance or burden for their family to look after.

Key terms

Chronic: an illness or condition that lasts longer than three months and is ongoing. It can be controlled but not cured.

Osteoporosis: causes a loss of bone density which weakens them and as a result they fracture easily.

Person-centred care means practitioners working together with an individual to plan their care and support to meet their unique needs at their particular stage in life. This cuts down the risk of inappropriate care or harmful treatment and neglect. The individual is put at the centre, able to choose and control how they want their care and support to be (Figure 8.4).

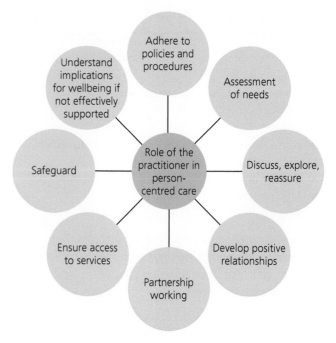

▲ Figure 8.4 The role of the practitioner in person-centred care

Active participation describes a way of person-centred working that makes sure an individual can take part in the activities and relationships of everyday life as independently as possible. They are an active partner in their own care and support, which should be provided with the person's best interests in mind.

Reflect

Make a list of the transitions and life events that you have experienced.

Using your list, describe some short- and long-term impacts you experienced as a result of three of these transitions.

A8.5 The key values of the healthcare sector when providing care and support

NHS core values (from NHS constitution)

The NHS core values were developed by patients, the public and staff. They consist of six statements that all staff, whether consultants, nurses, physiotherapists, paramedics, gardeners, porters or administrators, are expected to demonstrate in their work with patients at all levels in the NHS. They form part of the NHS constitution.

Compassion

This means providing care that demonstrates kindness, empathy, respect and consideration for the individual receiving treatment or using health services. It means being able to put yourself in the patient's shoes and show understanding.

Improving lives

This involves finding treatments and aids that help individuals have a healthier and better life. It also includes the personalisation agenda (see section A8.6, page 128) where individuals and communities are helped to take responsibility for living healthier lives.

Respect and dignity

It is important to respect an individual's views, opinions and choices to show that they matter, that they are valued as an individual. They should never be treated in a harmful or degrading way, for example, curtains round a hospital bed or hospital gowns should always be arranged to preserve someone's dignity and to not cause any embarrassment.

Commitment to quality of care

The NHS carries out clinical audits to review standards of care and implements changes where needed. Healthcare staff have to be revalidated every few years (see page 121); this demonstrates that their knowledge and skills are kept up to date. Feedback from patients and their families is used to identify areas where improvements are required.

Working together for patients

This value means that staff in all parts of the NHS work together to support the care of individuals using health services. Good communication between different care services to provide person-centred care is essential to provide 'joined-up' care that meets individual needs.

Everyone counts

No one should be discriminated against on any grounds of prejudice, including their age, ethnicity or gender, as per the Equality Act 2010 (see page 2). Treatment should be provided based on clinical need, not on prioritising one group of individuals over another, such as older people, and everyone should be valued equally.

6 principles produced by the People and Communities Board

The **People and Communities Board (PCB)** is the NHS England organisation that was commissioned to promote person-centred care between 2015 and 2017. The board developed six principles for engaging people and communities in this:

1 Care and support are person-centred (being personalised, coordinated and empowering). For example, if someone is very unfit and takes no exercise, the local practice nurse may give the individual a voucher for use at the local swimming pool. This may encourage them to take action to improve their poor level of fitness.
2 Services are created in partnership with citizens and communities so that they are relevant to local needs.
3 The focus is on equality and narrowing inequalities in the community.
4 Carers are identified, supported and involved in delivering care.
5 Voluntary, community and social enterprise and housing sectors are involved as key partners and enablers, focusing on enabling individuals to take an active part in their own care.
6 Volunteering and social action are recognised as key enablers to a healthier future. An NHS report published in September 2020, 'Rolling out **social prescribing**: Understanding the experience of the voluntary, community and social enterprise sector', describes successful projects and identifies areas for improvement.

> ### Key term
>
> ***Social prescribing:*** when individuals are referred to support and help from the community in order to improve their health and wellbeing. Sometimes referred to as 'community referral', it involves a range of local, non-clinical services. Examples include local support groups where meeting people with the same problems provides peer support; local activity groups such as for walking, knitting, swimming to improve mental health and general health and wellbeing. (See Chapter A9 for more on promoting health and wellbeing via signposting.)

A8.6 The purpose of the Personalisation Agenda 2012 and the importance of using holistic approaches in order to place individuals, their carers and significant others at the centre of their care and support

Purpose of the Personalisation Agenda 2012

This Agenda is designed to put the individual first in the process of planning, developing and providing care. Under this, individuals should be able to access support tailored to their individual needs and desires when treated for long-term illnesses and conditions.

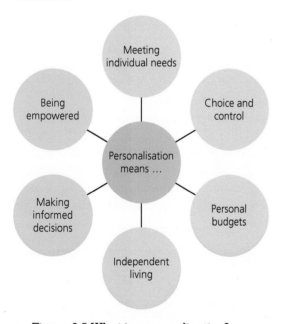

▲ Figure 8.5 What is personalisation?

Traditionally, care has been provided using a 'service-led' approach. Individuals were treated by services available rather than having care tailored to their individual needs, which was certainly not designed for giving them choice and control.

Person-centred care ensures the individual is involved in decision-making by discussing their care needs and then giving them, for example, information about different options that will meet their needs. The individual can then choose care that they prefer. This is enabling and empowering, ensuring the individual is at the centre of their care and has choice and control (Figure 8.5).

The introduction of personal budgets supports person-centred care as it is an amount of money the individual is awarded by the local authority to spend on the help they need. This helps them to achieve what is important to them and supports their choice and control. The emphasis is on individuals being able to choose the services they want rather than having a fixed range of standard services, a 'one size fits all' approach, which may not meet their needs as successfully.

Holistic approaches

Using a holistic approach is taking account of the whole person and their life, not just the part that needs treatment or care, for example, mobility difficulties. It takes everything into account, from their social situation and emotional feelings to culture and beliefs, background and family situation, in order to inform and determine the best ways to meet their needs.

Person-centred planning (PCP)

This holistic approach to planning places the person at the centre of their care and enables them to have a package of care put in place to support them, as an individual, to live as independently as possible.

Steps to person-centred planning are:
▶ the person is at the centre of the planning process, which is based on their individual preferences and identified needs
▶ family and friends can be partners in the process
▶ the plan will identify what is important to the person, both in the present and in the future, helping them to make informed choices
▶ the plan helps the person to achieve what they wish for individually and in the community, e.g. continue to work with adjustments to accommodate their needs because of a physical disability
▶ the plan is reviewed and adapted over time as required to continue to meet the person's changing care needs.

Person-centred care (PCC)

Read the case study on Amir on page 129 which gives an example of a person-centred care plan and person-centred planning in practice. Then answer the question.

Case study

Person-centred care for Amir

Amir is 89 years old; he lives on his own. Amir is thinking of going to live in a care home because his mobility is not what it was. He doesn't really want to go into a care home but he finds it very difficult to manage the stairs in his house and struggles with food shopping because he cannot walk very far. His daughter, who is his only child, works full time and lives too far away to help him regularly. His daughter is worried about the future for Amir and has contacted social services to discuss the situation.

Sundip, a social worker, arranges to visit Amir to have a chat about his possible move. Sundip uses a person-centred approach, ensuring that Amir is supported to make his choices and is involved and in control of his care.

As Amir's key worker, after their chat, Sundip plans the following care package:

▷ An occupational therapist to visit Amir's house to carry out a risk assessment and to see if any adaptations are needed to help with his mobility.
▷ A walking frame to be purchased and delivered as soon as possible, to help Amir keep his independence.
▷ Help with going shopping to be available from the following week, so Amir will be able to continue shopping himself.
▷ A week's stay is booked, at the end of the month, at a residential home Amir is interested in so that he can try it out and see if he likes it. This is to help inform his choice of whether to stay at home or move into residential care.
▷ The situation is to be reviewed by Amir and Sundip when Amir returns home from his care home stay.

Explain how Sundip has put Amir at the centre of his care plan and supported his choice, control, independence, needs and preferences to deliver person-centred care.

Hierarchy of the individual's needs (Maslow's hierarchy of needs theory)

Psychologist Abraham Maslow used a **humanistic** approach, which is person-centred, focused on the individual and their needs and development throughout life. His theory created a **hierarchy** of human needs, which is a theory of human motivation (Figure 8.6).

An individual's basic, physiological needs that must be met in order to survive, such as food, water and shelter, are shown at the bottom of the pyramid. Maslow's theory states that only when those basic physical needs have been met will a person have the motivation and capacity to progress to the next level of the pyramid.

When safety and security followed by emotional needs are met, a person will have the motivation to progress to trying to fulfil the higher-order needs for their personal development and achievement. Only then will a person 'self-actualise', that is, become the person they want to be.

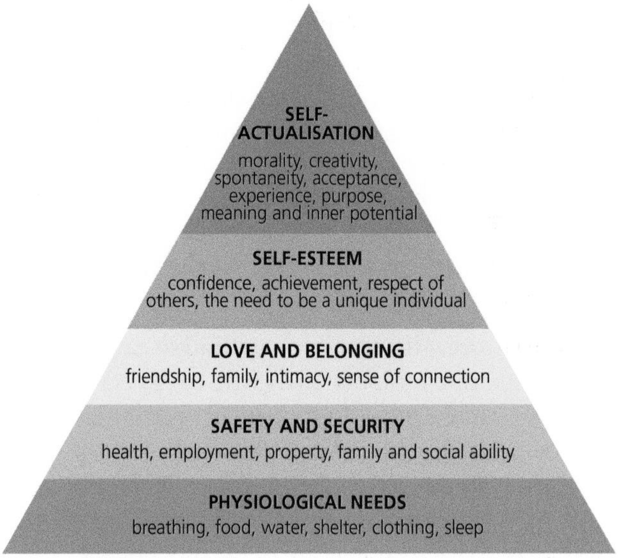

SELF-ACTUALISATION
morality, creativity, spontaneity, acceptance, experience, purpose, meaning and inner potential

SELF-ESTEEM
confidence, achievement, respect of others, the need to be a unique individual

LOVE AND BELONGING
friendship, family, intimacy, sense of connection

SAFETY AND SECURITY
health, employment, property, family and social ability

PHYSIOLOGICAL NEEDS
breathing, food, water, shelter, clothing, sleep

▲ Figure 8.6 Maslow's hierarchy of needs

Key term

Hierarchy: an arrangement of things in order of importance.

Case study

Maslow's theory into practice: Joan

Joan, who is aged 85, is facing a move into residential care. Joan knows she is no longer able to fully care for herself without help because of her arthritis. She knows that it would make sense to move into a care home, but she has mixed feelings about a possible move. She is worried about losing control over her life and losing all her independence as well as the fact that moving house is one of the most stressful times in life.

Following Maslow's hierarchy of needs, staff at the residential home should first ensure that Joan's basic needs are met, catering for her food preferences and giving her a comfortable, warm room with her own belongings to arrange as she wishes. This will give her a sense of control and empowerment.

However, Joan should also be welcomed and helped to meet other residents so that she feels a sense of acceptance and belonging developing. This will help Joan to feel respected and valued as a resident, and she will be more likely to be mentally, emotionally and physically healthy and comfortable in the new environment as her care needs are being met.

Can you think of any other practical things that the residential home staff could do or provide to help meet more of Joan's higher-level needs?

Advanced care planning (for example, end of life care)

End of life care, also known as **palliative care**, is personalised care for individuals who have been given a terminal diagnosis or are towards the end of their life. Specialist teams of professionals such as community nurses and sometimes also volunteers support the person to live as well as possible until they die. Alongside taking care of the individual's physical needs, a holistic approach is used to help with their emotional, spiritual and social needs. The team support carers, family members and close friends of the individual. This would also include any religious or spiritual figures such as an imam, priest or chaplain.

End of life care can be provided by **hospices**, which are specialist care settings that can provide a range of services to support individuals at this stage of life. Some hospice care is provided by charitable organisations such as Marie Curie Cancer Care and Sue Ryder services.

Do Not Resuscitate directive (DNR)

DNR stands for 'do not resuscitate' and means that the person has requested that they should be allowed a natural death without any attempt at CPR (cardiopulmonary resuscitation) if their heart stops beating. The person will usually have ensured that others – medical staff, social worker, family members – are aware of the DNR.

The importance of using holistic approaches

A holistic approach means looking at all the different needs of a patient. These include their medical condition and treatments, and whether they live alone or have any family or friends to look after them or become involved in their care if necessary. The approach considers how well the person understands their condition or illness and how they feel about it – are they feeling upset or depressed or feeling positive, for example.

Ensuring that any care provided is in the individual's best interest

'Best interest' relates to taking into account an individual's circumstances, needs and preferences before a decision or choice is made. Before decisions about care are determined, individuals should be given full and accurate information in a format they can understand. The pros and cons of each option will assist them to actively participate in the decision-making and will facilitate reaching an informed decision.

If an individual is assessed as lacking capacity, the Mental Capacity Act 2005 provides five key principles to follow for 'best interests' decision-making:
1. A presumption of capacity.
2. Individuals being supported to make their own decisions.
3. Unwise decisions.
4. Best interests.
5. The less restrictive option.

See sections A8.1 and A8.8 for details.

Complying with autonomous practice

Care planning and person-centred care must follow best practice guidelines and be based on professional **ethics** and practitioner expertise.

Practitioners such as community nurses and social workers should support individuals in making autonomous decisions. However, the decisions must be made so that people receive appropriate, safe and effective care.

All decisions must be based within the practitioner's scope of practice, that is, within their level of expertise, and they have a duty of care to manage risks to ensure the health, wellbeing and safety of the individuals in their care.

> ### Key terms
>
> *Ethics:* concerned with what is morally right or wrong.
>
> *Autonomous:* able to act independently, having control; not being forced to do something.

Encouraging engagement with healthcare professionals

Regular contact with healthcare professionals is important for monitoring an individual's health and wellbeing. Access to relevant services will not only promote individuals' health but will also develop their self-reliance and reduce their dependency on services they may have required had their needs not been met. Involving people in their own health is an effective way of promoting health and wellbeing. See also 'Social prescribing' on page 127 and Figure 8.4, 'The role of the practitioner in person-centred care' on page 126.

> ### Test yourself
>
> 1 Describe what personalisation of care means.
> 2 Describe three features of person-centred planning.
> 3 List the five types of needs identified by Maslow. Give an example of how three of the needs could be met for a care home resident or a hospital patient.

A8.7 A range of verbal and nonverbal communication techniques, potential communication barriers and how to overcome them to support an individual's condition

An important aspect of a person-centred approach to care is to recognise that all individuals have their own particular way of communicating. Eye contact,

body language and spoken language skills (where applicable) can all impact how someone communicates.

Range of communication techniques

Verbal (for example, spoken word and sound)

This includes:
- face-to-face conversations
- phone calls
- asking questions
- recorded messages
- delivering a training session or presentation
- interviewing someone.

You will probably be familiar with these methods and they are relatively self-explanatory: they involve using spoken words to communicate. However, there is more to communication than this and many of these methods are not a good option (or an option at all) for certain individuals.

Nonverbal

This includes:
- gestures
- facial expression – interest, reassurance, agreement
- body language – positive/open, no crossed arms.

Some special methods used by individuals with sensory impairments are:
- Makaton – a simplified form of sign language where gestures are used alongside symbols/pictures and speech
- British Sign Language – using hand signs, facial expressions and gestures
- **PECS – picture exchange communication system**, a system that uses pictures that aid communication. The individual points to the picture that shows what they need (Figure 8.7)
- **Braille** – involves touching a series of raised dots and symbols that represent letters, punctuation and numbers; used by individuals who have visual impairments.

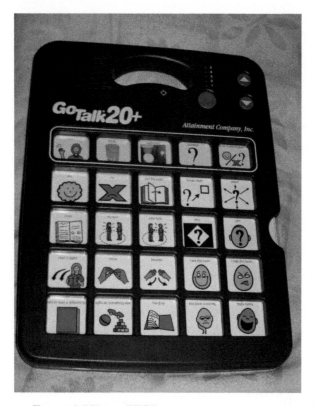

▲ Figure 8.7 Using PECS picture communication cards

Active listening is a communication technique that a care practitioner will employ to demonstrate an interest in, and responsiveness to, what a person is saying. It promotes good practice by showing respect and building trust with individuals.

Active listening skills include:
▶ open, relaxed posture
▶ eye contact – looking interested
▶ nodding agreement
▶ showing empathy, reflecting feelings
▶ clarifying.

Barriers to communication

To keep the person at the centre of their care, good communication with them is necessary. An individual's level of communication skills and how attentive they are, how well they can hear and see what is happening, and whether they are interested or motivated enough to make themselves understood can all be potential negative influences on communication.

Communication barriers can be a significant impediment to an individual receiving the care or treatment they need. If appropriate alternative methods of communication are not available to meet the individual's communication needs, they may not be able to communicate well enough to fully use the services available.

Sensory disorder

Barriers to communication for visually impaired individuals could include:
▶ information not available in different formats, e.g. Braille, large print.

Potential barriers for deaf and hearing impaired people:
▶ **hearing loop** not available in the building (Figure 8.8)
▶ no staff available who have been trained in sign language/Makaton so the quality of communication is impaired
▶ special methods such as **PECS** are not available
▶ the individual can't lipread and so has difficulties understanding what is being said in a conversation.

Speech impairments:
▶ an alternative method is not available, e.g. writing responses
▶ stroke/dementia patients may not be physically able to speak.

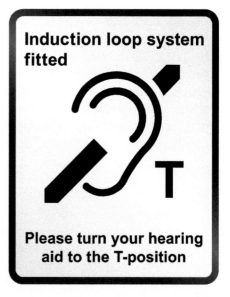

▲ Figure 8.8 Adapting the environment to overcome barriers to communication – hearing loop

Key terms

Hearing loop: a special type of sound system to assist people with hearing aids. The hearing loop provides a magnetic wireless signal that is picked up by the hearing aid and can greatly improve the quality of sound while reducing background noise.

PECS: stands for 'picture exchange communication system'; developed for use with children who have autism, it helps them learn to start communicating by exchanging a picture for the item they want.

Mental health condition

▶ Someone with dementia may not be able to answer questions, they may not remember what has happened or where they are.

▶ An individual with a learning disability may not have the ability or vocabulary to communicate effectively and so it can sometimes be difficult for them to explain how they are feeling and for others to establish what the problem is.

▶ In these situations, it is still important to give the patient opportunities to communicate, rather than assuming, and to do what we can to facilitate it.

Language barriers

Not everyone speaks or understands English well or at all, and this can pose significant challenges when discussing health and medical care and treatment with them. This barrier can take the form of:

▶ information not available in different languages

▶ no interpreter or 'language line' (telephone translation service) available, so staff can't understand and the patient can't explain their symptoms

▶ someone may have a very strong accent or use dialect that is difficult to understand for those not used to it

▶ practitioners can find themselves using technical terminology or medical jargon only they understand.

Time pressures

Some individuals will take longer than others to describe their symptoms or problems. Some may be lonely and just want to talk with someone and so are more demanding in terms of time. Unfortunately, with an appointment system, practitioners may have constraints limiting how long they can spend with each individual; they may keep others waiting if they spend too long with someone.

Noisy environment

It can be distracting if there is a lot of background noise when trying to have an important conversation and it can cause people to miss important information because they can't hear the person talking properly. It can be especially problematic when trying to communicate with, for example, someone with autism or who is impaired hearing. Some individuals with autism have sensory sensitivity and cannot ignore or block out background noise. Finding somewhere quiet and private can be difficult in care settings. However, many will have noise-cancelling headphones for certain situations.

Positioning of the individual from the healthcare professional (for example, proximity)

Free spaces for meetings may be too small so individuals invade each other's personal space or cannot sit facing each other in the position they would like. Often in offices a large desk is situated between those attending a meeting and so it becomes rather formal, which may not be appropriate for what a patient and a healthcare professional are going to discuss. It is also better for effective communication if people are at the same level as the practitioner, speaking with them to reduce the risk of feeling someone is 'talking down' to them. This is particularly important when speaking with children.

Tension or conflict

There may be tension because the individual is angry or upset following an argument, circumstances in their life or even their health, and this carries through into their responses to a practitioner asking questions. A young adult may be uncooperative if they feel they are being patronised or not taken seriously, or someone may not understand what is being said but not want to admit it. An individual may be dissatisfied with how long they have had to wait or with the standard of treatment they have received.

Overcoming barriers to communication

General ways of overcoming barriers to communication include:

▶ actively listen to the individual about their communication needs/preferences – show that they are valued

▶ active involvement from the individual – ask them how/when/where and in which way they are communicated with to meet their needs

▶ access to information that is understandable to the particular individual – correct language, avoiding specialist terminology

▶ offer a choice of communication aids or supports that match the needs and preferences of the individual

▶ offer the individual access to a range of support options and choices.

It is important that health and social care practitioners work to find a way to communicate despite difficulties, and that they do not create communication barriers themselves. They should ensure that they use their communication skills effectively to avoid creating barriers to care. The list above of general principles and the table below show some specific ways they can do this.

	Ways of communicating effectively
Using vocabulary that can be understood by all	Avoid jargon
	Explain any specialist terminology
	Use age-appropriate vocabulary
	Use simplified language, especially with, for example, young children, individuals with learning disabilities or patients with dementia
	Use interpreters or translators
Use communication that is appropriate to the individual	Use positive body language, such as nodding agreement and making eye contact
	Avoid sarcasm and do not talk down to the person
	Be polite
	Make the service user feel they are being taken seriously
	Be patient, especially when listening to repetition
	Do not ignore the person's views or beliefs just because they are different from yours
Listen to individuals' needs	Use active listening by demonstrating interest in response to what a person is saying, using body language to show a positive reaction
	Ask the person rather than assuming you know what they want, need or prefer
	Concentrate on what the person is saying – this can encourage them to communicate their needs
Adapt communication to meet individuals' needs or the situation	Emphasise important words
	Slow the pace of conversation if necessary
	Increase the volume of your speaking voice but do not shout
	Use repetition where appropriate
	Use gestures or flash cards/pictures if appropriate
	Make use of aids to communication such as a hearing loop system
	Use specialist communication methods such as Braille or signing
	Use technological aids, such as **Dynavox** or a **Lightwriter**

A8.8 The application of relevant legislation, including Mental Capacity Act (2005) plus Amendment (2019) and Liberty Protection Safeguards (LPS) on the provision of person-centred care

See also section A8.1.

Mental Capacity Act (2005) plus Amendment (2019), including the five principles

'Capacity' is the ability to make a decision, including understanding information and remembering it for long enough to make a decision, and to be able to communicate it to others.

This Act is in place to provide a legal framework setting out key principles, procedures and safeguards to protect and empower those who are unable to make some of their own decisions. This could include people with learning difficulties, dementia, mental health problems, strokes or head injuries.

The Mental Capacity (Amendment) Act 2019 has five statutory principles:

1 A presumption of capacity – every adult has the right to make their own decisions and must be assumed to have capacity to do so unless it is proved otherwise. So, a care worker must not assume someone cannot make a decision for themselves just because they have a particular condition or disability.

2 Support individuals to make their own decisions – a person must be given all practicable help before anyone treats them as not being able to make their own decisions. This might include presenting information in a different format for those with physical or learning disabilities, for example.

3 Recognise that unwise decisions do not mean lack of capacity – just because an individual makes what might be seen as an unwise decision, they should not be treated as lacking the capacity to make that decision. People have the right to make what others may regard as an unwise or eccentric decision. Everyone has their own preferences, values and beliefs which may not be the same as those of others – they cannot be treated as lacking capacity for thinking differently.

4 Best interests – action taken or decisions made under the Act on behalf of a person who lacks capacity must be done in their best interests. So, care workers should provide reasons showing the decision they are making is in the individual's best interests. They should try to involve the person, or consider whether the decision could be put off until the person regains capacity.

5 Less restrictive option – anything done for or on behalf of a person who lacks capacity should be the least restrictive of their basic rights and freedoms. A care practitioner must always consider whether a decision can be made in a way that is less restrictive of an individual's freedom. So, while it would be reasonable for a care worker to accompany an individual with learning disabilities who lacks capacity on a visit to the shops or to see friends, it would not be reasonable to lock them in their room to prevent them from going out. This would be an unacceptable deprivation of liberty.

Research

1 Use the link to view a video clip about each of the five 'best interests' decision-making principles: www.scie.org.uk/mca/introduction/mental-capacity-act-2005-at-a-glance#principles
2 In your own words, write an explanation, with examples, of each of the five 'best interests' decision-making principles.

Liberty Protection Safeguards (LPS)

The 2019 Amendment to the Mental Capacity Act replaces the Deprivation of Liberty Safeguards (DoLS) with the Liberty Protection Safeguards (LPS). This amendment aims to improve and simplify the process of assessing mental capacity and the care that is required, and to increase the individual's protection against losing their freedom unnecessarily or inappropriate decisions being made for them.

The LPS ensure that individuals are only deprived of their liberty or freedom in extreme situations, in order to protect them and keep them safe. The safeguards would apply when:

▶ the person lacks the capacity to consent to care arrangements
▶ the person has a serious mental disorder
▶ the arrangements are necessary to prevent harm for the individual
▶ the arrangements must be proportionate to the likelihood and severity of harm.

They seek to make the process simpler and more efficient, and to reduce the burden on individuals, their families, carers and local authorities. They also remove the requirement for repeat assessments when moving between healthcare settings, e.g. between hospital and a care home.

Test yourself

1 'A presumption of capacity' is one of the key aspects of the Mental Capacity Act. What is the meaning of 'capacity' here?
2 Describe two situations when the Liberty Protection Safeguards would apply.
3 What is the aim of the Liberty Protection Safeguards?

A8.9 The considerations when providing person-centred care to people with pre-existing conditions or living with illness

Conditions or illnesses

Serious illness (for example, cancer)

The term 'cancer' is a general description of a condition that can affect most parts of the body. Cells in a particular place reproduce uncontrollably to form a growth called a tumour. This can then invade healthy tissue, organs, blood cells or bones. Metastasis is when the cancer spreads from one part of the body to another.

There are many different signs and symptoms of cancer depending on the type. Treatments include surgery, radiotherapy and drug therapy called chemotherapy. The Macmillan cancer support website explains the types of cancer and the treatments available (www.macmillan.org.uk/cancer-information-and-support/cancer-types).

Neurological conditions (for example, dementia)

There are several different types of dementia but all result in memory loss, confusion, disorientation and communication difficulties. The disease usually

135

progresses over a number of years, gradually resulting in a loss of brain function and ability.

Respiratory conditions (for example, chronic obstructive pulmonary disease (COPD))

Respiratory conditions affect breathing, often involving problems with the lungs and airway.

COPD is the name for a collection of lung diseases including chronic bronchitis, emphysema and chronic obstructive airways disease. People with COPD have breathing difficulties due to the narrowing of their airways.

Physical disabilities (for example, a wheelchair user)

An individual may be a wheelchair user for a variety of reasons. They may have been born with a disability or involved in an accident later in life which caused injuries that left them without the use of their legs or with limited mobility. Cerebral palsy and spina bifida are disorders that affect movement, muscle tone and balance. Conditions such as multiple sclerosis and motor neurone disease affect the ability to walk over time. It is important to note that many people use a wheelchair only some of the time.

Considerations

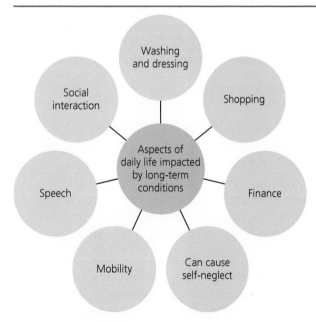

▲ Figure 8.9 Aspects of daily life affected by long-term conditions

Ongoing treatments

Some conditions can be treated with surgery, such as replacing a knee joint or removing a tumour. However, ongoing treatments are usually necessary for most serious conditions.

Treatments	Description
Medications/ drug therapy	Used to treat symptoms or combat the effects of an illness such as pain or to delay the progress of a condition. Medication can take many different forms, such as tablets, medicine, chemotherapy, inhalers. Injections are also used, such as insulin for Type 1 diabetes.
Occupational therapy	An occupational therapist will assess an individual to identify if they are having any difficulties with tasks such as dressing, bathing or shopping. The aim is to help the person maintain independence by providing equipment and adaptations to the home to make tasks easier.
Dietary changes	Advice on a healthy diet may be appropriate for some conditions where this is beneficial, such as arthritic knee joints and COPD, or controlling intake of certain things such as fat, sugar and alcohol. Some diseases may require vitamin or mineral supplements. A healthy diet may reduce the risks of some cancers and heart disease.
Relaxation techniques	These techniques can be used to relieve stress, anxiety or depression, for example, or to help with sleep problems, pain and headaches. All relaxation techniques combine breathing more deeply with relaxing the muscles. Yoga or tai chi are sometimes recommended.
Counselling	Talking therapy allows an individual to talk about their problems and feelings in a safe and supportive environment. The counsellor will listen with empathy and will help an individual to deal with negative thoughts and feelings. Cognitive Behaviour Therapy and psychotherapy approaches may be used.
Complementary therapies	Sometimes referred to as CAMs (complementary and alternative medicines). Covers a range of treatments and medicines, such as acupuncture, homeopathy, chiropractic, herbalism, meditation, colonic irrigation and aromatherapy. The NHS has recommended the use of the Alexander Technique for Parkinson's disease, acupuncture and massage for persistent low back pain.

Overall wellbeing

Often treatments for a serious disease or condition may cause side effects. These can include pain, trouble sleeping, fatigue, vomiting and hair loss, for example. These effects may be temporary but the person may need support from their family or carers, as well as through the health and social services, to get through the effects of their treatment.

For a person with significant mobility issues or who requires a lot of care or assistance at home, going on a trip to a day centre or a day out, for example, gives the individual a break and change of scene. Often third-sector organisations can arrange days out and activity days; this is an opportunity for the person to meet new people and make friends. They can share experiences with other individuals with similar experiences. This type of activity benefits the overall wellbeing of both the individual and the family or carers. The focus here is on enjoyment rather than just coping with daily tasks or treatment.

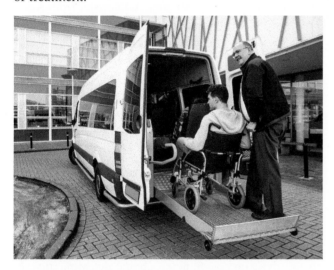

▲ Figure 8.10 Overcoming physical barriers

Someone with COPD, cancer and/or dementia or any other condition should always be encouraged to look after their general health as much as possible. This will make them feel more involved and in control, especially as they may need help with many aspects of daily life (Figure 8.10) which could leave them feeling dependent on others a lot of the time.

Follow the person-centred plan

An **holistic needs assessment** will be carried out to inform the person-centred planning, with the aim of ensuring adequate support is provided for both the carer and the person who has the illness. Often the assessment is completed by a social worker who will meet with the individual and their family or friends to discuss care needs, though it can be done as an online or telephone assessment in some cases.

The assessment would include establishing any help the individual may require with daily living activities such as showering, or whether adaptations, such as handrails, are needed in the home to promote independent living, or if the individual needs help with keeping the home clean. It could include help with transport to visit a family member or to attend a place of worship, for example. All aspects of an individual's physical, social and emotional needs will be taken into account. This person-centred planning will involve a multidisciplinary approach, including community services. As always, the ill person should be as fully involved as possible with the choices and decisions so that they remain at the centre of the care.

Co-morbidity and the impact on the individual and their family

Co-morbidity is the presence of two or more diseases or medical conditions occurring in a patient at the same time. Examples are cancer and dementia, COPD and heart disease. Co-morbidities are usually chronic (long-term) illnesses.

For example, Macmillan Cancer Support provides an advice and guidance booklet for individuals with cancer and dementia, and for carers of individuals with these diseases: **https://cdn.macmillan.org.uk/dfsmed ia/1a6f23537f7f4519bb0cf14c45b2a629/4007-source/mac16831-dementiacarers-e02-p04-20210309-mslowres?_ga=2.232460509.333146070.1627817819-1228785946.1627817819**

This includes details of the care required for dementia and cancer and detailed advice for carers about how to look after themselves as well as the person who is ill. Taking the time to eat well and keep active is encouraged and may help the carer to cope with the stress and demands of the situation. Most charities for serious illnesses have helplines and leaflets with advice for family carers who may be upset, angry or frightened about the illness their family member has developed.

Some charities can provide respite or short breaks care to give the main carer some time away from their caring duties, even just a day off, or they may offer a meeting with someone to talk it over, which can make a huge difference and give fresh perspective, improving their ability to cope.

The Alzheimer's Society has produced a guide for carers: www.alzheimers.org.uk/get-support/help-dementia-care/looking-after-yourself

Support groups led by carers or online support groups consist of individuals who have experienced the demands of caring for someone with a serious illness or condition, so they will understand exactly what a carer is going through. Joining one of these groups will enable a carer or family member to share their experiences, and they will gain advice, guidance and practical help. For example, if a carer has work problems, they can get advice about flexible working or going part-time, or if they are a full-time carer, advice on benefits is available.

Case study

Choose one of the real-life case studies which you can access using the following links:

Coronary heart disease: www.nhs.uk/Conditions/Coronary-heart-disease/Pages/Debbies-story.aspx

Deep brain stimulation treatment for Parkinson's: www.parkinsons.org.uk/sites/default/files/2018-10/B123%20Surgery%20for%20Parkinson%27s_WEB.pdf

Arthritis: www.versusarthritis.org/

Read the case study, then answer the questions.
1   Describe the illness or condition.
2   What are the possible mental health impacts on the person, and on their family and friends, of the illness or condition?
3   Why might the person fail to comply with prescribed treatments?

A8.10 How mental health conditions, dementia and learning disabilities can influence a person's needs in relation to overall care

Increased support requirements

Physical support requirements (for example, care support worker)

Attending regular specialist hospital appointments or doctors' appointments might require support. The individual may not have a car or may not be able to drive due to their condition. Public transport may not be frequent and it may be expensive. The individual may need someone to accompany them if they have a mental health condition. A care support worker may be needed to assist the individual to attend appointments for monitoring or treatment.

Communication support requirements

'Easy read' versions of documents would help the individual to understand more easily. When speaking with an individual with dementia or certain learning disabilities, it helps to speak clearly and slowly, using straightforward vocabulary with no specialist terminology. It is important to give them time to think and respond. At the same time, you should not patronise them, and always let them speak for themselves whenever possible.

In a formal situation an advocate may be needed if the individual has a meeting, for example, with a social worker to produce a person-centred care plan or when applying for disability benefits. A volunteer from Age UK or MIND, for example, or a trusted family member, would be needed to represent a person's best interests.

Reduced ability to self-care

Individuals with dementia (and learning disabilities) sometimes forget to eat or drink, may suffer from dehydration and/or eat an unbalanced diet because they don't realise they are hungry or thirsty. To combat this, memory aids can be stuck on cupboard doors to help the person to find things. It might be necessary for them to have someone to do the shopping for them due to confusion when decision-making. They may forget regular personal care such as showering and brushing teeth. Contacting a dementia charity can be a good idea to get advice on how to make a home 'dementia friendly'.

Increased monitoring requirements

The impacts of health conditions such as dementia vary greatly – each individual requires different types of care and support for their particular needs, whether keeping the house clean, cooking meals or remembering to take medication. People with a learning disability sometimes have poor physical and mental health due to health issues not being recognised or conditions not being noticed. The NHS encourages individuals who are on their GP's learning disability register to have an annual health check – see www.nhs.uk/conditions/learning-disabilities/annual-health-checks/

Behavioural factors

Refusal of treatment

Refusing to acknowledge their illness can lead some individuals to not go to the doctor or seek medical help, preferring to ignore any symptoms or treatment they would benefit from receiving. Alternatively, an individual with a mental health condition may think there is absolutely nothing wrong with them and so refuse any treatment or check-ups.

Behaviour that challenges (for example, violence or aggression)

Sometimes an effect of a learning disability or conditions such as dementia is aggression, especially if the individual is in a situation where they feel distressed, threatened and do not understand what is happening.

Use the link below to hear about Gerald's story from his wife. He has been diagnosed with dementia and is struggling to accept what is happening to him.

Gerald's story: **www.patientvoices.org.uk/ flv/0858pv384.html**

The charity Mind has created a detailed advice guide about how friends and family can learn to cope with someone who is angry and aggressive, and to help defuse the situation. Use the following link: **www.mind.org.uk/information-support/types-of-mental-health-problems/anger/for-friends-and-family/**

Comprehension factors

There is a range of factors that may affect someone's ability to understand a situation where they are in need of care (Figure 8.11). They may not realise that they need care at all.

▶ Anxiety around care can be an issue – if someone has never been in the situation of needing a care package, it can be a very stressful time for them. They may worry that they are losing control of their life and decisions by agreeing to receive support.
▶ Lack of understanding of the care to be provided – this can be a problem for someone with learning disabilities, dementia or any mental health condition, who may not even recognise that they need any special care.
▶ Impaired rationality around the condition or support requirements – sometimes individuals are in denial and cannot, or do not, accept that they have a particular condition.
▶ Some mental health conditions (**dissociative conditions**) can affect a person's sense of who they are, they may have a feeling of being disconnected

from reality and so can't understand or relate to what is going on.
▶ Awareness of possible abuse – this may cause a lack of trust and co-operation. The person will want to be self-reliant and not want to receive any care from others.

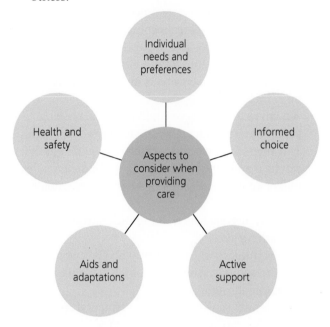

▲ Figure 8.11 Aspects to consider when providing care

A8.11 How to promote independence and self-care and the positive impact on the healthcare sector

How to promote independence and self-care

▶ Individuals should have involvement, choice and control over their self-care, achieved by using a person-centred approach to care planning. For example, organising the replacement of a bath with a shower and fitting 'tap turners' to help grip the taps can enable an individual to independently take care of their personal hygiene.
▶ Individuals should have access to support networks, appropriate information, a range of learning and development opportunities, and should be able to understand the range of options available to them. The individual's key worker should ensure they provide enough information to enable the individual, and their family, to make informed choices about their care and what matters to them.

- Support in risk management and risk taking will maximise independence and choice. Taking planned risks is confidence- and resilience-building and individuals should be encouraged and empowered in this.
- Individuals should be supported to identify their strengths, assess their needs and gain the confidence to self-care. Encouraging independence can only have a positive impact – choosing the type of care is much better for individuals than just being told what care to have and is much more likely to meet their unique needs.
- **Assistive technology** should be made available to support an individual's ability to live independently. This refers to any device or piece of equipment that can help an individual remain independent and less reliant on others. Examples of assistive technology are:
  - basic help such as walking stick or frame
  - bathing aids
  - electronic location devices with GPS which let carers know if someone has left the building
  - automatic lighting
  - 'telecare' sensors that detect temperature, smoke, movement and falls and send a signal via the telephone line to notify a carer.

Research

The Alzheimer's Society explains how assistive technology can help and puts carers' minds at rest, but there are ethical issues around monitoring every move a person makes in their own home.

Read the discussion at the site www.alzheimers.org.uk/about-us/policy-and-influencing/what-we-think/assistive-technology

What do you think?

There is a positive impact on the healthcare sector of promoting independence and self-care:

- Improving self-esteem and independence of the individual – being fully involved in decision-making gives individuals choice and control. They are less likely to be dissatisfied with their care if they have been involved in planning it and they will feel empowered.
- Improved partnership working – it encourages services and practitioners to work together to deliver the care an individual actually needs, not what the professionals think they should have in place.

- Improved efficiency of staff time within the healthcare service – there are likely to be far fewer complaints if the care is planned using a person-centred approach as the care is what the person prefers, wants and needs. This will lead to efficient use of resources and less time and resources wasted on care not wanted or not being appropriate.

Research

1 Use this link to read more detailed information from the NHS about involving people in their own care, including some case studies: www.england.nhs.uk/wp-content/uploads/2017/04/ppp-involving-people-health-care-guidance.pdf

2 Produce an information handout that covers the following:
   - ways of involving people in their own health and care
   - how it improves health and wellbeing
   - how it improves care and quality.

A8.12 The range of terms used in the healthcare sector in relation to death and bereavement, including their meaning

Terms used in relation to death and bereavement

End of life care

This refers to the care provided when the efforts made to successfully treat or control a disease have ceased. This care is provided when death is imminent and usually refers to the last year of life. This might include giving the individual medication or treatment for symptoms – to improve comfort or offer pain relief – rather than to treat the illness. For some people it might include a home assessment by an occupational therapist to inform them about the provision of aids, such as a stair lift, to enable them to stay in their own home until the end.

Palliative care

This is similar to end of life care but relates to symptom management and improving the quality of life for those with a serious illness.

It is personalised care provided by specialist teams of professionals such as GPs, community nurses and sometimes also volunteers. Palliative care supports the person to live as well as possible until they die. Alongside taking care of the dying individual's physical needs, a holistic approach is used, helping with their emotional, spiritual and social needs. The team support carers, family members and close friends of the individual.

Hospice

This is the place or organisation that provides care for people who are dying. Hospice care can be offered at the place of the individual's choice, for example, at home, in a hospice room at a hospital, in a nursing home or at a Marie Curie hospice.

Alongside taking care of the dying person's physical and spiritual needs, hospices support carers, family and friends, both while a person is dying and with the resulting bereavement. Hospices can provide a range of services in addition to pain and symptom control, such as complementary therapies, counselling, respite care, and practical and financial help.

Some hospice care is offered by charitable organisations such as Marie Curie Cancer Care (**www.mariecurie.org. uk/?msclkid=f5bb18ccc14d1269403379cb1adacd7a**) and Sue Ryder services (**www.sueryder.org/how-we-can-help/find-a-local-care-service**).

Expected death

This is the result of acute or gradual deterioration in an individual's health, often due to advanced disease or terminal illness. While the death may have been anticipated and the family may be prepared for it, they are likely to still be upset by the reality and experience feelings of grief.

Sudden or unexpected death

This refers to death without warning, for example, an accident, heart attack or act of violence. Family and close friends may be extremely distressed and shocked in this situation.

Grief

Grief is a response to loss of an important person in your life and is often described as intense sorrow.

The term is used in the context of having lost a person who has died and the feelings attached to this experience.

> See section A8.13 for information about the stages of grief.

Bereavement

This is the term used to describe the sense of loss when someone close passes away. This is a major life event that can affect all aspects of someone's life.

A8.13 The role of healthcare professionals in providing person-centred care for the individual during the active dying phase

Provide support to both the individual and to family/carers

Healthcare professionals should provide information about what the family/carers might be likely to expect during this time, so that they are prepared. The NHS provides extensive guidance and detailed examples of what families need to understand and expect: **www.nhs.uk/conditions/end-of-life-care/changes-in-the-last-hours-and-days/**

Practitioners should take time to be an active listener (see section A8.7). Being available to answer questions and address concerns honestly is a very important part of support required at this stage, as is providing emotional support or advice.

There are many theories that explain the emotional journey and it can be helpful for healthcare professionals to understand the stages of grief, for example, the Kubler-Ross model explained in Figure 8.12.

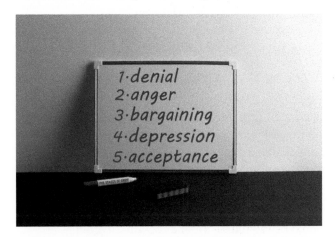

▲ Figure 8.12 The five stages of grief (Kubler-Ross)

- Stage 1: Denial and isolation – disbelief, shock, feeling numb, can't believe this has happened.
- Stage 2: Anger – feeling enraged, asking why this has happened.
- Stage 3: Bargaining – struggling to find meaning in the situation, questioning 'what if …' and 'if only I had … then it might not have happened'.
- Stage 4: Depression – realisation of the bleak reality of the situation, a sense of hopelessness.
- Stage 5: Acceptance – a feeling of coming to terms with what has happened and accepting your new reality and beginning to re-engage with others.

Source: Adapted from Elisabeth Kubler-Ross (2014) *On Death and Dying*. New York: Scribner

The stages do not necessarily progress in a linear way – some people will experience them in a different order or may experience only two or three of the stages. However, it is considered that the five stages represent most people's experience of grief. Knowledge of these stages can help to recognise how a person is feeling and the type of emotional support and advice they might need.

More detailed information about the stages of grief and the symptoms of grief in general can be found using this link: **www.psycom.net/depression.central.grief. html**

Recognising when someone may be entering the last few days and hours of life helps to prepare for loss but also helps to recognise what can be done for the individual to make their last few hours of life as comfortable as possible. Expert information about this is offered by Marie Curie Cancer Care, including video clips of families sharing their experiences: **www.mariecurie.org.uk/help/support/terminal-illness/preparing/final-moments**

Involving the individual and families in decisions about their care and wishes

Individuals may have specific wishes in relation to culture and religion. It is important to consult with the individual and their family concerning their particular requirements in this area.

People of different religions have unique requirements relating to prayer, diet and food preparation which should be catered for as far as possible. Different cultures and religious groups also hold differing beliefs in relation to life and death and these may apply both before and after a person has died. The person's religious rites must be upheld following death and

every effort should be made to ensure that the body is handled in line with the person's cultural and religious beliefs.

Involvement of multi-agency teams where required in the care of the individual

The advance care planning process allows people to have control of their end of life care, making it fully person-centred to the end. They can, for example:

- identify where they wish to die
- state their priorities
- make choices about types of treatment they want
- decide the types of treatment they do not want
- reduce the risk of conflicting decisions later in the care process
- make professionals aware of their wishes.

Involvement and communication with multi-agency teams such as community care services, the person's GP, practice nurse, social worker, occupational therapist and hospice staff supports the person to live as well as possible until they die.

Research

Choose two service users who have different faiths. Examples could include a Buddhist and a Jewish person.

Find out about and explain the factors that you would need to take account of when providing support for them and their families in relation to their beliefs, religion and culture.

A8.14 How to support people with bereavement and how to communicate with families

When a loved one dies, a whole range of emotions is released, which may be difficult to control. There are many ways to support bereaved people and their families, such as:

- providing a safe and comfortable environment and suitable resources, including, for example, tissues, refreshments, somewhere that offers privacy
- providing emotional support – this could be listening, allowing the person to talk and cry, for example (Figure 8.13)
- using active listening techniques to show your support and understanding

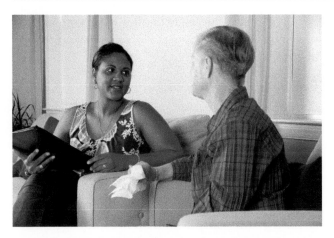

▲ Figure 8.13 A counsellor providing emotional support

▶ understanding that families may have an emotional reaction. Ensure that you know how to handle those situations, which may feature, at times, anger or aggression. Use empathy to support them and defuse the situation

▶ remembering the duty of candour to be honest and open about the provision of care and treatment, for example, accurately representing the situation or what has happened

▶ acknowledging cultural/religious rituals with a bereaved individual – see section A8.13

▶ signposting to applicable services, for example, bereavement care, national charities for bereaved people. A relevant booklet or leaflet will give contact details which people can take with them, or they can be given a link to a website or the name of an app.

Research

Carry out research into support groups in your local area that can assist people who are experiencing grief and loss.
▶ How can they be contacted?
▶ Note down examples of the types of support they offer.

A8.15 What the 6Cs are in relation to person-centred care

The 6Cs are key principles that underpin person-centred practice:

Care – a care worker should do all they can to maintain or improve an individual's health and wellbeing.

Compassion – being able to provide care and support with kindness, consideration, respect and empathy.

Communication – essential to developing good relationships with service users, their families and also with colleagues. Being able to listen carefully and speak in a way that individuals receiving care and support can understand.

Courage – being brave and able to speak up about concerns; doing the right thing and having the courage to try something new, such as new ways of working.

Commitment – a care worker is dedicated to providing care and support to meet individuals' needs.

Competence – refers to the ability of a care worker to provide high-quality, effective care by applying their knowledge, skills, understanding and expertise to meet an individual's care needs.

The Care Certificate sets out the standards that should be covered by induction training before members of the healthcare and social care support workforce are allowed to work without direct supervision.

Reflect

▶ Think about the daily tasks you do at your placement organisation.
▶ Write a description of two different tasks you carry out on a typical day.
▶ For each task, identify any of the 6Cs that you have applied and give examples of how you did this.

A8.16 The importance of practising and promoting the 6Cs in relation to demonstrating person-centred care skills, through own actions and promoting the approach with others

Practising and promoting the 6Cs

Providing choice and gaining consent

All individuals are entitled to make their own choices. Choice is empowering and this is a feature of person-centred care. Individuals should be offered a range of care options, for example, and given enough information about them to make an informed choice.

Consent must be obtained before any treatment or support is given. It must be informed consent and given voluntarily or it is not considered to be valid. The person giving consent must have 'capacity' so that they understand the information they have been given as a basis for informed consent.

Ensuring privacy and dignity

Many procedures in healthcare and social care require privacy, for example, showering and dressing someone or carrying out intimate procedures. It is vital to respect and protect the individual's privacy. This includes not talking about an individual with anyone who is not involved in providing their care.

Respecting individuals

This refers to:
▶ equality, diversity and inclusion
▶ sexuality
▶ faith, cultural needs and preferences – see section A8.13
▶ rights
▶ confidentiality – see Chapter A6 for more about confidentiality.

The people using healthcare and social care services are very diverse, that is, different and individual. The Equality Act 2010 identifies nine protected characteristics, and it is illegal to discriminate against any of the characteristics (see Chapter A1, page 2). Any unfair treatment, exclusion or discrimination against individuals on the basis of these characteristics is unethical and against the law.

Following the duty of care

Duty of care refers to the legal obligation professionals have to protect individuals they care for and support by protecting them from danger, harm and abuse. You must always act in the best interests of the individuals when carrying out your responsibilities and ensure they are kept safe from any harm.

Dealing with conflicts between rights and duty of care

An individual's right to take risks may conflict with the duty of care. The way to deal with this is not necessarily to avoid the risk but to find ways of handling the risk to reduce the potential consequences. So, for example, if a care home resident with arthritis in her hands wants to cook her own snack which involves use of the oven, the risk of a burn is high. Encouraging the resident to have a different snack that can be cooked in the microwave would enable her to prepare it independently with a reduced risk of burns.

Ensuring partnership working

This involves different professionals, services and agencies working together to provide the most effective care for an individual requiring treatment or support.

Ensuring honesty

Being honest about what went well and what didn't when reflecting on your work is important for professional development. Be honest with yourself – if you are unsure of something, always seek advice from your manager or supervisor.

Honesty is also very important when providing care for individuals. If you are unable to answer a question, admit it and find the information from a reliable source.

Prevent discrimination

This can be achieved through promoting inclusion and developing an inclusive environment, ensuring equal opportunities for all. Ways of valuing diversity in care settings include posters and displays that present positive role models from different genders and cultures, and respecting individual differences such as faith and language. Customs can be supported by providing prayer rooms, information in different languages and formats such as Braille or large print, ensuring access with ramps, lifts. These are all actions that help to promote equality and diversity and reduce the risk of discrimination against any particular group occurring in care settings.

Escalating concerns

The meaning of **'escalating'** something is to take an issue very seriously and to take further action, usually by involving more senior staff. Often just speaking with them and explaining the issue will be enough for them to improve their practice. However, in some cases the issue is very serious and could lead to (or may already have led to) consequences such as abuse or harm. If this is the case you have a duty to escalate the situation to a senior manager.

A8.17 The concept of safeguarding in relation to providing person-centred care

Safeguarding means the measures taken to protect people's health, wellbeing and rights, enabling them to be kept safe from harm, abuse and neglect. Practitioners in health and social care organisations must all be aware of the need for safeguarding.

All health services and healthcare professionals have a duty to safeguard all service users and protect their human rights. It is a key aspect of providing high-quality person-centred care in the health and care sector and must be taken seriously as a responsibility.

Some individuals may be more at risk of abuse, maltreatment or neglect than others. Examples include individuals who have a learning or physical disability, have a sensory impairment (visually or hearing impaired) or who lack mental capacity due to dementia or being unresponsive, in a coma, for example.

For many reasons these individuals may not want to, or be able to, report poor care or abuse. They are dependent on carers and may not want to upset them as their treatment might get worse. They may not know or understand their rights and possibly not even realise they are being abused. They may not see or hear who is abusing them. Staff have a duty of care to report concerns of suspected abuse or poor care to the organisation's safeguarding lead.

> See Chapter A11 for more on safeguarding.

A8.18 The importance of managing relationships and boundaries when providing person-centred care

Professionalism refers to carrying out a job role in a skilful and knowledgeable way and behaving in a manner that is appropriate and acceptable for the job role. Practitioners are expected to carry out their tasks to a high standard and professional conduct is integral to their role at all times. Contribution to teamwork is an important part of professional practice.

The importance of managing relationships and boundaries

Boundaries are the limits an individual must work within when carrying out a job role. Professional boundaries set limits for safe, acceptable and effective behaviour by practitioners. The job description indicates the scope and type of work involved and this will be reflected by the qualifications and experience required.

Working within boundaries:
- protects those providing and receiving care
- avoids misinterpretation of roles
- helps prevent potential abuse.

Practitioners must work within their own competence; they must understand the limits of their role and of their personal capabilities and know when to refer an issue to their supervisor or manager.

Practitioners must also always be aware of professional boundaries in terms of not having inappropriate relationships with patients. This would include, for example, oversharing personal information or discussing opinions of other members of staff. Being too friendly might lead to being seen as favouring some individuals over others, and you should not share your worries or personal problems, which would not be considered professional behaviour.

How to work within those parameters

- It is important to adhere to regulatory bodies' standards of professionalism. For more about regulatory bodies see section A8.3.
- Professional conversation is part of performance management. It is a planned, focused conversation between an assessor and a student, concentrating on a discussion of progress and development.

Project practice

Ben's day

Ben lives in a small residential home with five other people. Ben has physical and learning disabilities. He requires full support for his physical, social and emotional wellbeing. This is his description of a typical day in his life.

'I spend the morning sitting in the lounge watching TV. I watch the news every day because it is what is on.

At lunchtime I am taken to sit in the same seat every day, next to the same people, so they must be my friends. I have the same type of meal every day – something soft and easy to swallow. I spend most days like this. It would be nice to go out for the day and meet some new people, but the staff really are very busy and so it would be difficult for them to take me out.

At teatime I am given some soup and a cup of tea. They are both lukewarm. I am told that I can't have hot liquids because of a risk assessment, but I don't know what that means. Some of the others have biscuits with their tea, they look nice, but I don't get offered any.

At bedtime two carers help me into the shower and it is interesting to hear about their night out at the pub. I can't remember when I last went out to a pub.'

1 Ben is **not** receiving person-centred care. Identify and explain how his care is not appropriate for his needs.
2 Carry out some research:
   - Discuss Ben's situation and care needs with a care professional.
   - Internet research – find organisations/charity groups or third-sector organisations that may be able to help Ben, for example, with support groups or days out.
   - Using a multidisciplinary approach, who else could help?
3 Evaluate the care Ben is receiving and identify where his needs are not being met.
4 Produce a person-centred care plan that puts Ben at the centre of his care.
5 Consider the National Occupational Standards for supporting individuals to eat and drink. Create and deliver a presentation about aspects of Ben's poor care and details of his new person-centred care plan.
6 If possible, carry out an evaluation meeting with a care professional. Evaluate your care plan and your presentation.

Assessment practice

1 Explain the meaning of 'registration' for a care professional.
2 Describe **four** benefits of regulation and inspection of services.
3 Jamal is 16, he has a learning disability. He wants to get a job collecting trollies at the local supermarket. His mum does not want him to do this, she is worried he will not cope working on his own and may have an accident in the car park. His mum contacts Jamal's key worker to help dissuade Jamal from taking the job.

   Explain how **two** of the six key principles of the Care Act 2014 could be used by the key worker to reassure his mum and support Jamal in a person-centred way to help him to become more independent.
4 Explain how the CQC helps to improve standards in care settings. Your response should include:
   - details of the role of the CQC
   - examples of action the CQC can take if care is not up to the required standards.

5 Describe the meaning of social prescribing and suggest some examples.
6 What is meant by the personalisation of care?
7 Explain Maslow's hierarchy of needs and how it can inform the care that is to be provided.
8 Outline methods that could be used to overcome communication barriers for practitioners caring for individuals with sensory impairments. Your response should include:
   - examples of the communication barriers
   - details of how to overcome the barriers.
9 Draw a spider diagram to show the people who would be part of the care team for an individual approaching the end of their life.
10 Write a definition of the 6Cs and describe an example of how each is used in practice.

A9: Health and wellbeing

Introduction

Everyone wants to be healthy. It is easy to take being healthy for granted until something goes wrong and the individual becomes ill. Health comes from the Old English word meaning 'whole' and the term includes physical, emotional, intellectual and social wellbeing. The holistic way of looking at health and wellbeing is when all factors contribute to the health of the individual. It is difficult to collect information about wellbeing as it is harder to define, often taken for granted, and relates to how individuals feel about themselves and their personal experiences. A person can contribute to their own wellbeing through their efforts at keeping fit and healthy. People's basic health needs do not change. The differences are in the ability of the individual to provide for their own needs. Individuals need different amounts and types of support to meet their needs throughout life.

This unit covers the person-centred approach to health and wellbeing. Working to stay healthy is a lifestyle choice – people can make a conscious effort to do this – but modern patterns of life often make it difficult to follow a lifestyle that is healthy. This unit allows the exploration of good health as a choice in life, through all the life stages.

Government policies and resulting legislation have a big part to play in the promotion of good health. The introduction of screening programmes to prevent ill health has been a useful tool for catching problems before they develop. Even so, many personal factors affect health, some of which a person has little control over. Health promoters, too, have a significant role to play in helping individuals using services to make the right choice about health and wellbeing. Their choice of presentation approach can make or break a health promotion campaign.

Learning outcomes

The core knowledge outcomes that you must understand and learn:

A9.1 changes in the approach to healthcare and how to support a person's health, comfort and wellbeing

A9.2 how to recognise the signs and symptoms of a person who is experiencing pain and discomfort and/or whose health and wellbeing is deteriorating

A9.3 how to work in a person-centred way, to ensure adequate nutrition, hydration and care are provided to prevent deterioration in the individual's wellbeing

A9.4 the prevention agenda and the concept of preventative approaches for moving towards good health and wellbeing

A9.5 the ways in which health promotion is used to support the prevention agenda to support good health and wellbeing

A9.6 the overarching principle of the opportunistic delivery of health promotion through the Making Every Contact Count (MECC) initiative and the risk factors this initiative targets

A9.7 how lifestyle choices impact good health and wellbeing

A9.8 a range of methods of taking a holistic approach to healthcare

A9.9 the purpose of signposting individuals to interventions or other services and how this can support their health and wellbeing

A9.10 the impact of the ageing process on health and wellbeing

A9.11 how aspects of care requirements change throughout various life stages

A9.12 methods of supporting individuals to look after themselves at various stages of life.

A9.1 Changes in the approach to healthcare and how to support a person's health, comfort and wellbeing

Changes in approach to healthcare

Policy changes to focus on the promotion of health and wellbeing and prevention of ill health

The NHS Long Term Plan is a blueprint for the future of the NHS. It was published in January 2019 after consultations with patient groups, frontline NHS staff and national experts. The idea is that good health is about more than treating individuals when they are ill; it is about prevention of the illness in the first place. According to this plan, problems with ill health can be avoided by tackling **health inequalities** and by encouraging individuals to review their lifestyle choices. The NHS Long Term Plan sets out these health inequalities as:

▶ poor living environment
▶ poverty
▶ lack of life chances
▶ poor educational opportunities.

These health inequalities cost the NHS more because people in deprived areas make greater use of hospitals due to increased need. For example, people who live in poor housing which is difficult to heat in winter are most at risk of respiratory illnesses. Furthermore, if they have poor educational opportunities, they may be on the minimum wage or be unemployed and find it difficult to cover their expenses. Thus, apart from the negative impact of poor health and inequalities on individuals, it is also in the interests of the NHS to reduce these inequalities in order to save money.

The NHS intends to address these inequalities and make sure that everyone has the best start in life by providing continuity of care through pregnancy to birth and beyond. See Figure 9.1 for some of the ways the NHS plan will improve care for patients.

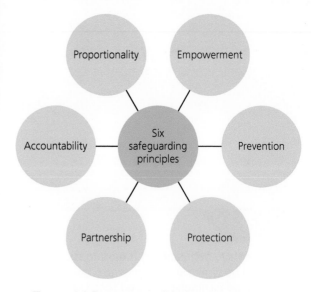

▲ Figure 9.1 Best start in life for everyone

Furthermore, the aim of the NHS Long Term Plan is that there will be world-class care for everyone throughout their lives, saving many thousands of lives and improving many more. See Figure 9.2 for examples of the world-class care which is to be offered.

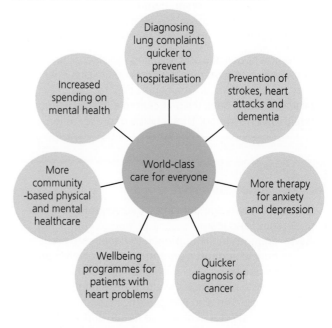

▲ Figure 9.2 World-class care for everyone

People will also be helped to age well. For example, there will be more money available for **primary care**, meaning that patients will have treatment from their own GP if possible, instead of having to go into hospital. Figure 9.3 lists examples of how the NHS aims to help and support people to age well.

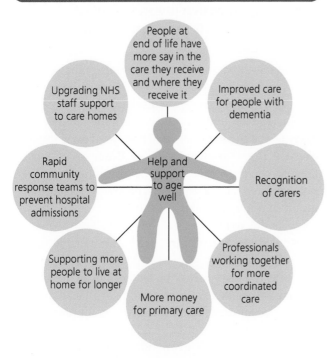

▲ Figure 9.3 Help and support to age well

The benefits of giving up smoking are enormous for the individual as they will feel healthier and be able to stay out of hospital. Every individual who follows preventative advice such as giving up smoking ultimately saves the NHS a huge amount of money compared with the cost of treating resulting, e.g. smoking-related, illnesses.

Change in approach from treating illness to promoting wellbeing

This is about encouraging and helping individuals to choose a healthy lifestyle. For example, if a patient consults their GP about a chest complaint, they will be asked about their smoking habits. If they smoke, they will be directed onto the NHS prevention programme to help them quit smoking. Giving up smoking significantly reduces that individual's risk of further illnesses developing, such as chronic obstructive pulmonary disease (COPD), heart disease or lung, kidney or stomach cancer. Similarly, if a patient is obese and has a sedentary lifestyle, they will be encouraged to follow a healthy, balanced diet as well as to increase their exercise. This approach aims to help reduce the chances of some conditions developing, such as high blood pressure, diabetes and heart disease, as well as making the patient feel better about themselves.

However, health is not just about physical health but also about mental health. For example, if an individual feels depressed, they may harm their physical health by drinking too much or binge eating. Healthcare professionals are encouraged to look at the holistic health of a person. Holistic means whole, where the whole person is considered rather than the separate aspects of health. It recognises that each aspect of health impacts other areas. For example, if you are emotionally upset, your mental, emotional and physical health can be affected. This emotional upset can show itself, for example, in the inability to concentrate, lethargy (a lack of energy/not feeling like doing anything) or being unable to sleep. Obviously, sleeplessness causes physical effects of tiredness, but it can also disturb normal thought processes. Thus we can see it is difficult to separate the aspects of health as they are so interrelated and interdependent.

Patrick

Patrick goes to his GP because he has been suffering from regular migraine headaches which have been so severe that he has had to take time off work. This has upset Patrick as he has just been promoted to a managerial position in his company. He finds the new job stressful as he is now in charge of a large team of people and a huge budget. Patrick now takes little exercise as he is too busy with his new job role. He used to have time to go to the gym and went jogging several times a week but has had to give this up due to work commitments. He also eats a lot of fast food for convenience, with little fresh fruit or vegetables.

While he is at the medical centre, the GP takes his blood pressure, which is higher than it should be. The GP also weighs Patrick and tells him he is overweight and is in fact classified as obese. Having discussed this and his change in lifestyle, she suggests that Patrick should follow the Eatwell Guide and should also exercise more, and to try to lose weight. Patrick is very annoyed as he thought the GP would just give him medication for his headaches. He did not expect the GP to look at his lifestyle and give him unwanted advice.

▶ Explain why the GP feels she needs to discuss Patrick's overall lifestyle and not just his headaches.

▶ Although Patrick has gained a promotion and a much higher salary, do you think his health and wellbeing have improved? Discuss this with a partner.

How to support a person's health, comfort and wellbeing

Collaborative approaches across the healthcare sector

The World Health Organization defines a collaborative approach as 'multiple health workers from different professional backgrounds working together with patients, families, carers (caregivers), and communities to deliver the highest quality of care'. From this definition it can be seen that it is not just the NHS working in isolation but the whole community, including the government and businesses, pulling together. For example, a strategy to help a patient who has had a stroke return to their own home involves several professionals across the healthcare sector. While in hospital, the patient will be helped to walk and regain their strength with physiotherapy. The pharmacy will

deliver their medication and an occupational therapist will go out to their home to ensure it is suitable for them to return to. When they return home, their GP will visit them if there are any problems and the community nurse may assess their **continence** situation.

Encouraging active involvement of individuals to self-manage their health and wellbeing

Individuals must be encouraged to self-manage their health and wellbeing as they will feel that they are making the decisions for themselves. They will feel empowered by their choices, making them much more likely to change their negative lifestyle than if someone else tells them they need to do so. Examples of poor lifestyle choices include smoking, drinking alcohol, poor diet and lack of exercise. The lowest-income groups often make the poorest health choices. This could be due to the stress of living on a low income. Lifestyle choices affect **cardiovascular**, nutritional, **neurological** and **psychological** health. For example, smoking and heavy drinking lead to cancer, heart disease and stroke. Eating a poor diet can lead to malnutrition, cancer and heart disease. A sedentary lifestyle can lead to similar outcomes. Making healthy lifestyle choices can help an individual to live longer, helping them to avoid many serious illnesses.

Continence: the ability to control the bladder and bowel.

Cardiovascular: relating to the heart and blood vessels.

Neurological: relating to a disorder of the nerves and nervous system.

Psychological: relating to a person's mental and emotional state.

Patrick

Go back to Patrick's case study above. In view of Patrick's anger at the GP's advice on his lifestyle, explain whether you think Patrick will follow his GP's advice. Suggest another approach that the GP could have taken to get Patrick on board with changing aspects of his lifestyle.

Encourage individuals to make decisions about the care, support and treatment they receive

Making decisions about their own care, support and treatment is a right that individuals have in law as set out in the standard of **person-centred care**. It is critical to successful integrated care. While most will be able to make an informed decision about care on their own, some individuals may need a lot of support to manage their health and wellbeing as they may lack the **cognitive** ability necessary to understand the options on offer. Research has shown that when healthcare professionals work together with their patients, more appropriate decisions are made. It is important to recognise that only the patient (if they are of age and are mentally competent) can decide if they want to continue with further treatment. Once the medical staff have presented all the options to the patient, they can make an informed decision, which can include refusing to consent to recommended medical treatment. This may be because they do not want to endure or prolong more painful treatments or procedures which will not guarantee a cure.

Key terms

Person-centred care: to see the person as an individual, focusing on their needs, wants, goals and aspirations.

Cognitive: relating to the processes of perception, memory, judgement and reasoning.

Reflect

Visit: www.theguardian.com/society/2014/apr/16/palliative-chemotheraphy-incurable-cancer

Read Kate's story. In pairs, discuss whether you think Kate made the right decision to stop the chemotherapy because her quality of life was suffering? Or do you think she should have persevered with the treatment?

Adopting a person-centred approach to support an individual's physical, intellectual, emotional and social wellbeing

The person-centred approach is to see the person as an individual, focusing on their unique needs, wants, goals and aspirations (see Figure 9.4). This approach addresses the physical, intellectual, emotional and social needs of the individual as they become central to the healthcare process. The support the individual needs must be designed with the individual, their family and/or carers. Supporting an individual involves giving them relevant and accurate information so that they can make informed choices about their life, and this is an important part of a person-centred approach. It promotes empowerment and dignity. The individual must have all the information they need to come to a decision so that they understand the implications and risks of their choice. When providing support, staff must be clear on whether the individual has the **mental capacity** to make the decision. If the staff decide that the individual does not have the capacity to make the decision, the people who care for the individual, for example, carers and family, can be brought in to help.

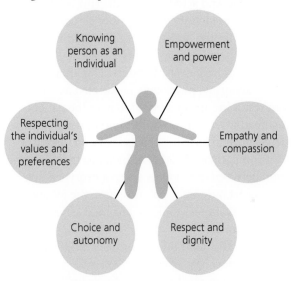

▲ Figure 9.4 Key concepts of a person-centred approach

A9.2 How to recognise the signs and symptoms of a person who is experiencing pain and discomfort and/or whose health and wellbeing is deteriorating

There are two types of pain – **chronic** and **acute**. Acute pain is a sharp pain that comes on suddenly, for example, toothache, burns, childbirth or appendicitis. It has a specific cause and usually disappears once the underlying cause of the pain goes. It is the type of pain which makes a person cry out and is a symptom of underlying disease or injury. Chronic pain is ongoing pain which can last for months even after the cause of the pain has gone, for example, back pain or nerve pain. This type of dull pain can nag on and on in the background.

Physical signs

Physical tics

Physical tics are involuntary movements which can include grimacing or frowning, blinking, jerking and coughing. The NHS says, 'They can also be fast, repetitive movements that result in sudden and difficult to control body jolts or sounds.' Anyone who has been in severe pain will relate to this feeling of being out of control of their body.

Altered baseline observations

Baseline **physiological** observations should be taken, recorded and acted on by staff. This is because it is important to identify early signs of clinical deterioration (i.e. the patient's condition getting worse). These physiological observations should be monitored at least every 12 hours. This should increase if abnormal physiology is detected as if left, this can result in further deterioration of the patient or even death. On admission, it is important to record a patient's normal baseline observations so there is a basis for comparison. This is necessary as there is some variation between individuals and not everyone has the same heart rate, etc. As a minimum, the following baseline observations should be recorded as part of routine monitoring:

▶ Heart rate: the heart rate is normally 60–100 times a minute. However, when a person is ill or fighting off an infection, the heart rate speeds up to help the circulation of oxygen and immune cells to help fight off the infection. Bacteria or infection that cause a disease and are accompanied by fever cause the heart rate to rise.

▶ **Respiratory** rate: the usual breathing rate for an adult is 12–20 breaths per minute but infections increase the rate. Breathing should be silent and easy, with the patient not working to breathe. Fast breathing is a sign that the patient has an infection such as pneumonia, heart failure or blood loss.

▶ Blood pressure: normal blood pressure for adults is in the range of 110/60 to 120/80. High blood pressure is defined as when the systolic reading is 140+ (top reading) while low blood pressure is when the systolic is below 100 (top reading). The top number given in a blood pressure reading is the systolic reading, which is the amount of pressure in the arteries during the contraction of the heart muscles to force blood around the body. The bottom number is the diastolic reading which is the lowest level of blood pressure as the heart relaxes between beats (see page 167). Blood pressure is often raised when a patient suffers from dehydration because of fever.

▶ Level of consciousness: patients can be alert with eyes open or confused with eyes open. As well as verbal responses if able, patients can respond to voice or pain stimulus, for example, pinching a toe or finger or shining a torch in the eyes. They are said to be unresponsive if there is no response to voice or pain, which could indicate a coma.

▶ **Oxygen saturation**: normal oxygen saturation is at least 90 per cent, with 94–100 per cent seen as normal, so if saturation levels fall it could indicate that the lungs are not functioning efficiently and may be filling with fluid. There could also be excess carbon dioxide as the lungs become inefficient at expelling it.

▶ Temperature: the average temperature of an adult is 36–37 °C. A higher temperature than this is called a fever or **hyperthermia**. Below 35 °C is called **hypothermia**. Coupled with an increased pulse and breathing, the fever is a sign of the body trying to fight off an infection. High fevers can damage the liver, kidney or other organs and can even cause death.

Key terms

Physiological: anything to do with the body and its systems.

Respiratory: related to breathing.

Oxygen saturation: level of oxygen delivered to red blood cells through arteries and delivered to internal organs.

Skin condition

In most emergency situations, the skin is one of the first organs to react to a dangerous condition. The healthcare professional can learn a lot about an individual's health and wellbeing by looking at their skin. Skin colour, temperature and moisture can reflect an individual's health.

Skin naturally comes in a variety of colours, from rosy to olive to very dark or white. Colour variations between individuals come from varying amounts of melanin, which is hereditary. Although there are many different pigments, if a person is unwell the colour under the skin can be pale for anyone, regardless of their natural pigment. This occurs because of limited blood flow: when there are not enough red blood cells flowing through the capillaries this means very little red and a general pale look. Thus people with very dark skin can also look pale when they have limited blood flow to their skin. (Symptoms for certain conditions may appear differently in those with darker pigment compared with those with naturally pale skin, however.)

Skin colour:

▶ If skin looks bluish or purple, this can indicate a problem with oxygen.
▶ Paler skin than normal can be a sign of shock or dehydration.
▶ Flushed skin can be an indicator of a fever or high blood pressure.

Skin temperature can indicate various health conditions:

▶ Skin that looks cool and wet can suggest a significant problem.
▶ Skin that feels hot could be an indication of a fever.

Moisture is also important:

▶ Wet skin should be noted if it is dripping or feels wet to the touch. Cold, wet skin can indicate an infection, hypoglycaemia, shock or a heart attack.
▶ Very dry skin is noticeable, especially when it is scaly. Ideally the skin should be supple, not scaly and not moist. Very dry skin can indicate dehydration.

Research

Mind the Gap is a handbook of clinical signs in black and brown skin being compiled by a team led by Malone Mukwende, a medical student based at St George's University in London. Visit: **www.blackandbrownskin.co.uk/mindthegap**

Using this or another suitable source, see if you can find out more about conditions which might present differently on brown skin to white skin.

Repeatedly touching or guarding part of the body

An individual may repeatedly touch the part of the body which is painful, almost as if they can protect the painful area from further pain or massage the pain away. Indeed, rubbing over a painful area of the body does sometimes help to reduce discomfort for a moment.

Moving slowly

Individuals with pain move slowly and carefully to reduce the impact of pain on their bodies. Imagine you have a headache and think how you move. A person may feel that if they move quickly, the pain will increase as they are putting too much stress on their body. The individual could be hunched over and shuffle along.

Wringing or clenching

Wringing the hands and clenching the fists can be a method that some individuals use to control pain. Clenching the jaw can also allow individuals to focus the pain elsewhere, with the idea that at least this discomfort can be controlled by the individual even if their other pain cannot.

Verbal signs

Self-report

A self-report of pain is when an individual tells a healthcare professional about their pain. However, a self-report from an individual with limited verbal and/or cognitive skills could be a gesture such as a hand squeeze or grasp or even a grimace. They may point to the area of their pain but be unable to say exactly where the pain is or what type it is, just that they are in great discomfort. They may not be able to say whether it is a pain or an ache. The healthcare professional can then further monitor and investigate the situation.

Crying out

Crying out and screaming can be an important indicator of pain, as can groaning and sobbing. Perhaps an individual has been on pain-suppressing medication and its effectiveness has started to wear off, causing the individual to cry out with the return of the pain. This can be involuntary, especially if the pain is sudden and sharp and the individual feels they cannot control it.

Groans/grunts

If individuals have limited verbal and/or cognitive skills they may express their discomfort by groaning or grunting as this could be the only method they have of alerting healthcare professionals to their pain. Again, the groaning or grunting could be involuntary.

Nonverbal signs

Facial expressions

Those individuals who are unable to verbally communicate their pain, such as older people with cognitive impairment caused by dementia or those who have had strokes, are totally dependent on others to be attentive to nonverbal signs of pain. The common facial expressions for these individuals who are in pain are grimacing, frowning, looking sad, closing eyes very tightly, clenched jaw, etc. However, these facial signs do not always indicate that the individual is in pain. They could indicate discomfort, anxiety, agitation or other causes.

Behavioural signs

Altered energy levels

When someone is experiencing significant pain or discomfort, their energy levels will drop as they will not feel like doing anything because they will not be able to stop thinking about their pain. Chronic or acute pain can make it difficult for someone to get out of bed in the morning, so individuals may want to conserve the little energy they have for tasks they may need to do later in the day. People may feel they cannot be bothered to do anything as everything is an effort. They may also not want to eat as they do not feel hungry. This in turn will affect their energy levels.

Altered character

Pain can alter a person's character by making them feel stressed, anxious, agitated and irritable. This is because if they are living with pain all the time, they may feel there is no escape from it. As a result, they find it harder to cope with everyday life and may be quick to lose their temper when normally they would be calm and unflappable.

Changes in usual eating/sleeping pattern

Pain can cause interruption of sleep and the effect on an individual is for them to wake up during the night. This means they will feel tired during the day and feel less able to deal with problems and issues. Pain is sometimes accompanied by nausea, which limits the amount and type of food the individual can eat. This can result in **malnutrition** (see page 212) as the individual is not eating the normal amount or variety of food that they would usually eat.

Test yourself

1 Explain the main focus of the NHS Long Term Plan.
2 Explain what is meant by a collaborative approach across the healthcare sector.
3 Describe how individuals can self-manage their health.
4 List the six minimum baseline observations.
5 Fill in the gaps to complete the following sentences:
   a If the skin looks bluish or purple this can indicate a problem with _____.
   b _____ can be an indicator of a fever or high blood pressure.
   c Very dry skin can indicate _____.

A9.3 How to work in a person-centred way, to ensure adequate nutrition, hydration and care are provided to prevent deterioration in the individual's wellbeing

Ensuring effective nutrition and hydration

Providing food and drink that meets individual needs

Good nutrition is essential for everyone. This means a good balance of nutrients such as proteins, carbohydrates, fats, vitamins and minerals. Poor nutrition can cause malnutrition and/or obesity as well as vitamin and mineral deficiency diseases (see Figure 9.5). When people receive any type of care or support (particularly long-term care), an assessment should be made about their nutrition and hydration. This should include food allergies as well as likes and dislikes. Their beliefs and the support they need to be able to eat and drink must also be considered. Medical conditions too must be taken into account. For example, if someone has **osteoporosis**, they need to eat foods rich in calcium and vitamin D. If the individual being cared for does not get enough nutrients, their medical treatment may not work as well.

Priya

Priya has recently given up her home after a serious stroke. She is living in a residential care home. Her BMI is over 30 and she has diabetes. This is partly because she had a poor diet before she moved into the home as she prefers foods and drinks with a high sugar content. Her care worker is carrying out an assessment about her nutrition and hydration needs. Priya tells him she does not like healthy food and would like to carry on with her usual high-sugar diet as she has a very sweet tooth.

Working in a person-centred way, explain why it may be in Priya's interests to eat less of her favourite foods. What strategies would you use to discuss the issues with Priya?

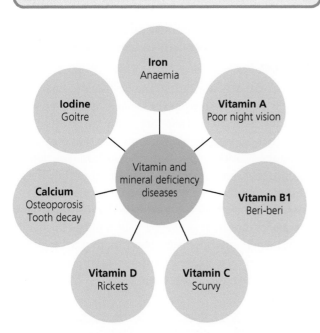

▲ Figure 9.5 Vitamin and mineral deficiency diseases

Ensuring food and drink provided does not have contraindications with any medicine the individual is taking

Food can affect some medicines taken by individuals depending what individuals eat or when they eat it. Taking a medicine at the same time as eating a certain food can cause the body not to absorb the medicine. Alternatively, certain foods may delay or decrease the absorption of the drug. For example, dairy foods such as milk, cheese or yogurt should not be combined with antibiotics (this is a **contraindication**). This is because the antibiotics combine with the calcium in the milk products to form an insoluble substance that the body is unable to absorb. Another example of food to watch out for is grapefruit, which has a negative impact when mixed with cholesterol-lowering medication.

Supporting individuals who might experience difficulties in eating or drinking

The care plan should tell the healthcare worker if an individual needs support in eating or drinking as well as the type of support needed. Never impose help or support on an individual; it is important that they are **empowered** by asking them if they require any assistance. Food should be tempting to the individual so the meal should look attractive and well presented. The healthcare worker should have a relaxed attitude. They need time to carry out the task without rushing the individual while they are eating. They may need to slow down if the individual is having difficulty coping with the amount of food. Individuals with dementia sometimes forget to eat or drink, especially as their appetite decreases and they lose interest in food. This confusion and loss of memory means they cannot remember whether they have eaten or what they have eaten that day.

Contraindication: a reason that makes it inadvisable to combine certain foods with particular drugs.

Empower: to give someone the authority or control to do something; the way a health worker encourages an individual to make decisions and to take control of their own life.

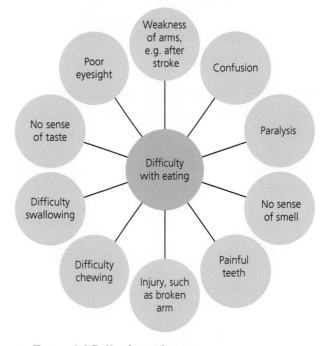

▲ Figure 9.6 Difficulty with eating

Providing equipment to support individuals in eating and drinking independently

There are many different aids available to help individuals feed themselves. These include different types of cutlery, plates, bowls, trays and drinking aids. Perhaps the simplest assistive aid is a drinking straw which allows the individual to drink without lifting the cup or glass. This would be useful for someone with a tremor or a poor grip (see Figure 9.6). Individuals with arthritis of the hand, which can cause poor grip, can have cutlery with thick handles. Plates with rubber bases to stop the plate slipping are useful for individuals who may have the use of only one hand. Two-handled mugs with a lid are useful as there is less likelihood of the individual spilling their drink and they have the security of being able to use both hands to hold it (see Figure 9.7). These assistive aids promote independence and self-confidence as well as safer eating. The important issue is to let individuals choose which assistive aids they would like to use.

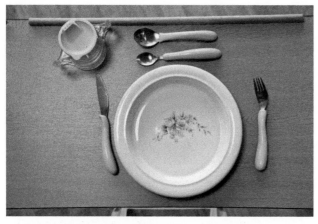

▲ Figure 9.7 Assistive aids

Ensuring individuals are provided with sufficient time to eat and drink

Keep calm and try not to rush the individual. It is important they do not feel hurried and they are given enough time to eat. Using assistive aids such as insulated bowls can help the individual finish their meal without it going cold. For some individuals, chewing is difficult and if they are rushed they may give up trying to eat.

Close monitoring of nutrition and fluid intake

Monitoring of food and drink eaten helps healthcare workers to ensure that the individual has the proper intake of fluid and other nutrients. It is important that the individual has nutritious food in order to

stay healthy. Monitoring of output helps determine whether there is adequate output of urine as well as normal **defecation**. If the individual is in danger of malnutrition and **dehydration**, the amount of food and fluid given and consumed by the individual should be recorded.

> ### Key terms
>
> **Defecation:** final act of digestion which removes solid or semi-solid waste material from the digestive tract via the anus.
>
> **Dehydration:** when the body loses more fluids than it takes in.
>
> **Constipation:** infrequent, irregular or difficulty with defecating.

Communicating with individuals to identify any barriers in relation to eating and drinking

If an individual is not eating, the best way to deal with it is to ask them what the issue is and then try to sort it out for them. There are many barriers to eating that could be to blame. It may be that they are having medication or a treatment which makes them feel nauseous, so they do not want to eat or they have lost their appetite. The medication could also cause **constipation**, so they feel too bloated to eat. They may have a sore mouth or problems with their teeth, so it is painful when anything is in their mouth. Lacking taste and smell can also cause a barrier as often the smell of food will make the mouth water and start the flow of gastric juices.

> ### Reflect
>
> Imagine you have a cold and cannot taste or smell your food. Explain how this situation affects your appetite.
>
> Imagine if you could not taste or smell your food permanently – would you enjoy food?

Promotion of the value and importance of effective nutrition and hydration to overall wellbeing

Effective nutrition and hydration is very important for everyone, young or old. Without good nutrition – which includes the right balance of protein for growth, repair and recovery; carbohydrates and fats for energy;

and vitamins and minerals to strengthen the immune system – individuals do not have good health. Good nutrition protects individuals from chronic diseases such as heart disease, diabetes, strokes and some cancers. It can lower cholesterol and reduce blood pressure. Vitamins and minerals help the immune system guard against illnesses and **immunodeficiency** problems. It is the duty of the healthcare professional to look after the health and wellbeing of the individual, so they should encourage individuals under their care to eat and drink healthily. The type and amount of food eaten affects the way the individual feels and how their body works. Good nutrition also helps individuals to recover from illness.

> ### Key term
>
> **Immunodeficiency**: a condition in which the body has difficulty protecting itself against disease.

Working in partnership with carers or family members to ensure effective nutrition and hydration of the individual

Family members and carers can help by reinforcing what the healthcare professional has said to the individual about their feeding habits. They can also plan a strategy to use with the individual so everyone follows the same plan to encourage good nutrition. For example, there could be a weekly menu for the individual so everyone knows what the individual will be eating every mealtime. This ensures consistency for the individual.

Obviously, the individual will play a big part in deciding what the menu will be. This will make them feel they are still able to make decisions about their own welfare. This is empowering for them and if they have had a choice, they will be more likely to eat the meal.

Working in partnership with other healthcare professionals to ensure effective nutrition and hydration of the individual

There is a wide range of professionals who could work together to help with effective nutrition and hydration. They can help sort out any issues that the individual may have with eating. For example, if the individual has problems with their mouth or teeth, the dentist can help. The dietician could make suggestions for alternative dishes if the original menu does not agree

with the individual, perhaps suggesting liquidising some food, e.g. turning vegetables into soup, if chewing is too difficult or takes too long, so they can still gain the nutrients found in vegetables. A GP could help to treat indigestion.

> ### Test yourself
>
> 1 List the four main groups of nutrients.
> 2 Explain what is meant by a contraindication.
> 3 Explain why it might be necessary to monitor nutrition and fluid intake.
> 4 Describe a strategy that a carer could use to ensure an individual has sufficient nutrition and hydration.
> 5 Suggest other healthcare professionals able to help with effective nutrition and hydration.

A9.4 The prevention agenda and the concept of preventative approaches for moving towards good health and wellbeing

Prevention agenda as set out by health and social care policy and reforms

'Prevention is better than cure' was published in November 2018 as the Secretary of State for Health's vision for a prevention agenda, with the aim that life expectancy would be increased by at least five years by 2035. This policy document works in conjunction with the NHS Long Term Plan discussed in section A9.1.

According to this policy paper, the choices the individual makes have a huge impact on their health and life expectancy. If the choices an individual makes reflect reliable health advice, then many illnesses and diseases are preventable.

The aim of the 'Prevention is better than cure' policy is to try to keep people healthy to prevent problems throughout individuals' lives from birth to death (see Figure 9.8). If a problem does occur, individuals will be supported and helped to manage it. The aim is to provide community support for older people to be independent and live in their own homes for as long as possible.

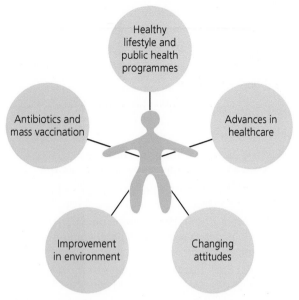

▲ Figure 9.8 Reasons for people living longer, healthier lives

The document identifies a range of challenges that need to be addressed by individuals, local and national government, communities, health and social care and employers all working together to remove the barriers to healthy lives. These challenges are shown in Figure 9.9.

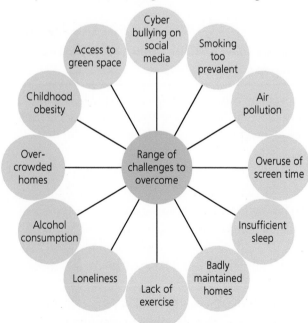

▲ Figure 9.9 Range of challenges to overcome to remove barriers to healthy lives

Preventative approaches

Help people to stay healthy and independent for as long as possible

Good health starts before birth. Pregnant women need access to good quality **antenatal** (before birth)

and **postnatal** (after birth) care services for both their own health and that of their child. New mothers are entitled to free dental treatment. The child then needs access to immunisations against childhood ailments and close monitoring to ensure they meet all the key development stages. Their home should provide them with good nutrition and they should have a healthy and secure upbringing in a house that is safe, warm and comfortable. They should have access to outside space for them to exercise in and enjoy, for instance parks or playgrounds. School should be a place where they can learn and develop to the best of their ability. It is also a place where they can socialise and make friends, which will help them to develop resilience and good physical and mental health. When the child grows into an adult, they can maximise good health by habits such as:

▶ not smoking
▶ drinking moderately
▶ looking after their mental health
▶ working or volunteering to improve a sense of self-worth
▶ attending regular screening appointments such as cervical smear tests.

As people grow older, they can help themselves by continuing the good habits for a healthy lifestyle developed in adulthood. They can look after their teeth and go for regular dental check-ups and visit their GP if they have any health issues. Once they are 40, they are entitled to a full health review where their blood pressure, cholesterol level, weight and sugar level are tested. This is available for the individual up to the age of 74. They can go to regular health screenings such as mammograms or carry out home tests such as bowel cancer screening. Screening can be a useful preventative tool. The idea behind screening is that a disorder can be detected before any outward signs or symptoms are evident. Early detection can mean quicker recovery for the individual and because of early treatment, the disease will not be so far advanced, therefore it should be less expensive to treat. Aids and adaptations to the individual's home can help the older adult to stay in their own home for longer. All these factors when combined will help the individual to stay healthy and independent for as long as possible.

Stopping problems arising in the first place, focusing on keeping people healthy

Stopping problems before they arise can be successful if the focus is on keeping the individual healthy and fit. Small choices taken every day can add up to healthy living, for example, choosing to drink water instead of a sugary drink. However, there are larger decisions to be made and messages reinforced time after time for physical health, such as exercising regularly, eating high-fibre foods including plenty of fruit and vegetables, and limiting added sugar and salt intake.

Individuals must be healthy mentally as well as physically. Small improvements in wellbeing can help reduce mental health problems. These are known as 'The Five Ways to Wellbeing':

▶ Be active – take part in an activity which is enjoyable for you.
▶ Keep learning – learning new skills can give a sense of achievement.
▶ Take notice of what's going on around you and be interested.
▶ Connect with people, neighbours and family.
▶ Give to people – even the smallest act can count, it could be a smile or kind word.

Provide people with knowledge and skills to make lifestyle choices that help them to stay healthy

Health and wellbeing are affected by lifestyle choices and these can have a positive or negative influence. People need to know all the facts so that they can make an informed decision. Therefore, health education is vital to improve the health and wellbeing of a person as they can weigh up the presented evidence and arrive at a conclusion. This would allow them to prevent some diseases from developing. If people are encouraged to take preventative measures, many lives could be saved and many individuals may not develop life-threatening conditions.

Professionals too have an increasing understanding of environmental factors that cause ill health. These factors may include services such as waste management, water supply, sanitation, affordable housing, pollution, energy sources, access to health and social care services, and access to leisure and recreation facilities. Some people cannot afford, or do not have time due to having to work long hours, to access leisure facilities. People who have to deal with poor housing and sanitation are more likely to fall ill. These are therefore major barriers to improving public health and preventing illness, and professionals and local authorities need to include fixing these problems as part of a holistic approach to public health. Professionals also need to help individuals to increase their skills to be able to take control of their own health.

A9.5 The ways in which health promotion is used to support the prevention agenda to support good health and wellbeing

National campaigns from government departments

On 18 August 2020 the UK government announced a new approach to public health by launching the National Institute for Health Protection (NIHP). The purpose of the NIHP is to protect the public against external threats to the UK, pandemics and infectious diseases. It was formed by uniting the organisations Public Health England (PHE), the Joint Biosecurity Centre and Track and Trace. The NIHP will continue PHE's health improvement and wider prevention work, supporting the government's stated aims of giving children the best start in life, tackling risk factors such as obesity and smoking (among others), and reducing health inequalities.

Before beginning any health promotion campaign, the Department of Health (DH) identifies the need for change of behaviour to reduce ill-health within communities across the country. The National Census, the Office for National Statistics (ONS) and data from hospitals across the country provide the sources of information for the DH. New health promotion campaigns are thought up in response to this information to ensure an accurate picture of the population. However, it is also essential that appropriate agencies, organisations and people with related expertise and up-to-date information on the proposed health promotion campaign are consulted before any action is taken or any decisions are made. For example, if a campaign aims to target older individuals to prevent falls, it would make sense to consult Age UK as the charity has experience with this age group and ideas about the best way to approach the issue.

A wide variety of resources is produced for national government health campaigns, therefore local authority health promotion units may decide to run their campaigns at the same time as national ones. (See page 161 for more on this.)

Examples of national campaigns

This Girl Can is a national campaign developed in 2015 by Sport England and a wide range of partnership organisations. It is designed to get women and girls of all shapes, sizes and abilities to exercise more. The idea is to inspire women to challenge cultural assumptions about female sport that prevent them engaging in sport and exercise.

> ### Reflect
>
> Go to www.thisgirlcan.co.uk and watch the video clip for the campaign.
>
> Now read the article at www.theguardian. com/commentisfree/2015/jan/16/this-girl-can-campaign-sex-sport-real-women-bodies-objectifying-female-flesh
>
> Do you agree with the comments from *The Guardian* that the This Girl Can campaign is 'all about sex, not sport'? Discuss with your classmates.

The idea of the public health campaign Change4Life, which started in 2009, is for individuals to make many small changes to their lifestyle which, when taken together, will add up to a significant change. Eating well, moving more and living longer form the basis of this campaign. The campaign has a recognisable look and feel and offers lots of tips for eating a healthier diet, simple exercising advice for everyday life, e.g. walk upstairs instead of taking the lift, swapping sugary snacks for fruit and how to cut down on alcohol.

In December 2013, Public Health England, the Department of Health and the Cancer Research Campaign working together in partnership launched Smokefree, which is a service to help individuals to give up smoking. It offers an app, Quit Kit, email, SMS and face-to-face guidance.

Cardiovascular (heart and circulatory) disease causes more than a quarter of all deaths in the UK (Source: British Heart Foundation). As a result of this there have been many different health campaigns linked to heart disease. All healthy eating programmes, exercise regimes, sensible consumption of alcohol and smoking campaigns are related to reducing deaths from heart disease. Change4Life emphasises the dangers of heart disease because of obesity, and that eating a diet high in sugar can lead to Type 2 diabetes.

Alcohol has featured in many health campaigns over the years. The Drinkaware website (www.drinkaware. co.uk) has factual information about all aspects of alcohol from units in drinks to dangers of children drinking, plus an app which can be used to help reduce alcohol intake. One of its latest campaigns is called 'You wouldn't sober, you shouldn't drunk'; its aim is to stop people committing sexual harassment on a night out while drunk.

> ### Research
>
> Are you aware of how many units of alcohol are in popular drinks? Find out how many units are in the following:
> - one pint of 5% draught lager
> - 500 ml can of 5.5% cider
> - 250 ml glass of 12% wine
> - 275 ml bottle of 4.5% alcopop
> - 25 ml shot of 40% spirit.
>
> Check your answers at: www.alcoholchange.org. uk/alcohol-facts/interactive-tools/unit-calculator
>
> Which drink did you think had the most units? Has this changed your perception of alcoholic drinks?

Opportunistic delivery of health promotion by all healthcare professionals

Usually individuals visit their local GP surgery or healthcare centre when they are not well. They may need a **consultation** (i.e. to be seen and possibly examined by a doctor) if they have a medical problem such as a problem breathing. This could be the ideal time to ask them if they smoke as they may be more likely to try to give up smoking if they feel this is what has caused their medical problem. It is not appropriate to pressurise the patient but merely a good opportunity to offer them access to the smoking cessation programme. Other follow-up procedures could include taking the patient's blood pressure.

Campaigns by specific groups and charities

Many different charities are involved in health promotion, e.g. the British Heart Foundation offers exercise classes on YouTube. It also supplies healthy eating information on its website and in leaflets. Voluntary organisations can make a huge contribution in helping the NHS and other public bodies to deliver improved services. Small locally-based charities and social enterprises often deliver preventative services that keep people away from hospital or GP appointments. They can offer community exercise groups, cooking healthy meals on a budget, mindfulness, etc. Even the national charities can offer localised services. They reinforce the message given by national government agencies.

Research

Research the different voluntary organisations in your local area which provide health and wellbeing advice and services. Explore the various services that they offer to the community. Explain how you think the services on offer contribute to making the individual healthier and happier.

Sharing examples of health promotion activities

Local health promotion teams base their campaigns around nationally set health events. Local teams choose their own particular targets depending on the health issues within their area. For example, one local area might have chosen the following as its health campaigns for 2021:

- World Cancer Day 4 February
- No Smoking Day 11 March
- National Walking Month 1–31 May
- Blood Pressure Week 7–13 September.

Another area of the country may have chosen entirely different events from the calendar, depending on local needs. The NHS will produce health promotion posters, leaflets, etc. to support the campaigns, which are supplied free of charge to the local areas which request them. Organisations can contact the NHS and request a date for their particular concern, and if there is a national health and wellbeing campaign that NHS staff will benefit from, this can be submitted for review. For example, in the 2021 calendar of events the British

Association of Dermatologists was given 6–13 May as Sun Awareness Week.

Research

1 Contact your local health promotion unit (which will be listed under your local council area) and find out its calendar of events for the year.
2 Look at the NHS website for the Health Events calendar for this year. Search for: 'Calendar of national health and wellbeing campaigns table - NHS Employers'.
3 Which local events match the national promotion? Research the reasons for this.

Test yourself

1 Discuss the creation of the National Institute for Health Protection (NIHP) by the British government in 2020. Explain the reasons for this decision.
2 Explain why sharing examples of health promotion is a good idea.
3 Describe what is meant by opportunistic delivery of health promotion.
4 Justify the involvement of organisations and charities in health promotion.

A9.6 The overarching principle of the opportunistic delivery of health promotion through the MECC initiative and the risk factors this initiative targets

Approach to preventative behavioural change which uses day-to-day interactions that individuals have with any healthcare professional

The Making Every Contact Count (MECC) initiative is an **evidence-based approach** to improving people's health and wellbeing by helping them change their behaviour. The NHS Long Term Plan cites the statistic that every 24 hours the NHS staff come into contact with more than a million people. But MECC also recognises that staff across local authority and voluntary sectors as well as health and social care have thousands of contacts every day with individuals and are ideally placed to promote health and wellbeing. If all these professionals worked together, they could help to change an individual's life for the better. The MECC approach encourages healthcare workers to talk to people about improving their health by addressing lifestyle factors such as diet, exercise and alcohol consumption.

> **Key term**
>
> **Evidence-based approach:** making better decisions by considering all the facts, statistics, etc. and using them as a basis for making a decision.

Using brief and very brief interventions whenever the opportunity arises

MECC states that the NHS is well placed for brief and very brief interventions which could help someone adapt their lifestyle. These interventions could be as short as 30 seconds but would be useful as healthcare staff could encourage and support patients, suggesting other services which could help the individual if necessary. Mental, physical and emotional health and wellbeing could be improved.

In practice, brief and very brief interventions can make a difference to an individual's health even though it may take seconds. The healthcare professional may be able to address two issues in one meeting. For example, a young mother brings her school-age child into a clinic or GP surgery for immunisation. The healthcare professional may notice that the child is slightly overweight and mention the fact to the child's mother. Having discussed their habits, the healthcare worker could suggest that a way of helping the child to lose weight would be to walk with them to school rather than drive if possible. This would be a very brief intervention as it might take only 30 seconds, but it could have a huge impact on the child's health if it could help to stop them becoming obese and developing serious health conditions. If, however, the mother needed more advice, she might have to be referred to the dietician or health visitor in the practice, which would take a little longer and would fall into the category of brief intervention.

NICE has stated that very brief and brief interventions are both cost effective and effective in changing behaviour, particularly in the areas of reducing smoking and alcohol consumption as well as losing weight and improving physical activity.

Highlighting risk factors

Some long-term diseases and illnesses in the UK are linked to the choices people make. This can lead to years taken off the average population's lifespan due to ill health caused by smoking, alcohol, high blood pressure, being overweight or lack of physical exercise. Making changes such as giving up smoking, increasing physical exercise, losing weight and cutting down on alcohol could help to reduce the risk of certain illnesses or poor health.

MECC focuses on lifestyle issues that, when addressed, can make the greatest improvement for an individual's health:

▶ stop smoking
▶ drink alcohol within recommended units
▶ eat healthily
▶ be physically active
▶ keep to a healthy weight
▶ improve mental health and wellbeing.

The risk of developing Type 2 diabetes can be reduced with a healthy diet and by keeping active, which will help to manage the blood sugar level and avoid the development of insulin resistance.

> **Reflect**
>
> Go to: www.youtube.com/watch?v=4SZGM_E5cLI
>
> Watch the short clip and educate yourself about Type 2 diabetes. Did you learn something new about this condition?

Signposting to additional support and resources available

As well as the resources available in their own place of work, healthcare professionals can refer to MECC links to websites and other resources to raise awareness and signpost people to help with improving their health and wellbeing. The MECC link gives a full range of information, including self-care, national and local support services.

Test yourself

1 Describe what is meant by an evidence-based approach.
2 Explain the idea behind Making Every Contact Count (MECC).
3 List the six lifestyle issues MECC states could make the greatest improvement to an individual's health.

A9.7 How lifestyle choices impact good health and wellbeing

Diet and body mass index

Obesity increases risk of developing a range of diseases

BMI or body mass index is a measure used to indicate whether an individual is under or overweight compared to the average of the overall population. BMI is calculated by dividing a person's weight by the square of their height. This number falls into one of five BMI groups, which have been designated as follows:

► underweight: BMI 19.9 and below
► normal: BMI 20–24.9
► overweight: BMI 25–29.9
► obese: BMI 30–39.9
► severely obese: BMI 40 and above.

Reflect

Work out the BMI for each person:
► Marsha female – aged 53, height 167.6 cm, weight 63.5 kg
► Darius male – aged 36, height 186 cm, weight 98 kg
► Bing male – aged 24, height 188 cm, weight 57 kg

Are they a healthy weight according to BMI? Check your answers: www.nhs.uk/live-well/healthy-weight/bmi-calculator

Are there other factors that should be considered (for example, Darius doing a lot of weight-training)?

Obese is a term used to describe an individual who is very overweight, who may have a lot of body fat. Around one in every four adults in the UK is estimated to fall into this category (which is defined as having a BMI of 30 or above) and around one in every five children aged 10–11 in the UK.

Source: www.nhs.uk/conditions/obesity/

As a general rule, obesity results from consuming more calories over time – particularly from fatty and sugary foods – than the individual burns off through physical activity. The excess energy is then stored by the body as fat. Obesity is an increasingly common problem because many modern lifestyles can involve increased access to cheap, high-calorie food and are sedentary (involve less movement), with the average person spending a lot more time sitting at desks, on sofas or in cars than previous generations have done. Regular exercise can reduce the chance of becoming obese.

Not everyone who has a BMI of over 30 is overweight. Those with muscular bodies such as athletes may have a high BMI and be clinically healthy. This is because muscle is denser than fat. This excess weight comes from muscle so does not have health-related risks associated with too much body fat.

If individuals follow a well-balanced, healthy eating plan such as the Eatwell Plate, they are less likely to become obese. A good diet involves plenty of fruits and vegetables, good sources of protein such as fish, and will not involve excessive amounts of saturated fat, refined sugar or salt. (See note on the CVD on page 164.)

It is important to note that this is general advice and that each individual's weight is the result of a complex range of factors and that the relationship between weight and health is not straightforward. A healthy lifestyle reduces the likelihood of a BMI in the obese category, however there may also be social factors that influence the individual's likelihood of obesity (for instance, poverty), and certain health conditions make losing weight very difficult (for instance, thyroid problems or limited mobility or other disability). Social stigma surrounding obesity can be damaging to mental health and make it more difficult to address health issues and risks in obese individuals, so sensitivity and a holistic approach to health are essential.

Being underweight is also detrimental to health. People who are 19.9 or below on the BMI scale risk:
► a weakened immune system and are therefore more prone to infections
► difficulty with temperature regulation
► nutritional deficiencies such as osteoporosis
► malnutrition.

Reducing obesity increases the likelihood of better outcomes in a range of conditions:

▶ **Lower chance of developing Type 2 diabetes:** Cells depend on a single simple sugar, glucose, for most of their energy needs. A healthy body has intricate mechanisms in place to make sure glucose levels in the bloodstream do not go too low or too high. When eaten, most digestible carbohydrates are converted into glucose and rapidly absorbed into the bloodstream. Any rise in blood sugar signals the pancreas to make and release insulin, which instructs cells to soak up glucose. Without it, glucose floats around the bloodstream, unable to slip inside the cells that need it. Type 2 diabetes occurs when the body cannot make enough insulin or cannot properly use the insulin it makes. What an individual eats is an important factor: the risk of developing Type 2 diabetes is increased by a diet full of quickly absorbed sugars and refined carbohydrates; their cells slowly become resistant to the effects of insulin so blood sugar or glucose will remain at a high level. Over time this can harm almost every organ in the body. (Note that people with lower BMIs can also have high-sugar diets and may develop Type 2 diabetes.)

▶ **Less chance of developing hypertension (also known as high blood pressure):** What an individual eats and drinks has a real effect on their heart and blood pressure. The healthier their eating habits are, the lower their blood pressure is likely to be (assuming no other relevant health conditions). If an individual does have high blood pressure, it is even more important to make healthy changes to their diet. If they take medicines for their blood pressure, then a healthy blood pressure diet can reduce the number of medicines they may need. For some individuals, following blood pressure-friendly eating habits may help them to avoid medicines altogether. Blood pressure can rise if an individual's diet contains too much salt. If the blood pressure remains high, over time there is a risk of the individual having a stroke.

▶ **Lower risk of cardiovascular disease (CVD):** This is a general term for conditions affecting the heart or blood vessels. It is usually associated with a build-up of fatty deposits inside the arteries (atherosclerosis) and an increased risk of blood clots. It can also be associated with damage to arteries in organs such as the brain, heart, kidneys and eyes. The risk of heart disease can be reduced by keeping to a healthy weight and by eating healthily. A low-fat, high-fibre diet is recommended, which should include plenty of fresh fruit and vegetables (at least five portions a day) and whole grains. Saturated fats are important, but the amount eaten should be regulated – these saturated fats are found in foods such as sausages, bacon, pies, butter, cream, hard cheese and anything made with lard. Too much saturated fat can produce high levels of cholesterol, which can lead to heart disease. The increase in cholesterol causes a build-up of fatty deposits called **atheroma**. However, unsaturated fats found in foods such as oily fish, nuts and seeds, avocados, etc. should be included in the diet, as should unsaturated oils such as sunflower, olive, rapeseed and vegetable oils.

Cancers

Lifestyle factors, including diet, can make a huge difference in helping to reduce cancer risk. Eating more fruits and vegetables can lower the risk of a variety of common cancers such as colon or breast cancer. High consumption of some foods actually increases the risk of cancer, while eating others will support the body and strengthen the immune system. Research shows that many cancer-related deaths are directly linked to lifestyle choices such as smoking, drinking, a lack of exercise and having had an unhealthy diet over a long period. Avoiding cigarettes, limiting alcohol, maintaining a healthy weight and getting regular exercise are what doctors advise to help prevent cancer.

Research

Read the NHS Eatwell Guide at: www.nhs.uk/live-well/eat-well/the-eatwell-guide/

Discuss with your partner the reasons why this guide and these simple diagrams might help an individual who is struggling to remember which foods they should eat and in what quantity.

Malnutrition risk of vitamin deficiency

Everyone has different nutritional needs and some individuals can cope with nutritional deficiencies better than others. The body is able to adapt to reduced food intake, but too little food can lead to ill-health through **undernutrition** (not getting enough energy from food). In extreme cases, starvation causes stunting of physical and mental development and wasting.

In the UK, starvation is less of a problem compared with certain parts of the world, but it can still occur, often due to poverty. People do go hungry in the UK, as the increase in number and usage of food banks demonstrates. Excessive amounts of food can also cause **malnutrition** (literally, poor diet), which may lead to conditions of ill-health such as obesity, heart disease or high blood pressure.

People on low incomes who work long hours may not have the time or money to buy fresh ingredients or cook highly nutritious meals so they rely on quick convenience foods. Fruits and vegetables can also be more expensive and less convenient than more calorie-dense foods such as biscuits.

Diseases such as **scurvy** (see table) and some forms of anaemia are caused by a deficiency (lack) of certain nutrients or by the body's ability to absorb them. The table describes why we need each vitamin and what effects are caused by not getting enough of it in our diet.

> **Key terms**
>
> **Beri-beri**: vitamin B1 deficiency that leads to a nervous system disorder.
>
> **Scurvy**: vitamin C deficiency which causes tooth loss, poor skin healing with sores, anaemia.

Vitamin	Necessary for	Deficiency causes
A	• fighting infection • healthy skin and blood • strong bones and teeth • good eyesight • growth of new cells	• night blindness • skin problems
B-complex essential B vitamins including: • B1 – thiamine • B2 – riboflavin • B3 – niacin • B6 • B7 – biotin • folate and folic acid • B12	• energy production • nervous system • blood production • healthy hair, skin, eyes, liver and mouth • muscle tone	• problems with nervous system • muscle weakness • skin problems • **beri-beri** • anaemia • mouth ulcers
C	• helping skin to heal • production of red blood cells • fighting off bacterial infections • helping iron to be absorbed • helping to prevent infections	• **scurvy** • wounds and cuts being slow to heal
D	• strong bones and teeth • helping to regulate the heart • contributing to good health • protecting against muscle weakness • helping calcium be absorbed	• rickets in children • weak bones and teeth • muscle weakness
E	• improving circulation • helping muscles use oxygen • helping normal clotting and healing • extending life of red blood cells • keeping eyes healthy • helping prevent heart disease	• possible weakening of light receptors in the eye and loss of vision over time
K	• blood clotting • normal liver function • helping calcium be absorbed	• easy bruising • excessive bleeding in babies

▲ Vitamins: how they benefit the body and the results of their deficiencies

Smoking

One of the biggest causes of death and illness in the UK/increases the risk of lung cancer

Smoking is the biggest factor in deaths and illnesses in the UK. Every year 78,000 people in the UK die from the damage caused to their bodies by smoking and from debilitating smoking-related illnesses (source: NHS). Smoking leads to a significantly increased risk of many different cancers such as lung, oesophagus, larynx, throat, kidney, bladder, liver, pancreas and stomach. Smoking is the biggest preventable cause of cancer. Toxins, e.g. tar and carbon monoxide, in cigarette smoke can weaken the body's immune system, making it harder to kill off cancer cells. These can also damage or actually alter a cell's DNA so the cell can begin to grow unchecked, creating a tumour.

Increased risk of heart disease

Smoking-related deaths are mainly due to cancers, **chronic obstructive pulmonary disease (COPD)** and heart disease. Smoking increases the risk of **cardiovascular disease**, which includes very serious symptoms such as **stroke** and heart attack. Smoking leads to a build-up of fatty material (atheroma) which narrows the artery. The **carbon monoxide** inhaled in tobacco smoke reduces the amount of oxygen taken into the blood, meaning the heart has to pump harder to supply the body with the oxygen it needs. Exercise becomes difficult as the individual gets short of breath more easily. The nicotine in cigarettes stimulates the body to produce adrenalin, which makes the heart beat faster and raises the blood pressure, making the heart work harder. The blood is more likely to clot because smoking causes the blood platelets to stick together, which increases the risk of a heart attack or stroke.

> **Key terms**
>
> **Chronic obstructive pulmonary disease (COPD):** the name for a collection of lung diseases which make breathing increasingly difficult.
>
> **Cardiovascular disease:** general term that describes a disease of the heart or blood vessels.
>
> **Stroke:** serious and life-threatening medical event that occurs when the blood supply to part of the brain is cut off.
>
> **Carbon monoxide:** odourless, colourless, tasteless toxic gas.

Low physical activity

Risk factor for a range of long-term conditions, including heart disease and/or hypertension

According to current NHS advice, adults should do at least 30 minutes of moderately intense exercise for 5 days each week if they wish to improve their general health. Physical inactivity over a period of time can lead to increased risk of chronic disease and obesity. Exercise can help an individual to maintain lean tissue. As discussed on page 163, overweight and obese people have a higher risk of developing heart disease, hypertension, stroke and Type 2 diabetes. An inactive lifestyle is one of the top risks for heart disease, but it is one that is remedied by taking exercise.

Regular exercise can strengthen the heart and improve the circulation, so the body uses oxygen more efficiently. Lungs benefit from increased capacity as aerobic exercise makes the lungs work harder. The result is greater lung efficiency, which improves stamina and overall health. Exercise also has the advantage of increasing energy and endurance and helping to lower blood pressure. When exercising, the heart muscle contracts more often and more powerfully so it increases in size and strength. **Cardiac** (heart) output increases, so more blood is pumped out to the body by the heart. As a result, the individual who exercises regularly will generally have a lower resting heart rate than those who do not, with a quicker recovery time from exercise. Exercise can help to prevent certain diseases such as bowel cancer as exercise can speed the path of food through the colon, so preventing constipation. Regular exercise coupled with sensible eating is the recipe for good health.

Each time the heart beats it pumps out blood into the arteries. Blood pressure is highest when the heart contracts and this is called the **systolic** pressure. When the heart is at rest between beats the blood pressure falls, which is known as the **diastolic** pressure. Blood pressure is given as systolic pressure over diastolic such as 120/80 mm Hg. Studies show that regular aerobic exercise over several months can lower blood pressure.

The table shows the different readings used for blood pressure. Only one of the readings needs to be too high to put an individual in a hypertension category. For example, if an individual's reading was 149/85, they would be classified as having high blood pressure; even though the diastolic reading is in the normal range, the systolic figure is in the stage 1 mild hypertension category.

Systolic	Diastolic	
Less than 130	Less than 85	Normal blood pressure
130–139	86–89	High–normal blood pressure
140–159	90–99	Stage 1 (mild) hypertension
160–179	100–109	Stage 2 (moderate) hypertension
180–209	110–119	Stage 3 (severe) hypertension
210 or higher	120 or higher	Stage 4 (severe) hypertension

▲ Blood pressure readings

Linked to increased anxiety and depression

Exercise can promote good sleeping habits and reduce stress and depression as it can boost feel-good endorphins. If an individual takes part in team sports or games, they can help their emotional and **social health** as well as their physical health. Exercise can be enjoyable and help people feel good. When an individual exercises, their body releases chemicals called endorphins which trigger a positive feeling in the body. This is usually accompanied by a positive and energising outlook on life. Exercise helps deplete stress hormones and releases mood-enhancing chemicals which help individuals to cope with stress better. While taking part in exercise, individuals may be able to forget about their problems for a while and feel physically and mentally stronger and more resilient. Exercise can help individuals with depression and may reduce the occurrence of depression in the first place.

Key terms

Adverse: harmful or unfavourable.

Social health: the ability to form friendships and meaningful personal relationships with other people.

Older adults who are physically active can reduce their risk of falls

Being active in older age, where possible and in ways appropriate to an individual's ability and health, can help to slow down the rate at which muscles deteriorate. As people age, their muscle strength and balance reduce, which can lead to them being more likely to have a fall. Exercises designed to improve muscle strength can reduce the risk of a fall by improving posture, coordination and balance. Training can build strength and improve balance. These exercises can make a person steadier on their feet and more in control. They are especially helpful for older people who have already had a fall or who have problems with balance or walking. Getting sufficient energy is important in keeping up strength and preventing falls. A nutritious, well-balanced diet is therefore essential; if an individual is weak and shaky through lack of food, they are more likely to fall.

Consumption of alcohol

Long-term effects include organ damage, including heart, liver and pancreas

When an individual drinks beer, wine or another alcoholic drink, the alcohol quickly enters the bloodstream. The alcohol then gets broken down and distributed throughout the body, affecting the brain and other tissues.

Alcohol can have an **adverse** effect on all the body systems. Health risks of high alcohol consumption include higher risks of the following conditions:
- various cancers such as mouth, throat, oesophagus, larynx, breast and liver
- a stroke
- heart disease
- liver disease
- pancreatitis
- reduced fertility
- diabetes
- depression and anxiety.

If an individual regularly drinks more than the recommended weekly amount of alcohol (14 units over the week for adults) over a sustained period, they risk damaging their health. There is no guaranteed safe level of drinking and if consumed occasionally and in moderation, alcohol may not be a problem, but the more an individual drinks, the greater the health risks.

Organ damage – the heart

The heart muscles are weakened by the toxicity of large amounts of alcohol and cannot pump the blood efficiently around the body. The lack of blood flow disrupts all the body's major functions. This is known as cardiomyopathy and it can lead to heart failure.

Organ damage – the liver

The liver has many functions that are essential to health, such as:

▶ breaking down drugs, alcohol and other potentially toxic substances
▶ producing bile to aid with the digestion of fats
▶ storing nutrients like glucose in the form of glycogen, as well as certain types of vitamins
▶ making proteins that are important for blood clotting.

Various substances can damage the liver. While liver tissue can regenerate, continued damage, such as constantly having to break down alcohol, can lead to the build-up of scar tissue. This is because the liver cells die and do not have the chance to regrow. As scar tissue forms, it replaces healthy liver tissue. This can impair the liver's ability to carry out its vital functions. Alcohol consumption is one of the leading causes of liver damage. When liver damage has happened due to alcohol, it is called **alcohol-related liver disease (ARLD)**. Alcohol-related liver disease does not cause any symptoms until the liver has been severely damaged. There are three stages of ARLD:

▶ Alcoholic fatty liver disease – this is when drinking large amounts of alcohol even for a few days can result in fatty deposits in the liver.
▶ Alcoholic hepatitis – this is when the liver has been abused by drinking large amounts of alcohol over a longer period of time.
▶ Cirrhosis – this is when the liver cells have died off and been replaced by extensive scar tissue and is the sign of long-term abuse.

Organ damage – the pancreas

The pancreas is responsible for producing pancreatic juices called **enzymes** which break down fats, sugars and starches in food and drink during digestion. The pancreas also helps the digestive system by making hormones such as insulin which helps to maintain safe blood sugar levels (see diabetes on page 343). Alcohol causes the pancreas to produce toxic substances, leading eventually to pancreatitis, which is a dangerous inflammation of the blood vessels in

the pancreas that prevents proper digestion. Regular drinking over the recommended weekly limits of alcohol can cause acute **pancreatitis**.

> ### Key term
>
> **Pancreatitis:** pancreas becomes inflamed over a short period of time.

Increased risk of hypertension and heart disease

Drinking more than the guidelines regularly and over a prolonged period of time can lead to a bigger risk of heart disease. This is because drinking large quantities of alcohol raises the blood pressure, causing hypertension which can lead to a heart attack or stroke. (See page 166 for more on hypertension and strokes.)

Weakens immune system, increasing risk of infections

Excessive alcohol can suppress the immune system, making an individual more vulnerable to infections caused by viruses and bacteria. The immune system may take longer to recognise and respond to an infection. As a result, it takes longer for the body to fight off the infection, meaning it has more time to develop and is more likely to become dangerous. Additionally, the consumption of alcohol impairs the function of B-lymphocytes, which produce **antibodies** in the blood. These antibodies ward off viruses and other diseases that may attack the body. Excessive alcohol can also damage the immune system as the alcohol prevents nutrients from feeding the immune system. The alcohol is absorbed into the bloodstream through the stomach. Once in the bloodstream, alcohol will reduce the white blood cell count in the body.

Weakens bones, increases risk of fracturing and breaks

When an individual drinks over the recommended limit, alcohol acts to block calcium, preventing this mineral from being absorbed from the food they eat. Heavy drinking disrupts the bone-building cells from doing their job. This means that not only do bones become weaker, but when a bone breaks, alcohol can interfere with healing. People who drink heavily are more likely to have frequent bone fractures, which could lead to osteoporosis in later adulthood.

Effects on the brain including cognitive function, neurotransmitters and brain tissue

As soon as alcohol enters the bloodstream it begins to affect the individual's brain. In an individual with a healthy liver, this organ will start to filter the alcohol. However, when a person drinks heavily, it is too much for the liver to deal with quickly. This has an immediate effect on the brain. With continued excessive alcohol consumption, lasting damage will be the result. Excessive alcohol consumption can affect the neurotransmitters (see pages 314–315) in the brain, decreasing their effectiveness. Brain cells are destroyed and brain tissue contracts. Too much alcohol can change the shape and structure of the brain. These changes are the result of the toxic effects of alcohol and lack of vitamin B1 (thiamine). Alcohol stops the body absorbing vitamins, so vitamin deficiency is a common problem for heavy drinkers. Alcohol-related cognitive impairment refers to the damage that repeated excesses of alcohol consumption can have on the brain's ability to function. Cognitive impairment can include difficulties with memory, learning new concepts, reasoning, concentration and problem solving.

Substance abuse and addiction

Effects on health may occur after one use

Drugs are chemical substances that can affect the body in different ways. Some drugs, even those legally acquired such as alcohol, nicotine and over-the-counter drugs, can even change the body and brain, sometimes permanently in ways that last long after the individual has stopped taking drugs. Many deaths, illnesses and disabilities stem from substance abuse. Individuals who live with substance dependence have a higher risk of bad outcomes, including unintentional injuries, accidents, medical problems and death. Methamphetamine, or crystal meth, is a highly addictive illegal drug. It is possible for an individual to become addicted to crystal meth after just one use.

Longer-term effects include risk of heart disease, cancer and hepatitis

Possible side effects of drug abuse include heart dysfunction, which can even occur in young people with no history of heart disease. Common side effects are arrhythmia or irregular heartbeat. There can be a change in blood pressure, a heart attack or a stroke if illegal drugs are taken in large quantities.

▶ Often drugs such as heroin and cocaine are mixed with cancer-causing additives to stretch out the amount of drugs for sale. These are cheap substances including talcum powder, wood dust, horse tranquilliser and strychnine (a substance found in rat poison). It is estimated that 80 per cent of cocaine is cut with phenacetin, an illegal painkiller which leads to bladder cancer.

▶ Smoking crack cocaine or marijuana can lead to the same cancerous conditions as smoking tobacco.

▶ Hepatitis B and C are regularly transferred through sharing needles. These diseases are spread by contact with the blood of infected individuals, so reusing needles increases this risk.

Test yourself

1 Explain the factors that increase the risk of a person developing Type 2 diabetes.
2 Describe how an individual's eating habits can affect their blood pressure.
3 Explain what is meant by cardiovascular disease.
4 A deficiency of the following vitamins causes:
   Vitamin A: _____; Vitamin B-complex: _____; Vitamin C: _____.

A9.8 A range of methods of taking a holistic approach to healthcare

Treating the person not just the condition

As discussed earlier in this chapter (page 149), a holistic concept of health considers the whole person rather than just the separate aspects of health. It recognises that each one of the aspects of health impacts the others. It is very difficult to separate the aspects of health as they are interrelated and interdependent. For example, if a person is emotionally upset, their mental and physical health can be affected. So too could their emotional and **spiritual health**.

Key term

Spiritual health: having a sense of purpose, a clear set of morals and values, and living life according to those morals and values. This is different for different people. It is not religion.

Case study

Hasim

Hasim is a 33-year-old man who runs a successful business and has a comfortable lifestyle with his wife and two children. Physically he looks after himself as he watches his food intake, he does not smoke or drink alcohol. He goes to the gym three times a week. Sometimes he feels worried about his business but he does not discuss this with anyone as he was brought up to be self-sufficient and independent. He has lots of friends and he is very popular. He believes in looking after his immediate and extended families; his parents and his parents-in-law visit every week. As they are living on a state pension and have few savings, he pays for them to go on holiday and often helps them to pay bills.

Applying the concept of holistic health to Hasim, decide whether he has a healthy lifestyle. Explain your answer.

Bespoke treatment plans that meet the personal choices and needs

A personalised care and support plan is developed following an initial holistic assessment around the person about their health and wellbeing needs. The individual is central to the process. The person, or their family, work hand in hand with their health and social care professionals to complete this assessment, which then leads to producing an agreed personalised care and support plan with people who use the services. When drawing up bespoke treatment plans, the healthcare professional must consider:

► empowerment and power
► the person as an individual
► respecting the individual's values and preferences
► choice and autonomy
► respect and dignity
► empathy and compassion.

Understanding the individual's lifestyle

This is about recognising and considering an individual's other commitments such as family. For example, a young mother who has to have kidney dialysis finds it very stressful. This is mainly because she has to leave her young children for a full day every week to go to hospital for her treatment. Her blood pressure is too high when in hospital and she cannot relax during her treatment as she is constantly anxious. She discusses her concerns with the hospital staff who arrange for a renal nurse to go out to her home once a week for one hour. This removes the stress as the mother does not have to leave her children. In this instance the hospital staff recognised that the young mother knew she needed the treatment for her physical complaint but they also considered her emotional and mental state. This is about designing the treatment around the young mother's needs. People want to be treated as individuals and one size does not fit all.

Understanding the individual's mental health needs

There are many services available for individuals who have mental health needs. The GP is usually the first healthcare professional that the individual would see. Common examples may be a new mother with post-natal depression or a student with anxiety or a retired person who is depressed. Other conditions include obsessive compulsive disorder (OCD), schizophrenia, bipolar, anorexia and bulimia. Anyone can suffer from a mental health condition – mental health charity Mind UK states that one in four people will have a mental health condition in their lifetime.

From an appointment with the GP there may be a referral to a psychiatrist or clinical psychologist or counsellor. Further on in the treatment for their condition they may see an occupational therapist or a drama, art or music therapist. These creative therapy professionals help people on a one-to-one or group basis. Creative activities could address the need to:

► socially interact and communicate with others
► express emotions in a safe environment
► build a strong, robust self-image
► provide intellectual understanding of yourself and your relation to the world around you.

Depending on practical needs such as providing food for their children or respite care for a dependent relative, a social worker or a community support worker may also help. There could be several different practitioners working with the individual at any time.

Integrated working

Integrated care can go right across the life stages from baby to old age and involves a range of professionals and specialists working together in a connected way. For example, in the case of an adolescent having significant issues with behaviour there could be a social worker, police officer, educational welfare officer (EWO) and educational mental health professional all working together in partnership to meet the needs of the young person. A young person truanting from school would need the input of the EWO to get them into school and improve their attendance, or if they have been caught shoplifting while truanting, the police would be involved. If, when their parents are contacted by the school, they say that they cannot cope with their child's behaviour, a social worker will help them. A mental health professional could help with a child's phobia of going into school and they might offer counselling.

An older person who has been admitted to hospital with a stroke will be looked after by nurses and doctors. They may need a speech therapist if they need help with talking again. The occupational therapist may go out to the person's home to suggest adaptations to help them live alone. Social services would then be involved in carrying out these adaptations.

> **Key term**
>
> *Integrated care*: provides people with the support they need across local councils, the NHS and other partners. The idea is that barriers between GPs, hospitals and council services have been removed, meaning people no longer have disjointed care.

Health and wellbeing boards

Health and wellbeing boards are a formal committee of the local authority whose role is to promote greater integration and partnership between bodies from the NHS, public health and local government. Their aim is to facilitate individuals experiencing more 'joined-up' care, particularly in changing from healthcare to social care. For example, when an individual is discharged from hospital back to their own home, they may need help to be organised by social care before the discharge can happen as they may be unable to cope on their own.

> **A9.9** The purpose of signposting individuals to interventions or other services and how this can support their health and wellbeing

Signposting individuals

Purpose: to determine the most appropriate service for the individual, including considerations given to the most cost-effective approach

Community-centred approaches are seen as successful by Public Health England NHS in tackling ill-health. They provide value for money in that there will be less use of both GP and hospital services as well as a reduction in the use of prescription drugs. Community-centred approaches help people to feel part of society and empowers them to access services and social resources. They may be particularly suitable for members of marginalised communities who feel less able to access traditional healthcare settings or face barriers in doing so. If individuals engage with others in their community, they are more likely to follow the direction given to them by people they know and trust.

> **Research**
>
> Visit: www.gov.uk/government/publications/health-matters-health-and-wellbeing-community-centred-approaches/health-matters-community-centred-approaches-for-health-and-wellbeing
>
> Read the further information on community-centred approaches and write an explanation of community health assets.

How it can support an individual's health and wellbeing

Provide awareness on a wider range of services available

GPs and healthcare professionals can refer people to a wide range of local, non-clinical services supported by link workers. These link workers are non-clinical social practitioners who aim to address socio-economic or personal issues such as debt, unemployment, housing and provide support for people's specific needs. This is known as social **prescribing** and addresses people's needs in a holistic way. There are many different community-centred schemes running right across the country, from mental health support to running clubs, gardening groups to breastfeeding support, prostate cancer groups and so on. People can be signposted to the club that best meets their needs, where they can find support from individuals who have similar experiences and needs and/or who are professionals working with these groups.

Provide alternative options

Providing alternative options such as community-centred non-clinical services can be surprising for some individuals as they may think that only healthcare professionals can help them to improve their physical health and wellbeing. While this may be true of some acute conditions such as heart attack, other areas of their wellbeing can be addressed through a variety of techniques and approaches, including non-clinical support. The addition of these link workers means they can focus on the wider needs of individuals, not just physical health needs. Many patients have visited medical practices with no physical symptoms but rather emotional and social needs that the medical team have not had the time to address.

These non-clinical workers can arrange their time to suit patients because they are giving them a personalised service. As the non-clinical workers are not part of a formal appointment in a GP surgery, individuals may find it easier to talk to them and say what is really troubling them. This meeting can be reassuring for the individual as the worker is able to focus their attention on the individual's needs, whatever they may be, and may help to reduce loneliness and inequality. This is because they can direct individuals with practical advice about issues such as money, or they may help get someone back into education so they can gain qualifications, or they may help an individual fill in forms to apply for jobs or more suitable housing. The link worker can also direct individuals to community groups and new activities, helping them with emotional and social issues.

Opportunities to discuss specific complaints or experiences with specialists or peers

As well as peer mentoring, there is the opportunity to discuss experiences with individuals from the voluntary sector. Healthcare professionals are available if issues are not resolved, though it is hoped this will not be necessary. Having link workers to discuss issues with patients is efficient as the link worker will be aware of voluntary, statutory and private organisations that will be able to offer relevant help and support for the individual. For example, if a man has been diagnosed with prostate cancer, the link worker will be able to direct him to a cancer support group such as Macmillan. There he will be able to discuss issues with others who are in the same situation as himself; he will feel comfortable about asking them questions about treatments, side effects, etc. as he knows they will have experienced them. He will also have access to the expertise of the specialist Macmillan nurses. If he needs nursing at home, Macmillan will also provide nurses who will visit and offer advice, equipment and even grants for low-income families and respite care. The link worker will also be able to direct the family to hospice end-of-life care.

> ### Research
>
> Research the community-centred schemes that are available in your area. Hint: you should be able to find information on the local council website about community-centred approaches. Can you find out how any different schemes are available? Are they across all age groups? What would you recommend for a 65-year-old man who has recently retired and feels he has lost his sense of purpose?

> ### Test yourself
>
> 1 Explain what holistic means in the context of healthcare.
> 2 Explain why the use of community-centred approaches by the NHS can be beneficial.
> 3 Describe what is meant by integrated care.

A9.10 The impact of the ageing process on health and wellbeing

Impact of ageing on physical health

As people age, they become aware of physical changes that become more obvious with old age. The table summarises the effect of ageing on physical development.

Part of body	Physical development due to ageing
Skin	• wrinkles • looseness because of loss of elasticity • dryer skin
Hair	• thinning • growth slows • men may go bald
Hearing, smell and taste	Senses deteriorate: • ability to hear diminishes • smell and taste decline • may lose appetite
Eyesight	• long sightedness may develop • cataracts and glaucoma may develop and cause blindness if not treated
Teeth	• decay and gum disease may occur if dental hygiene has been neglected
Lungs and respiratory system	• lungs become less elastic (become stiff and less likely to expand and fill with air) • respiratory muscles weaken • less able to take part in strenuous exercise due to reduced lung capacity • more likely to be affected by disorders such as influenza, pneumonia or COVID-19 so should be vaccinated against these
Heart and blood vessels (cardiovascular system)	• heart efficiency decreases • blood pressure may be raised • blood vessels are less elastic (they become narrower and less flexible) • can lead to cardiovascular disease such as strokes, heart attacks, etc.
Digestive system	• saliva and digestive juices decrease with age so may have indigestion or heartburn • food takes longer to go through the system as muscles are weaker and less efficient; this can lead to constipation
Urinary system	• kidneys become less efficient at filtering waste products • may need to pass urine more frequently • may be prone to urinary infections
Reproductive system	• menopause marks end of reproductive capacity for women
Skeleton and muscles	• people shrink in height • total bone mass is reduced • in women, osteoporosis may result (after menopause due to reduced oestrogen) in fractured and broken bones. Men can have osteoporosis but it is less common • knee and/or hip problems can cause mobility issues • muscles become less flexible • balance can be affected • posture and mobility likely to alter

Age-associated diseases

Not all people experience age-associated diseases. Similarly, some diseases can occur in adults of any age, for example, diabetes, heart disease and cancer can affect younger people. However, the ageing body is increasingly subject to **degenerative diseases**. These are diseases that gradually worsen over time.

Age-associated disease	Caused by
Parkinson's disease	loss of nerve cells in the brain
Alzheimer's disease	brain cells dying off
Age-related macular degeneration	deterioration of central part of the retina (within the eye)
Arthritis	joints becoming inflamed
Osteoporosis	bones weakening; prone to fractures
Osteoarthritis	joints becoming inflamed
Rheumatoid arthritis	body's immune system becoming overactive and causing inflammation that affects the joints
Rheumatism	joints and muscles stiffening and becoming painful

▲ Examples of age-associated disease

Research

Choose one of the age-associated diseases listed in the table and research the condition. Use the information you collect to prepare a presentation and deliver it to the rest of your group. Make sure you present an overview of the condition, the symptoms, the diagnosis and the treatment.

Impact of ageing on cognitive health

Memory

Forgetfulness is a common complaint among older adults. As people age, they experience physiological changes that can cause slowness in brain function. It takes longer to learn and recall information. People often mistake this slowing of the mental processes for true memory loss. Many mental abilities are unaffected by normal ageing. If an individual continues to make an effort to learn new things and engage in cognitive activities, this can minimise ageing effects on cognitive health.

The causes of age-related memory are:
▶ The hippocampus, a region of the brain involved in the formation and retrieval of memories, often deteriorates with age.
▶ Hormones and proteins that protect and repair brain cells and stimulate **neural growth** also decline with age.
▶ Older people often experience decreased blood flow to the brain, which can impair memory and lead to changes in cognitive skills.

It is important to understand that not all older people will develop dementia.

Key term

Neural growth: refers to any growth of the nervous system.

Research

Research dementia and find out what the symptoms are. Visit: www.ageuk.org.uk/health-wellbeing/conditions-illnesses/dementia/what-is-dementia

Case study

Colin

Colin is 69. His partner has noticed that he has difficulty getting washed and dressed in the morning. He has started to repeat stories several times during the same conversation. Last week he set off to his daughter's house and got lost. He had his sat nav and tried to use it but couldn't follow the directions.

Jane is 72. She occasionally has difficulty finding the right word to use in conversation but has no problem with following and holding a conversation. However, she recently forgot her wedding anniversary.

Decide which person is likely to have dementia and which one has memory loss. Explain why.

Attention

Older adults retain the ability to pay attention and concentrate on tasks. However, if they try to divide their attention between two or more different tasks at the same time, this is when they face difficulties. They may need to concentrate on one task at a time if they wish to achieve a satisfactory outcome.

Reasoning and problem solving

Long-established ways of approaching solutions are maintained in older people; just because they are ageing does not mean they lose all their reasoning or problem-solving skills. However, a new, unencountered problem may take extra time for them to work through to a solution.

Information processing

Ageing does affect the speed of processing information as cognitive and motor processing slow down. This does not mean that older individuals cannot carry these out, just that they may take longer.

Impact of ageing on emotional wellbeing

Transitions and significant life events

Many older people are not retiring at 65 but are working for longer. For some this may be an economic necessity, while others feel they lose their status and a sense of who they are when they retire. For example, a headteacher is no longer a headteacher or a factory manager is not a factory manager anymore and they feel they have lost their place in society. People often feel the loss of their purpose in life as well as their income, which can fall significantly, perhaps by half or even more. They may also lose friends as they no longer see their work colleagues every day. For some, those who are in relationships and live with a spouse/partner who does not go out to work, there could also be stress in their relationship with their spouse/partner who may be used to being at home by themselves during the day.

When a partner dies, as well as the upset and sorrow there can be confusion about, for example, financial matters or how to run the home. The remaining partner could feel lonely and isolated, particularly if they depended on their partner to take them shopping or accompany them out and about. This can be especially acute if their late partner had been their primary carer. They may feel they do not have anyone to go out with. If the couple were together for many years, the remaining partner may become depressed and not want to leave the house.

People with long-term medical conditions can also suffer from depression and other mental health conditions. They may experience shock when they are initially diagnosed with a condition and have difficulty coming to terms with the implications this might have for them, e.g. having to take daily medication, make lifestyle changes or the realisation that there may be no cure. They may feel a range of emotions, including fear of what the future may bring, frustration, anger and resentment, and loss of self-esteem because they are more reliant on other people, the condition changes their view of themselves or the way others see them. Families too may feel upset and perhaps resentful.

Own mortality

If people have lost a partner because of death, they often start to think about their own mortality. As people age, colleagues they worked with die, as do family and friends. Older people often say, 'I'm the only one left in my family.'

Loneliness/social isolation

This may happen for a variety of reasons among older people. They may be isolated in their own home as they may be unable to get out due to poor mobility. They may live alone or they may not have many visitors, or perhaps their family live far away. It is also possible for people to feel extremely lonely even if they live among a lot of others in a residential home. They may find it difficult to form new friendships with other residents or staff.

A9.11 How aspects of care requirements change throughout various life stages

Life stage of human development and potential care requirements

Birth and infancy, 0 to 2 years

One important responsibility for those caring for babies is to ensure they are vaccinated. As the tables show, it is not only babies who require immunisation, but they do have the most vaccinations within a short window of time. It is the responsibility of parents or guardians to ensure that children receive all their vaccinations. Parents and carers will automatically receive letters from their NHS Trust a few weeks before each vaccination appointment is due.

Age	Vaccines	Diseases protected against
8 weeks	• 6-in-1 vaccine • Rotavirus vaccine • MenB	• diphtheria, hepatitis B, polio, tetanus, whooping cough (pertussis), Hib (Haemophilus influenzae type B) • Rotavirus: a highly infectious stomach bug • MenB: meningococcal infections (meningitis B and blood poisoning) • Pneumococcal pneumonia (a disease affecting the lungs)
12 weeks	• 6-in-1 vaccine (2nd dose) • Pneumococcal (PCV) vaccine • Rotavirus vaccine (2nd dose)	
18 weeks	• 6-in-1 vaccine (3rd dose) • MenB (2nd dose)	

▲ Vaccines offered to babies under the age of one

Source: www.nhs.uk/conditions/vaccinations/nhs-vaccinations-and-when-to-have-them

Mothers and babies are monitored after they leave hospital by the community midwife for a period of between 10 and 28 days after birth. The midwife will check the mother's physical and emotional recovery. They will carry out various checks on the baby such as weight, feeding, whether they have jaundice, how they are sleeping, whether the umbilical cord is healing, and will carry out the heel prick test to check their blood for various conditions such as cystic fibrosis and sickle cell. The midwife will then discharge the mother and baby if all is well. At six weeks after the birth, the GP will give both mother and baby a health check-up.

Every family with children under five years has access to a named health visitor who will check things such as:
▶ the baby's growth and development
▶ teething
▶ feeding
▶ any health concerns.

They will also be there for the parents to provide support with parenting, family planning, any health concerns about themselves as well as health promotion.

Children may need paediatric care from birth if they have a congenital condition such as cerebral palsy, spina bifida or hydrocephalus. These are long-term conditions that cannot be cured but the symptoms and complications can usually be controlled with treatments. Parents will need a lot of support from healthcare professionals as these can be challenging conditions for both the child and the family who look after them. If a parent/carer feels they need extra support, they could speak to their health visitor or GP who could refer them to their local council for a needs assessment. This could lead to extra family support.

Early childhood, 3 to 8 years

Children at this age may be assessed as having **special educational needs and disability (SEND)** and may need an individual learning plan, also known as an **individual education plan (IEP)**, to allow them to access education in a way suitable for their needs. An IEP builds on the curriculum that the child is following and sets out the strategies being used to meet the child's specific educational needs. However, a child may need an **education and healthcare (EHC) plan** if they need more than just educational support at school. This is when there is involvement from different professionals in education, health and social care. The local authority reviews the needs assessment and decides whether to issue an EHC plan or not. Where possible, this is drawn up with the young person's involvement. The local authority has a legal duty to secure educational provision detailed in the EHC plan. The local healthcare provider has a legal duty to arrange healthcare provision. However, although social care can be specified on the plan, there is no legal duty to provide this except for care provided under the Chronically Sick and Disabled Persons Act 1970.

Age	Vaccines	Diseases protected against
1 year	• Hib/MenC (1st dose) • MMR (1st dose) • Pneumococcal (PCV) (2nd dose) • MenB (3rd dose)	Hib/MenC: Haemophilus influenzae type B (Hib) and meningitis C MMR: measles, mumps and rubella
2 years to 10 years	• Flu vaccine every year	Seasonal flu
3 years and 4 months	• MMR (2nd dose) • 4-in-1 preschool booster	4-in-1 preschool booster: diphtheria, tetanus, whooping cough and polio
12 years to 13 years	• HPV	HPV (human papillomavirus): cancers caused by HPV
14 years	• 3-in-1 teenage booster • MenACWY	3-in-1 teenage booster: tetanus, diphtheria and polio MenACWY: meningitis and septicaemia

▲ Vaccines offered to children aged 1 to 15

Source: NHS vaccination schedule

Adolescence, 9 to 18 years

Due to their rapidly changing physical, sexual, cognitive and emotional development, adolescents pose different challenges for healthcare services. A wide range of healthcare professionals are involved in their healthcare at primary and referral level. Adolescents may suffer from mental health conditions such as anxiety, depression, suicidal thoughts, self-harm and panic attacks. They may need referrals to Children and Adolescent Mental Health Services (CAMHS). Beyond puberty and into late teenage years, individuals may also need to be directed to advice about sexual and reproductive health, such as sexually transmitted infections (STIs) and contraception.

Early adulthood, 19 to 45 years

Parenthood is often a focus for adults in this age range. Pregnant women are offered two ultrasound pregnancy scans, one at 8–14 weeks and another at 18–21 weeks, the appointments for which also involve various checks on their health and that of the foetus. For instance, they have blood tests for hepatitis, HIV and syphilis and will be screened for sickle cell and thalassaemia. Antenatal classes are offered by the NHS and can take place in health centres where information about pregnancy, keeping healthy, labour and birth, and pain relief methods are covered. These classes include breastfeeding workshops. Partners are welcome to attend these classes to learn how to provide support.

Women will be offered cervical screenings from the age of 25 until they are 64. This is a test to detect cancer of the cervix, which is the opening to the womb from the vagina – a sample of cells is taken from the cervix. Just as women check their breasts for lumps, men are recommended to examine their testicles for lumps or swellings regularly.

When offered	Vaccines
During flu season	Flu vaccine
From 16 weeks pregnant	Whooping cough (pertussis) vaccine (offered so mother can pass on immunity to her baby)

▲ Vaccines offered to pregnant women

Middle adulthood, 46 to 65 years

During this middle adulthood period, women between the ages of 50 and 70 will be offered breast screening to check for any abnormalities such as lumps. Men at the age of 65 will have abdominal aortic aneurysm (AAA) screening. This screening checks for swelling in the aorta, which is more common in men than in women. Between the ages of 60 and 74 people will have the opportunity to have a bowel screening. People should also have regular eye tests once they are over the age of 40, particularly if they have any sight problems.

Later adulthood, 65 years onwards

Many people remain remarkably fit into extreme old age, staying physically strong and mentally agile. According to Age UK, '"frailty" is a term that's used a lot for older people when assessing their overall health but is often misunderstood. When used properly, it refers to a person's mental and physical resilience, or their ability to bounce back and recover from events like illness and injury.' A single injury or illness can lead to older people being labelled as frail, for example, a fall or a urinary infection. People living with frailty can lead a full and independent life; to achieve this they need joined-up services which are planned to meet their needs – 10 per cent of over 65s live with frailty (the risk of falls or illnesses which may necessitate admission to hospital), which rises to between 25 per cent and 50 per cent for over 85s.

Age	Vaccines
65 years	Pneumococcal (PCV)
65 years and every year after*	Flu vaccine
70 years	Shingles vaccine

▲ Vaccines offered to adults

*Some younger individuals with certain health conditions may also be offered this

Source: NHS vaccine schedule

Test yourself

1 List three examples of age-associated diseases.
2 Describe how retirement can affect an individual.
3 Explain why pregnant women are offered a vaccine for flu and whooping cough.

A9.12 Methods of supporting individuals to look after themselves at various stages of life

Young people

Self-awareness is an important skill for anyone to have regardless of age. It is the ability to tune into your emotions, feelings, thoughts and actions as well as abilities and preferences. It is also about recognising that how you act affects yourself and others. The World Health Organization (WHO) recognises self-awareness as one of the 10 core life skills. Young people should be encouraged at an early age to have good habits which will help them throughout their lives, including eating healthily and good sleep habits. School educates young people through a programme of PSHE.

Healthy adults

High self-esteem helps individuals to relate more easily to the people they meet, such as family, friends and colleagues. A person who has a high self-concept will often view life very positively and value themselves as a person. If a person thinks they are valuable, they will expect others to value them. An individual with low self-esteem will not feel good about themselves. They will not like the image they have of themselves and as a consequence may not be able to relate well to others. They may feel that others do not value them and that they are unable to make a worthwhile contribution to society. The overall result will be that such people have a very low opinion of themselves and a poor self-portrait. This could cause individuals to become isolated from other people and have few friends.

Hopefully by adulthood, individuals will have developed good habits such as regular exercise, a healthy, balanced diet and good sleep habits. They will know how to keep themselves healthy by brushing their teeth, not smoking or overindulging in alcohol, etc. If they have any health issues it is good practice to follow them up promptly. For example, any unexplained bleeding or lumps could be a sign of cancer and if diagnosed early can be dealt with before it spreads to other parts of the body. This is the reason regular uptake of screening is so important. It is recommended that adults have a dental check-up at least every six months. It is important for people to unwind at the end of a working day and if they have problems, to be able to talk them over with trusted friends.

Unfortunately, following all the good advice on being healthy does not guarantee that the individual will not have any health issues as some aspects are out of an individual's control. For example, they may have reproductive issues such as a problem with conception or an inherited genetic condition.

Adults who have health or wellbeing concerns

Negative stereotyping about age highlights sickness, dependency and not being able to be sociable. Some may see older people as slow or inefficient, due to ageism, which is a form of discrimination and should not be tolerated. Adults who have disabilities may also face discriminatory attitudes. With the right support, individuals from both groups should be able to live fulfilling lives.

Disabled individuals will be supported through statutory services if they are assessed by the local authority as eligible. They may receive a personalised budget to meet their needs, and provisions such as home care or respite or day services may be made. In the UK there is a Blue Badge scheme to enable eligible individuals to use disabled parking bays and a Radar key scheme for access to public bathrooms.

It is important to remember that not all disabilities are visible. For instance, some people may face harassment or suspicion for parking with a disability permit and then walking from their cars. However, just because a person is not in a wheelchair does not mean they are capable of walking any distance without pain or discomfort. Certain conditions may also mean that an individual's mobility varies – some days they may be able to walk and others they may not.

Old age 65+

Any adult over the age of 40 can have an NHS health check-up. This is a preventative measure as when people age, they are more likely to develop signs of common conditions such as stroke, heart attack, Type 2 diabetes or dementia. The health check-up is designed to detect early signs of these conditions so they can be treated before they cause serious harm.

People are increasingly living for longer. This is the result of new technology such as screening, improved standards of living and greater awareness of what contributes to a healthy lifestyle. Many are able to carry on working after the traditional retirement age and many contribute to the communities in which they live. For example, they may be members of committees, volunteer in charity organisations or participate in sports activities. Some will develop health problems during this stage of life, but it is the process of helping them manage and cope with the problems that is important. For older adults who do develop health problems, a wide range of services are available to help, each designed to encourage as much independence as possible so that individuals feel in control of their lives. Examples of such services include:

▶ handyperson services
▶ lunch clubs
▶ day centres
▶ exercise and physical activities
▶ social activities
▶ advice lines on pensions, insurance, etc.

End of life

An **end-of-life care plan** is a written plan that sets out an individual's preferences, wishes, beliefs and values regarding their future care in circumstances where they are likely to be near death. This is where they can express their wishes about where they would like to receive care (say, at home or in a hospice rather than in hospital) and where they would like to die. The plan can contain an advanced decision (so if their condition deteriorates, they have already recorded their choices) or living will in case the individual cannot communicate their wishes if they become too ill. They can document that they wish to refuse a certain type of treatment in the future. For example, they may wish to refuse chemotherapy in favour of quality of life, or have a '**Do not resuscitate**' instruction on their plan. Having this kind of care plan can empower the individual to know that their wishes will be respected, help to guide professionals working with them and take away difficult decisions from their family.

This plan may include **power of attorney**. This is a legal document which gives someone the authority to act on behalf of another person. For example, if a parent's mind is deteriorating through dementia and they recognise that they will not be able to make decisions in the future, they may appoint their daughter/son as their spokesperson who will make decisions for and about them. They know the family member will act in their best interests.

Project practice

Choose two health professionals from the following list:
▶ health education specialist
▶ health visitor
▶ school nurse
▶ community nurse
▶ GP
▶ sexual health adviser.

1 Write a message requesting an interview with the chosen health professionals and/or invite them to your centre. Ask them for a thorough description of their role in promoting health.
2 Ask the professionals about the skills and qualities they require to meet the needs of individuals.
3 In their time working in the industry, have they noticed any changes in the approach to healthcare?

Assessment practice

1. The NHS advice is that an adult should do 30 minutes of moderately intense exercise for 5 days each week if they wish to improve their health. Barney is a 31-year-old male who does 50 minutes a week in the gym. He thinks this is sufficient exercise to keep him healthy. Explain to Barney why this may not be sufficient.

2. Kourosh is in hospital after a minor stroke. He tells you he has a friend who has an end-of-life care plan and he wants to know more about this for himself. Outline how you would explain what an end-of-life plan is to Kourosh.

3. Samadara drinks two glasses of wine (approximately half a 750 ml bottle) every evening when she gets home from work. Over the weekend she drinks two more 750 ml bottles of wine. She does not think she drinks too much as she never feels drunk.
   a. Work out the units Samadara consumes over a week.
   b. Outline the long-term damage that drinking over the recommended amount of alcohol will do to her liver.

4. Will is 42 years of age. He has severe learning disabilities and has recently moved into residential care after the death of his father. His healthcare worker Mandi has decided that Will is overweight and needs to cut out sweets, chocolates, etc. which he loves. Portions of cakes and puddings are reduced. Will is very upset and does not understand what has happened, as nothing was discussed with him. Mandi did give Will a booklet on healthy eating. Discuss whether this was the right approach for Mandi to take.

5. Aadesh is an intensive care nurse looking after a patient with pneumonia. He is taking the baseline observations of this patient. Choose **three** of the baseline observations and explain why these are important for the patient's welfare.

6. Sara is 55 and has had a stroke. She has lost the use of her left side and feels very depressed. Which assistive aids for eating might you recommend for Sara? How else could you support her in this situation?

7. Mark goes to his medical centre for a full health check-up. He is shocked when the nurse tells him his blood pressure is 163/99. The nurse tells Mark he will have his blood pressure checked again next week. Explain how Mark could reduce his blood pressure without taking any medication.

8. Summarise the main points of the NHS Long Term Plan.

9. Explain how ageing affects the memory.

10. You are looking after the nutrition of Emily who is in hospital with a broken hip. She is not making the progress she was expected to as she does not eat the meals provided because she does not like the food. Describe what you could do to help her and what advice you could give her to persuade her to eat her meals.

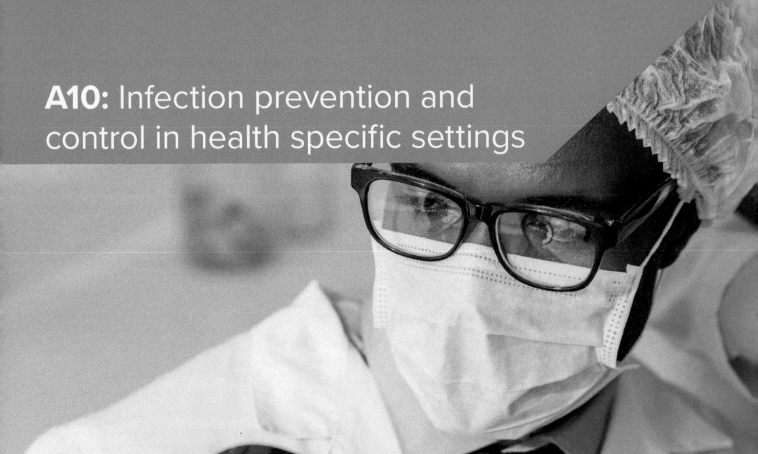

A10: Infection prevention and control in health specific settings

Introduction

Infection control is very important for good health, especially in large organisations such as hospitals, schools and residential homes where an outbreak of an infectious disease can affect hundreds of people, sometimes causing death. The recent outbreak of COVID-19 across the world caused many excess deaths and increased the public's awareness of the importance of hygiene measures.

In March 2012, NICE (the National Institute for Health and Care Excellence) produced guidelines, revised in May 2019, *Healthcare Associated Infections: Prevention and Control in Primary and Community Care*, which laid out infection prevention and control measures that should be taken by all healthcare workers involved in care of patients. It applies to care in the community, such as in **general practice** (GP surgeries) or **residential care settings**, as well as in patients' homes or **domiciliary care**.

The guidelines state that, as a minimum, any healthcare workers in these settings should be educated about standard principles of infection prevention and control. They must also be trained in hand decontamination, the use of personal protective equipment, and the safe use and disposal of sharps. This chapter details these considerations and also discusses microbial resistance and how to respond to this issue.

Learning outcomes

The core knowledge outcomes that you must understand and learn:

A10.1 the techniques for infection control and why they are important in stopping the spread of infection

A10.2 the importance of good handwashing techniques and personal hygiene and how to practise this in relation to infection control

A10.3 the scientific principles of cleaning, disinfecting, sterilisation and decontamination

A10.4 the differences in procedures for cleaning, disinfecting and sterilisation

A10.5 the meaning of impact of antimicrobial resistance, including how this can potentially impact infection control and the ways in which to reduce microbial resistance.

A10.1 The techniques for infection control and why they are important in stopping the spread of infection

Techniques for infection control

The best way of preventing infection spreading in the **home** or anywhere is to keep the hands clean by washing frequently with warm water and soap. The hands can pass on an **infection** and can pick up germs from one place and transfer them to another. The importance of this basic step should not be underestimated and should become part of your and everyone's routine.

Use of personal protective equipment (PPE)

Personal protective equipment – known as **PPE** – is used to protect healthcare workers while performing specific tasks that might involve them coming into contact with infectious materials. Disposable gloves are worn when performing or assisting in a procedure that involves a risk of contact with body fluids, broken skin, dirty instruments and harmful substances such as chemicals and disinfectants. This includes procedures that involve:

- ▶ a risk of being splashed by body fluids (blood, saliva, **sputum**, vomit, urine or faeces, for instance)
- ▶ contact with the patient's eyes, nose, ears, lips, mouth or genital area, or any instruments that have been in contact with these
- ▶ contact with an open wound or cut
- ▶ handling potentially harmful substances, such as disinfectants.

Aprons are not needed to carry out many normal aspects of day-to-day care with patients, such as helping them to go for short walks, but they will be needed for:

- ▶ performing or assisting in a procedure that might involve splashing of body fluids
- ▶ performing or helping the patient with personal hygiene tasks such as washing
- ▶ carrying out cleaning and tidying tasks in the patient's living space, such as bed-making.

Healthcare workers routinely use face masks as part of their PPE. However, these do not protect the wearer from inhaling small particles that can remain airborne for long periods of time. Face masks are effective barriers for retaining large droplets which can be released from the wearer through talking, coughing or sneezing. They are useful in many patient care areas as they may reduce wound site contamination during surgical or dental procedures. But face masks cannot be used as protection from many hazardous airborne materials. Often these face masks are used in conjunction with a face shield.

Since the COVID-19 pandemic, Public Health England (PHE) has updated its advice for the protection of healthcare staff. It said, 'Any clinician working in a hospital or primary care within 2 metres of a COVID-19 patient should wear an apron, gloves, surgical mask and eye protection.'

Key terms

Residential care setting: where long-term care is given to adults or children who live in a residential (designed for people to live in) setting rather than their own home.

Domiciliary care: care offered to any individuals living in their own homes to help them stay there rather than go into residential care. This can include help with personal tasks such as bathing, getting out of bed, dressing, and breakfast and other meals.

Infection: the process of bacteria, viruses or other micro-organisms (such as fungi or parasites) invading the body, making someone ill or diseased.

Sputum: mucus or coughed-up material (phlegm) from lower airways (trachea and bronchi).

Practice point

Practise putting on and removing PPE. The chart from the NHS Infection Prevention Control website will help you: Correct-order-for-putting-on-and-removing-PPE-July-2020.pdf (www.infectionpreventioncontrol.co.uk/content/uploads/2020/07/Correct-order-for-putting-on-and-removing-PPE-July-2020.pdf)

Use of cleaning and disinfecting agents

Cleaning must be carried out before disinfecting begins. Cleaning will remove contamination (blood, vomit, faeces, etc.) and many micro-organisms using **detergent**, for example, washing-up liquid and warm water. Disinfection can then take place. Care must be taken as misuse and overuse of chemical **disinfectants** may result in damage to the user, patient or equipment and may also result in the development of antimicrobial resistance.

When using any cleaning or disinfecting agent the healthcare worker must be sure to:

▶ follow the manufacturer's instructions for dilution
▶ never just guess how much to dilute a disinfectant
▶ wear personal protective equipment
▶ ensure adequate ventilation
▶ never use two disinfectants together
▶ not add anything to a disinfectant (including detergent) as this may result in a dangerous chemical reaction
▶ discard disinfectant solution after use
▶ not 'top up' solutions of disinfectant with anything but dispose of any unused solution.

Best practice for disinfection is to use a diluted chlorine-based product such as household bleach.

Area contaminated with blood or blood stained
Household bleach 10 parts per million (ppm) available chlorine
Dilution of 1 in 10. For example, 10 ml of household bleach to 100 ml of water OR 100 ml of household bleach to 1 litre of water

Area contaminated with body fluid (not blood or blood stained)
Household bleach 1000 ppm available chlorine
Dilution of 1 in 100, for example, 10 ml of household bleach in 1 litre of water

▲ Dilution guidelines for disinfection

Key terms

Detergent: purifying or cleansing agent which increases the ability of water to break down grease or dirt. Detergents act like soap but unlike soap they are derived from organic acids rather than fatty acids. Common examples are laundry detergent, e.g. soap powder or liquid, and dish detergent, e.g. washing-up liquid.

Disinfectant: a substance that destroys, inactivates or significantly reduces the concentration of pathogens such as bacteria, viruses or fungi.

Aseptic: free from contamination caused by harmful bacteria, viruses or other micro-organisms; surgically sterile or sterilised.

Effective handwashing techniques

The World Health Organization introduced the '5 moments of hand hygiene' in an attempt to reduce the occurrence of healthcare-associated infections. Many NHS trusts in England have adopted this model of hand hygiene, which prompts healthcare workers to clean their hands at five distinct stages of caring for the patient. Cleaning hands is the simplest, cheapest and most effective way of preventing germs being passed from one person to another. According to WHO, there are five moments for hand hygiene.

Moments	When	Why
1 Before patient contact	Always clean your hands before touching a patient.	To protect patient against germs on the healthcare worker's hands.
2 Before a clean/aseptic procedure	Clean hands immediately before any clean/aseptic procedure as this prevents contamination. An aseptic procedure could be a change of dressing or bandage for the patient.	To prevent harmful germs from both healthcare worker and patient entering the patient's body if dressing is not kept sterile.
3 After body fluid exposure risk	Clean hands immediately after exposure to body fluids (and after glove removal).	To protect healthcare worker and environment from harmful patient germs.
4 After patient contact	Clean hands when leaving patient's side, after touching the patient and their immediate surroundings.	To protect healthcare worker and environment from harmful patient germs.
5 After contact with patient surroundings	Clean hands after touching any object or furniture in the patient's immediate surroundings, when leaving – even if patient has not been touched.	To protect healthcare worker and environment from the patient's germs.

▲ Five moments for hand hygiene

Source: Adapted from www.who.int/gpsc/tools/5momentsHandHygiene_A3.pdf?ua=1

Good personal hygiene and uniform requirements

To prevent infection among patients, it is essential that uniforms are clean. The Royal College of Nursing advises that sufficient uniforms must be provided to enable freshly laundered clothing to be worn for each shift or work session, with access to spare items if staff clothing becomes contaminated (for example, splashed with blood and/or body fluids). It also suggests that uniform fabrics must be capable of withstanding water temperatures of at least 60 °C (which is high enough to kill bacteria and viruses) and tumble drying.

Tying hair back, where it is long enough, is essential in health and social care as it can contain bacteria which could cause infection. Furthermore, cross infection (transferring infections from one place to another) could occur if the hair is allowed to trail into body fluids when a healthcare worker is cleaning up a patient or serving food on the ward. Besides this, long hair which was not tied back would get in the way of many tasks, risking getting caught or impairing vision.

Safe disposal of sharps/appropriate waste segregation and disposal

Clinical waste for disposal should be separated into different containers which indicate how hazardous or infectious the waste might be. A colour-coding system has been developed to indicate to everyone dealing with the waste just what is in each container and how it needs to be disposed of to prevent the possibility of the spread of infection, either to the people handling the waste or to the environment. For example, if highly infectious waste were to be sent to a landfill site instead of to an incinerator, the material could leak into the water table, e.g. polluting rivers and sewers, and could cause disease. See the table for details on the colour coding of waste containers/plastic bags.

Colour	Type of waste	Disposal method
Sharps bin with purple lid	Sharps used to administer cytotoxic or cytostatic (used in the treatment of cancers) medicinal products	Incineration
Red clinical waste bin	Body parts, organs, blood bags, blood preserves	Incineration

Colour	Type of waste	Disposal method
Sharps bin with yellow lid	Sharps and syringe bodies with residual medicinal product	Incineration
Yellow waste bags	Highly infectious waste plus anatomical waste from theatres and diagnostic specimens	Incineration
Blue clinical waste bin	Waste medicines, out-of-date medicines, medicine liquids in bottles, blister packs of pills	Incineration
Orange plastic bags	General infectious waste, soiled dressings and autoclaved laboratory waste	**Autoclave** (to treat with high temperature steam – see page 190 later in this chapter)
Sharps bin with Orange lid	Sharps not contaminated with medicinal products, typically phlebotomy (blood test) sharps	Either incineration or autoclave
Tiger/ yellow-and-black striped bags	Offensive/hygiene waste which is not infectious	May be recycled, incinerated or landfilled in suitably permitted/licensed facilities
Black plastic bags	General waste such as packaging, plastic containers, tissues, flowers, sandwich wrappings	Requires disposal by landfill

▲ Colour coding of waste containers/plastic bags

For the safety of everybody who will handle the waste after it has left the clinical area, it is important for the person disposing of the waste to put it in the correct container. This avoids accidental infection such as being injected by used needles, which could have serious health implications. Also, as clinical waste is extremely expensive to dispose of, it is essential that any other type of waste is not put in with the clinical waste, which would result in the healthcare organisation paying a very high price for disposing of non-clinical waste.

Importance in stopping the spread of infection

Prevent harm caused to both individuals and healthcare workers

As mentioned above, good standards of personal hygiene are essential to ensure the health and welfare of individuals and healthcare staff. Poor personal hygiene causes the spread of more diseases than anything else. For example, influenza and colds are spread by people coughing and sneezing without covering their face. Unwashed hands after using the lavatory spread germs such as **norovirus**.

Poor infection control is responsible for **healthcare-associated infections (HCAIs)**, which can develop either as a direct result of healthcare interventions such as medical or surgical treatment or from being in contact with a healthcare setting. The term HCAI covers a wide range of infections, including those caused by methicillin-resistant Staphylococcus aureus (MRSA) and Clostridium difficile (C. difficile). HCAIs pose a serious risk to patients, staff and visitors as these diseases are easily spread from one person to another. They can result in significant extra costs and workload for the NHS and cause significant **morbidity** (likelihood of disease) to those infected. As a result, infection prevention and control is a key priority for the NHS.

> **Key terms**
>
> **Norovirus:** very infectious virus common in the winter which causes diarrhoea and vomiting.
>
> **Healthcare-associated infections (HCAIs):** infections which can occur as a result of having treatment in hospital or after surgical or medical treatment.

> **Test yourself**
>
> 1 Explain the importance of using the correct colour waste bags or bins.
> 2 Choose two pieces of personal protective equipment and explain how they can protect the healthcare worker.
> 3 State why healthcare workers' uniforms must be washed at 60 °C.
> 4 Explain the meaning of aseptic.
> 5 Explain three of the '5 moments of hand hygiene' as a method of infection control.

A10.2 The importance of good handwashing techniques and personal hygiene and how to practise this in relation to infection control

Importance of good handwashing techniques and personal hygiene

Help prevent the control of disease, infection and as a result, illness

The purpose of handwashing is to remove or destroy any bacteria picked up on the hands. Bacteria and viruses can easily be spread by touch. They may be picked up from contaminated surfaces, objects or people, then passed on to others. Effective hand **decontamination** (see page 183) – either by washing with soap and water or with an alcohol-based hand rub – is recognised as crucial in reducing avoidable infection. From the beginning of the COVID-19 pandemic, the government's Chief Medical Officer has urged people to wash their hands frequently as one part of the slogan in Figure 10.1. Shops and other public buildings now provide sanitiser for people to decontaminate their hands before and after entering.

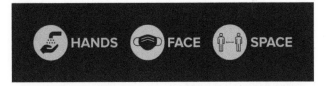

▲ Figure 10.1 Hands, face, space logo from the NHS

Reduce the risk of disease, infection and illness being passed on through cross contamination

Handwashing with soap and water is effective in removing most micro-organisms from the hands and can go a long way towards preventing cross contamination (where food is contaminated by contact with other food) and **cross infection** (where infection is passed from one person to another, which occurs when microbes are passed between them). This is especially the case in health settings where more harmful organisms might be picked up from infected individuals and passed onto others if hand hygiene is ignored. In clinical areas, soap should be supplied as liquid soap in disposable containers or containers that are washed and dried before refilling. The containers should never be topped up or added to but must be cleaned out before re-use. Cross infection can happen in many ways from:

▶ healthcare workers' clothes
▶ their hands if unwashed or when using the same pair of gloves for more than one individual
▶ droplets of infection in the air (breathing it in)
▶ inadequately sterilised equipment or instruments
▶ inadequately washed bed linen (e.g. bed sheets, pillowcases).

Simple precautions such as washing hands between individuals, wearing the uniform only at work and ensuring all equipment and linen are adequately sterilised, will contribute to the control of cross infection. Cleaning, disinfecting and sterilising (see page 190 later in this chapter) are essential components in an infection-free environment.

Key term

Cross infection: the process by which bacteria or other micro-organisms are unintentionally transferred from one person to another, with harmful effect.

Case study

Chelsey

Chelsey, a student nurse, goes onto a ward that has an outbreak of norovirus. She is in full PPE as she helps tend to one of the affected patients who is in an isolation room on the ward. She finishes her task without removing her PPE and goes to help another patient go to the toilet.

Explain to Chelsey the likely outcome of her actions. What would have been good practice in this instance?

Legal requirements

The **Health and Safety at Work Act 1974** places responsibility on both the employer and individual employees to do what is reasonable to adequately control the risks of infection for staff and others. Under this legislation, all employees have the responsibility to co-operate with the employer on matters of health and safety and in the context of healthcare, particularly regarding the reduction of

risks from HCAIs. Instruction should be given on the use of appropriate PPE as part of this. It is also the employees' responsibility to identify any issues and report them.

The **Control of Substances Hazardous to Health (COSHH)** Regulations 2002 require employers to prevent or control exposure of employees, patients, visitors, etc. to biological hazardous substances, such as certain micro-organisms, at work. In hospitals and residential care homes, risks may arise from the handling of clinical waste and soiled laundry, which can be contaminated with a variety of pathogenic organisms. Such hazards should be identified and assessed under the provisions of the COSHH Regulations 2002. Procedures for safe handling, segregation, storage, spillage control and disposal should be laid down and staff should be trained accordingly. Staff should be protected against hazardous substances they may have to deal with as part of their work activities, for example, staff in residential care homes and hospitals are particularly at risk from clinical waste, including soiled laundry. Therefore, staff should be trained in safe working procedures and hygiene standards, as well as being given appropriate protective equipment.

As well as protecting staff from biological hazards, the requirements of COSHH affect the use and storage of hazardous materials. The regulations state that all settings must have a COSHH file, which is kept up to date, listing all the hazardous substances stored on their premises. Hazardous substances in healthcare settings include some cleaning materials, disinfectants and micro-organisms from soiled laundry and clinical waste. All cleaning materials, for example, bleach, should be kept out of reach of vulnerable individuals. This can be achieved by keeping the substances in a locked cupboard when not in use. When working with any hazardous substances, the healthcare worker should ensure precautions listed in the COSHH file are followed. Guidance for storage of hazardous substances is also given in the COSHH file.

The Reporting of Injuries, Diseases and Dangerous Occurrences 2013 (RIDDOR) is concerned with certain types of injury, occupational ill-health and dangerous occurrences within the workplace. These include serious incidents that involve any individual present, including non-employees, for instance visitors or patients. As well as reporting these, the employer has the responsibility of reporting certain notifiable diseases (see Figure 10.2). It is important that such diseases are reported to the relevant medical authorities so that the wider community can be protected.

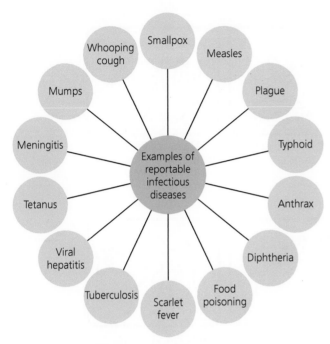

▲ Figure 10.2 Reportable infectious diseases

How to practise good handwashing techniques

Follow workplace guidance

Ayliffe handwashing technique/5 moments/12-point technique

The Ayliffe handwashing technique was developed in the 1960s by Professor Graham Ayliffe to reduce the spread of infection. It was adopted by hospitals in Britain, followed by the WHO in 2009. The 12-point technique shown in Figure 10.3 is the NHS version based on the Ayliffe model of cleaning the hands thoroughly. The 5 moments defines the key moments when healthcare professionals should wash/clean their hands (see the table on page 183). To facilitate effective hand hygiene, healthcare workers should:

► cover cuts with waterproof dressings to prevent harmful bacteria that may be present in the cut from being transferred to surfaces, patients or food
► keep their arms bare below the elbow, i.e. wear short sleeves or sleeves rolled up to elbows
► remove wrist or hand jewellery (for example, a watch or decorative rings with/without stones). NB: slim plain rings such as wedding rings may still be worn as they have no crevices to allow an accumulation of bacteria
► keep nails short and clean, as long nails allow build-up of dirt and bacteria
► not wear nail polish
► avoid acrylic/artificial nails which can harbour micro-organisms.

1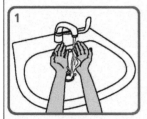
Wet hands
with water

2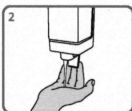
Apply enough soap
to cover all
hand surfaces

3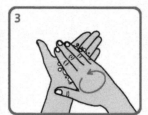
Rub hands palm
to palm

4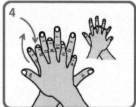
Rub back of each hand
with palm of other hand
with fingers interlaced

5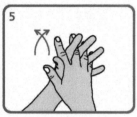
Rub palm to palm with
fingers interlaced

6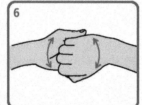
Rub with back of fingers
to opposing palms with
fingers interlocked

7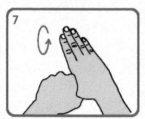
Rub each thumb clasped
in opposite hand using a
rotational movement

8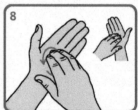
Rub tips of fingers in
opposite palm in a
circular motion

9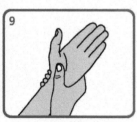
Rub each wrist with
opposite hand

10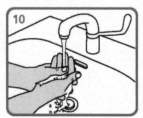
Rinse hands
with water

11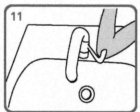
Use elbow to
turn off tap

12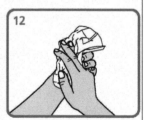
Dry thoroughly with
a single-use towel

13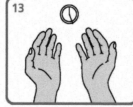
Handwashing should take
15–30 seconds

clean**your**hands®
campaign

NHS
National Patient
Safety Agency

© Crown copyright 2007 283373 1p 1k Sep07

Adapted from World Health Organization *Guidelines on Hand Hygiene in Health Care*

▲ Figure 10.3 Handwashing technique with soap and water

Research

Examine Figure 10.3. Do you use the correct method of washing your hands? Wash your hands the way you would normally. Then, if your school or college has one, use a hand inspection cabinet to see if your hands are really clean and free from bacteria. You may be surprised! Now repeat handwashing following Figure 10.3 and retest in the cabinet. Has this activity reinforced the importance of thorough handwashing?

Research

Find out about the provision of clean uniforms in your work placement. Does the organisation wash the uniforms or does the individual have to wash their own? What is the organisation's policy on uniform provision? Is the cleanliness of the individual's uniform checked? Present your findings to other students in your group and compare notes. What conclusions can you draw from all the information? Is it common practice for your placement to provide staff with clean uniforms? Is that the same for all placements?

How to practise good personal hygiene

Washing body and hair regularly

Healthcare workers need to ensure a high standard of personal hygiene. The skin has pores that need to be kept clean as this is where the body rids itself of grease and sweat. If skin is left unwashed then the smell is obvious. Extra care must be taken where sweat is trapped in folds of skin. Regular washing or showering will help prevent build-up of dirt and sweat. Regular use of deodorant and antiperspirant helps to prevent the build-up of stale smells and keeps the person feeling fresh. Some people need to wash their hair more than others because their skin and scalp are oilier. Dirty hair can spread infection, particularly if it is loose and hanging around the face.

Wearing clean uniform

As stated in section A10.1, the healthcare worker should wear a clean uniform every day in their place of work. The 2020 NHS guidance on uniforms and workwear suggests that ideally nursing staff should change out of their uniform before leaving work if there are changing facilities available. If there are no facilities, their uniform should be covered by a coat. This is because although there is no evidence of an infection risk from travelling in uniform, many people see it as unhygienic.

Cleaning teeth

Clean teeth mean healthy teeth and less chance of bad breath. Every time an individual eats, plaque starts to build up on their teeth. Teeth should be brushed at least twice a day – in the morning and before going to bed. Particular attention should be paid to the gumline as individuals often forget to brush their gums as well as their teeth. Anti-bacterial mouthwash can help to maintain oral hygiene. A visit to the dentist every six months is recommended to ensure any problems are spotted early.

Covering mouth and nose when coughing or sneezing

Covering the mouth and nose when coughing and sneezing helps reduce the spread of germs, including the highly contagious COVID-19 virus. The flu and other infections are spread through microscopic water droplets expelled from an infected person, commonly through coughing, sneezing and hand-to-mouth contact. Aside from washing the hands with warm water and soap, one of the most important and effective ways to stop the spread of germs is to cover the cough or sneeze. An uncovered cough or sneeze can send infected droplets up to six feet away and remain airborne for several hours. The live virus can also live on surfaces for up to 48 hours.

Maintaining short, neat and clean nails

Healthcare workers should have short, clean nails as dirt and bacteria can easily become trapped under long nails and contribute to the spread of illness and infection. Long nails are also more likely to snag or damage gloves worn as part of PPE.

A10.3 The scientific principles of cleaning, disinfecting, sterilisation and decontamination

Principles

Cleaning

Cleaning reduces the presence of micro-organisms on surfaces and instruments by removing visible foreign matter and this minimises the risk of the transfer of micro-organisms. The environment (e.g. door handles, toilet flush handles, taps) plays an important role in cross infection during outbreaks. Therefore, special attention must be paid to these fittings and anywhere that people have contact with, particularly during outbreaks of infectious diseases such as norovirus. In addition, accumulations of dust, dirt and liquid residues will increase infection risks and must be kept to a minimum by regular cleaning and by using good design features such as numerous, convenient handwashing sinks with automatic soap dispensers and toilet facilities that allow through access for cleaning in healthcare buildings.

A written cleaning schedule should be devised for each area, based on COSHH (see page 49), to include the regular removal of dust by damp dusting both high and low horizontal surfaces. As well as this, all health and social care settings should have in place a decontamination policy and cleaning schedule stating how and when to clean the different areas of the environment, fixtures, fittings and specialist equipment (for example, a hoist); what products and equipment to use when cleaning; what to do and what products to use if there is a spillage of blood or body fluids; what training staff need to implement the policy; and a description of individual responsibilities for cleaning.

Disinfecting

Disinfectant is used to reduce the number of micro-organisms on surfaces to a level that is considered safe, but which may not necessarily destroy some viruses or bacterial spores. Disinfection is usually acceptable for items that pose a medium risk of infection if these devices cannot be effectively sterilised. Chemical disinfection is not as effective as heat disinfection. Heat disinfectants such as dishwashers, washing machines and washer-disinfectors clean the item and then expose the items to hot water for the required time to achieve thermal disinfection:

- 65°C for 10 minutes
- 71°C for 3 minutes
- 80°C for 1 minute
- 90°C for 1 second.

While most chemical disinfectants are capable of inactivating bacteria and certain types of viruses (those which have an 'envelope', an outer layer), many are not so effective against some viruses, for example, the hepatitis viruses, cysts and bacterial spores.

Sterilisation

Sterilisation is used for food, medicine and surgical instruments, but some items are too fragile for sterilisation as the temperature is too high for them to withstand. To sterilise means to kill all microbes and their spores – whether harmful or not – present on a surface or object, and thus is more effective than disinfection. This can be done by using steam in machines called autoclaves which use steam heated to 121–134°C. Extreme care must be taken when using these machines as steam can scald the skin. Another method is to use direct heat, which can include incineration, boiling in water and dry heat, which inactivates and kills micro-organisms in objects such as glass and metals. Items that can get damaged by heat are subjected to chemical sterilisation, e.g. biological materials, fibre optics, electronics and plastics.

Irradiation, high pressure and filtration are other agents used in the sterilising process. Irradiation can be used for aseptic work areas and for sterilising surgical equipment. High-pressure sterilisation would be used to sterilise contaminated instruments. Filtration can be used to sterilise fluids such as drugs solutions which would be damaged by heat, irradiation or chemical sterilisation.

Decontamination

Decontamination is a process or combination of processes such as cleaning, disinfecting and sterilising that removes or destroys contaminants so that infectious agents cannot cause infection. As soon as a piece of equipment is contaminated with urine, blood, vomit, etc., it should be removed from service immediately. It must be decontaminated as soon as possible but best practice is to do it immediately, away from busy areas in the healthcare setting. Decontamination is essential to lower the number of cross infections between people and to prevent HCAIs.

Research

Research the cleaning schedule from your work placement, bringing a copy into your centre. Compare this with one used in another setting, e.g. if you are in a hospital you need to compare your cleaning schedule with that of another student who was in a different hospital setting, nursing home, etc. What are the similarities and differences?

Test yourself

1 Explain what disinfecting an item/area means.
2 Explain the most effective method of disinfection.
3 Explain what is meant by decontamination.
4 Describe the purpose of an autoclave.

A10.4 The differences in procedures for cleaning, disinfecting and sterilisation

Different procedures

Cleaning procedures

Cleaning tools/cloths and floor scrubbers

There is a national colour-coding scheme for hospital cleaning materials and equipment. All NHS organisations should have adopted this code for cleaning materials. All cleaning items, for example, cloths (re-usable and disposable), mops, buckets, aprons and gloves, should be colour coded according to where they are used. This also includes those items used to clean catering departments.

Colour	Application
Red	Bathrooms, washrooms, showers, toilets, basins and bathroom floors
Blue	General areas including wards, departments, offices
Green	Catering department, ward kitchen areas and patient food service at ward level
Yellow	Isolation areas

▲ National colour-coding scheme

Essential rules for safe cleaning procedures mean that healthcare workers should:
▶ use the correct colour for each area
▶ ensure cleaning equipment is stored away clean and dry
▶ change cleaning cloths at least daily
▶ change and launder mop heads daily
▶ use cleaning agents or detergents adhering to COSHH regulations.

Practice point

Thinking of your placement, notice if the cleaners are strict in following the national colour-coded scheme for cloths, cleaning tools and scrubbers, etc. Who checks if they are using the correct colours? Where is the policy document on this kept and are the cleaners aware of this? Have you noticed staff wearing different colour aprons for different areas?

Vacuum cleaners

Many hospitals require vacuuming of hard surface floors as opposed to dust mopping because vacuuming reduces the amount of dust and other bacteria such as spores that can become airborne. Vacuuming hard floors is considered highly effective in reducing the spread of infection in hospitals. Vacuum cleaners should be well maintained to minimise dust dispersal and be equipped with **HEPA filters**, especially for use in high-risk patient-care areas.

> ### Key term
>
> *HEPA (high-efficiency particulate air) filter:* a type of filter that can trap tiny particles that other vacuum cleaners would simply recirculate back into the air. HEPA vacuums are recommended for minimising dust and other common allergens.

The use of cleaning agents

Thorough cleaning with a neutral detergent and or biological cleaning solution and warm water (body temperature) will remove large numbers of micro-organisms from a surface, especially if the article can be rinsed. Micro-organisms reduce further as the surface dries. Devices cannot be effectively disinfected or sterilised without having first been thoroughly cleaned and dried.

Disinfecting (this involves the use of an agent known to destroy pathogenic micro-organisms)

Use of disinfectant agent

Sodium hypochlorite or bleach has a lot of clinical uses in healthcare, for example:

▶ cleaning environmental surfaces
▶ decontamination of blood spills
▶ disinfection of equipment
▶ disinfection of laundry.

It prevents the spread of infection among patients and healthcare workers. It is inexpensive and kills off micro-organisms which cause disease. When mixed with water, sodium hypochlorite becomes hypochlorous acid, which penetrates the normally resistant surfaces of micro-organisms and destroys them, along with any of their spores.

Sterilisation

Application of chemical

Sterilisation can be done by two main methods: physical and chemical. Physical methods include heat, irradiation and filtration (see below). Chemical methods involve using liquid and gaseous chemicals. Products that can get damaged by heat are subjected to chemical sterilisation, for example, biological materials, fibre optics, electronics and plastics. Though bleach solution is used as a disinfectant, it is much more concentrated in sterilisation, and the infected item is left immersed for a longer duration for effective sterilisation. Dry sterilisation process with chemicals is useful for sterilising plastic bottles which are used in medical and pharmaceutical applications.

Application of high pressure

This is a method of sterilisation that uses high temperature and pressure generated by water steam. It is a quick, effective and inexpensive method of eliminating dangerous micro-organisms. It is usually performed using a machine (an autoclave, see Figure 10.4) that can expose objects to high temperature, steam and high pressure. Autoclaves are often referred to as steam sterilisation machines. The moist heat works by **denaturing** the proteins that make up bacteria and viruses, making them unable to cause infection. The minimum exposure times in an autoclave are 30 minutes at 121 °C or 4 minutes at 132 °C. This method is usually used for sterilising surgical instruments.

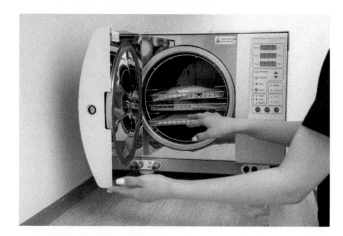

▲ Figure 10.4 An autoclave

> ### Key term
>
> *Denaturing:* protein structures are disrupted and changed so that they are no longer able to cause infection.

Application of heat

One method of sterilisation uses a high temperature in dry conditions without any water or steam to kill the micro-organisms. It works by oxidising the molecules, leading to the organism's death. The temperatures needed for this process are:

▶ 160 °C for 2 hours
▶ 170 °C for 1 hour
▶ 180 °C for 30 minutes.

Application of irradiation and filtration

Filtration does not destroy microbial contaminants (such as bacteria, moulds, yeasts, viruses, toxins) but removes them. The liquid or gas used in this process is passed through a filter with pores too small for the microbial contaminants to go through but the gas or liquid can pass through easily. It is common in pharmaceutical manufacture for products such as antibiotics and vaccines which are heat sensitive, and is used to prevent microbial contamination for patient safety. Fluids that would be damaged by heat, irradiation or chemical sterilisation such as a drug solution could also be sterilised by filtration. It can be used for clarification and sterilisation of liquids and gases.

Irradiation is the process of exposing surfaces and objects to different types of radiation for sterilisation. It is mainly electromagnetic radiation such as **ultraviolet light**, microwaves, **X rays** and **gamma rays** that is used for this purpose. Both X rays and gamma rays can be used for the sterilisation of medical equipment such as syringes, needles and cannulas. Microwaves can be used for the sterilisation of any medical instruments that do not melt. Ultraviolet light is usually used to sterilise patient rooms as well as operating theatres. If delivered at appropriate levels, all forms of ionising radiation can sterilise objects, including medical instruments. Irradiation works by disrupting the bacterial DNA of the micro-organisms, preventing bacterial division.

Key terms

Ultraviolet light: a form of radiation not visible to the human eye but present in sunlight.

X-ray: an electromagnetic wave of high energy and very short wavelength, which is able to pass through many materials, opaque to light.

Gamma radiation: a penetrating form of electromagnetic radiation arising from the radioactive decay of atomic nuclei.

Test yourself

1 Explain the importance of having a national colour-coding scheme for the NHS.
2 Within this colour-coding scheme, what should yellow-coded cleaning materials be used for?
3 Explain why HEPA filters should be used on vacuum cleaners within healthcare settings.
4 List the three categories of sterilisation methods.
5 Describe what is meant by irradiation.

A10.5 The meaning of impact of antimicrobial resistance, including how this can potentially impact infection control and the ways in which to reduce microbial resistance

The meaning of microbial resistance

Ability of a micro-organism to survive exposure to antimicrobial agents

An **antimicrobial** is something that kills micro-organisms or stops their growth. Antibiotics are antimicrobial agents used to treat infections caused by bacteria by inhibiting the growth of or destroying the bacteria. They do this in various ways, such as destroying the bacterial cell wall or making it harder to generate energy from glucose. **Microbial** or **antibiotic resistance** happens when bacteria develop the ability to survive exposure to antibiotics that were designed to kill them. Antibiotic-resistant bacteria will grow, multiply and cause infection even when exposed to antibiotics. Antibiotic resistance is a major obstacle in the treatment of infectious diseases caused by bacteria as it means that certain antibiotics can no longer be used to successfully treat some infections. This significantly affects the prevention and treatment of these diseases, increasing recovery time, time spent in hospital and death rates.

Impact of antimicrobial resistance

Overuse of antibiotics has reduced the overall effectiveness

Antibiotic or antimicrobial resistance occurs due to changes, or mutations, in the DNA of the bacteria, or the acquisition of antibiotic resistance genes from other bacterial species through **horizontal gene transfer**. These changes enable the bacteria to survive the effects of antibiotics designed to kill them. This means that when an antibiotic is used, all the bacteria that have not undergone a mutation are killed, while the antibiotic-resistant bacteria remain unaffected. The antibiotic-resistant bacteria continue to divide and grow, producing even more bacteria that are not affected by the antibiotic. The existence of resistant strains of bacteria means that these spread rapidly, posing a risk to public health.

The overuse of antibiotics has played a major role in increasing the prevalence of antibiotic-resistant bacteria. By frequently exposing bacteria to antibiotics, it makes the emergence and spread of resistance much more likely. Antibiotics are often prescribed for minor conditions that could easily get better on their own and patients often do not finish a course of antibiotics as prescribed by their doctor because their symptoms improve quickly. To help prevent further emergence of antibiotic resistance, steps are being taken to ensure that antibiotics are prescribed only when there is a clear need for them and that they are used properly (i.e. the full course is taken).

> ### Key term
>
> *Horizontal gene transfer*: the transfer of genetic material directly from one organism to another by various processes, without reproduction.

Overuse has led to the emergence of new strains of micro-organisms

The overuse of antibiotics in recent years means they have become less effective and this has led to the emergence of 'super bugs'. These are strains of bacteria that have developed resistance to many different types of antibiotics. The more antibiotics are used to treat less serious conditions, the more likely they are to become ineffective for treating more serious ones. Antibiotic prescribing and antibiotic resistance are linked. Areas with high levels of antibiotic prescribing also have high levels of resistance. The NHS and health organisations across the world are trying to reduce the use of antibiotics, especially for health problems that are relatively less serious.

Increase in super bugs (for example, MRSA and Clostridium difficile)

MRSA is one such super bug. Its full name is methicillin-resistant Staphylococcus aureus. The symptoms of MRSA depend on where the infection is. Most often, it causes mild infections on the skin, like sores, boils or abscesses. However, it can also cause more serious skin infections or infect surgical wounds, the bloodstream, the lungs or the urinary tract. MRSA is a type of staphylococcus aureus bacteria that has become resistant to the antibiotic methicillin and some other commonly used antibiotics. This means infections with MRSA can be harder to treat than other bacterial infections.

Clostridium difficile, also known as C. difficile or C. diff, are bacteria that can infect the bowel and cause diarrhoea. The infection most commonly affects people who have recently been treated with antibiotics. It can spread easily to others. C. diff bacteria are found in the digestive system of about 1 in every 30 healthy adults. The bacteria often live harmlessly because other bacteria normally found in the bowel keep them under control. But some antibiotics can interfere with the balance of bacteria in the bowel, which can cause the C. diff bacteria to multiply and produce toxins that make the person ill.

There are new super bugs evolving all the time and one of the most recent to emerge at the time of writing is called NDM-1. Bacteria that make an enzyme called NDM-1 can exist in different bacteria (for example, E-coli), making them resistant to the most powerful group of antibiotics. Another superbug is Klebsiella pneumoniae, which occurs naturally in the intestines without causing any problems, but if a person is unwell, it can infect the lungs, causing pneumonia and meningitis.

Reducing antimicrobial resistance

Antimicrobial stewardship coordinated program in the healthcare sector to promote appropriate use of antimicrobials

NICE, in collaboration with PHE, has developed clinical syndrome-specific guidance and advice offering evidence-based antimicrobial prescribing information for all care settings to help slow the development of antimicrobial resistances. This is part of an approach being promoted across the whole healthcare system and related organisations of **antimicrobial stewardship**, to ensure they continue to have some effectiveness in future. Clear guidelines are offered to prescribers on whether they should prescribe antibiotics or not. For example, they should:

▶ only prescribe antibiotics in line with NICE antimicrobial guidelines

▶ ensure medicines prescribed are clinically effective and cost effective.

Key term

Antimicrobial or antibiotic stewardship: the effort to measure and improve how antibiotics are prescribed by clinicians and used by patients. Improving antibiotic prescribing and use is critical in continuing to effectively treat infections.

Project practice

You are a student on the second year of your Health T Level. The ward manager has concerns about how staff use PPE. He has asked you to provide a straightforward handout with diagrams that any staff could follow to ensure the correct use of PPE.

You should cover considerations to do with:

▶ hands

▶ aprons

▶ gloves

▶ face masks

▶ face shields.

The handout should be succinct and easy to read.

Assessment practice

1 Bharti's partner is in hospital after heart surgery. Bharti goes to visit him every day. Today Bharti has had diarrhoea and vomiting. She now feels a little better and thinks she may be able to visit her partner this evening. Explain to Bharti why this is not a good idea.

2 Vinnie goes to his GP as he has a sore throat. His GP is reluctant to prescribe antibiotics for Vinnie as he has had two lots of antibiotics in recent months. Referring to advice from NICE/PHE, explain why his GP is concerned.

3 Explain the role that handwashing plays in infection control.

4 Name **two** super bugs that could be caught in hospital.

5 Patsy has responsibility for a ward in a large hospital. She has three new student healthcare workers starting next week. Explain three ways in which Patsy could encourage them to take care of their personal hygiene while on the ward.

6 Explain how the following legislation could be effective in infection control:

a The Health and Safety at Work Act 1974

b Control of Substances Hazardous to Health 2002

c The Reporting of Injuries, Diseases and Dangerous Occurrences.

A11: Safeguarding

Introduction

Everyone is entitled to be safe and protected from harm and abuse. This is the foundation of providing high-quality care, be it in hospital, residential care, nursing homes, schools and nurseries or community care. Safeguarding is the responsibility of everyone and all staff must do their part to look after the individuals in their care, many of whom will be vulnerable.

This unit covers the meaning of safeguarding and how government legislation helps to keep individuals safe. Learning about the different types of abuse and their signs and symptoms will help healthcare professionals to identify those who may be suffering. As well as the more well-known physical abuse, lesser-known types of abuse, including social and emotional, will be covered. These range from modern day slavery to honour-based abuse to forced marriage. Radicalisation and the Prevent strategy are also discussed as they are relevant. Of course, an important part of safeguarding is knowing what to do and who to contact if you suspect or if someone discloses abuse. Finally, the importance of healthcare staff acting in a professional manner throughout any interactions with patients, without stereotyping or leaping to conclusions based on little evidence, is considered.

Learning outcomes

The core knowledge outcomes that you must understand and learn:

A11.1 the meaning of safeguarding in the health sector and the key principles, including why safeguarding is important

A11.2 how to safeguard individuals in relation to legislation, policies and procedures

A11.3 factors that may contribute to an individual being vulnerable to harm or abuse and the vulnerable groups that require protection

A11.4 a range of different types of abuse and harm

A11.5 some of the possible signs of abuse or harm that may be identified in individuals using healthcare

A11.6 what action to take if abuse is suspected or disclosed

A11.7 actions that can be taken by individuals and organisations to reduce the chances of abuse

A11.8 the meaning of patient safety and clinical effectiveness, including why they are important

A11.9 what is meant by radicalisation, identifying signs of radicalisation and the purpose of the Prevent strategy (2011)

A11.10 the importance of positive behaviour, including a range of positive behaviours expected of a health professional

A11.11 the types of support for managing positive behaviour

A11.12 what is meant by a conflict of interest and how to deal with those while practising healthcare.

A11.1 The meaning of safeguarding in the health sector and the key principles, including why safeguarding is important

The meaning of safeguarding in the health sector

Protection of health, wellbeing and rights of individuals

Safeguarding means protecting an individual's health, wellbeing and human rights, enabling them to live free from harm, abuse and neglect. It is an essential part of providing high-quality healthcare and it is the responsibility of all staff working in any area of health.

Those most in need of protection according to the NHS include:

▶ children and young people
▶ adults at risk, such as those receiving care in their own home, people with physical, sensory and mental impairments, and those with learning disabilities.

Research

Ask your work placement or another setting for a copy of their safeguarding policy. Read the policy through and produce a summary of the main points. Compare policies between your classmates and look for common themes. Are the policies similar in their layout, contents and vocabulary? Are they easy to understand and follow? Draw conclusions from your comparisons.

The key principles of safeguarding in the health sector

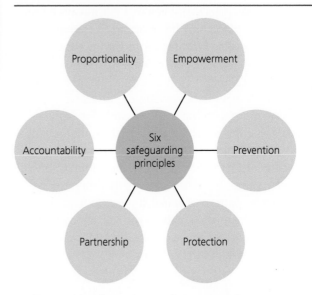

▲ Figure 11.1 Six safeguarding principles

Empowerment

The individual should be supported to make their own decisions based on the best possible information

One of six principles of safeguarding (see Figure 11.1) as defined by the Care Act 2014 is that anyone reporting their own abuse or neglect should be encouraged to make their own decisions about what happens next. They should be consulted and give their consent before any course of action is taken. Empowerment is to enable an individual to be in control of their life and able to make their own decisions. To do this, an individual must have access to all the information they need to help them come to a decision. The individual may need help and support from the healthcare worker to weigh up all the facts. It is about choice; giving this choice is central to the quality of care. It takes the power and control from the healthcare worker and places it where it belongs with the service user. Individuals should be encouraged to make their own decisions and to be involved as much as possible in making decisions about their own life as they know what they would like. In this way, people are empowered and allowed to keep their dignity and self-respect, and they also gain confidence.

Prevention

Better to take action before harm occurs

The prevention principle states that it is always better to take action before any harm occurs. It is vital that anyone responsible for safeguarding knows the red flags that may indicate abuse. Some are obvious and visible (physical marks or bruising) while others are not (slight changes in behaviour, e.g. an active child becoming more withdrawn). If a healthcare worker suspects that there may be abuse happening they must report their suspicions to their line manager. There will be a safeguarding policy to follow. Incidents of abuse may seem minor but when put together they could form a bigger pattern of abuse. It is better to raise a concern and be mistaken about the suspicion of abuse than to allow actual abuse to escalate and leave the individual at risk of further harm.

> **Case study**
>
> **Liam Fee**
>
> Go to: http://bbc.co.uk/news/uk-scotland-edinburgh-east-fife-36333032. Read the article on the abuse of toddler Liam Fee.
> ▶ Discuss how Liam Fee could have been protected from the abuse.

Proportionality

Actions should be proportionate to the risk, being overprotective can disadvantage service users to be able to make their own decisions

This principle states that those responsible for safeguarding should utilise preventative measures or respond to a safeguarding issue and provide the least intrusive response appropriate to the risk presented, not apply a one-size-fits-all response. This ensures that any decision takes the child, young person or adult into account when dealing with abuse. All risks are considered and addressed so that no further harm is done.

The action that is taken should be **proportionate** to the risk involved. If the risk is low, a large-scale overprotective approach can do more harm. It can make a child or young person feel uncomfortable and vulnerable, especially when a more restrained course of action would have been enough. For example, if one suspicious bruise were observed on an individual on

one occasion and there were no other signs of abuse, an appropriate response would be to note this with the date and time and keep it on record in case there were further suspicions of abuse.

Conversely, a serious case should be treated as such and if the individual is in immediate danger and the matter is urgent, dial 999. It can take a huge amount of effort and courage for someone to report instances of abuse or physical harm. They should feel that appropriate action is being taken. Otherwise, they might feel ignored or as though they are not believed. Feeling this way can have a significantly negative impact on a vulnerable person and discourage future disclosures from them or others.

To make the safeguarding processes proportionate, it is important to involve the vulnerable adult when making decisions. They can give input on what actions, in their mind, have the least impact on their quality of life and dignity. Reacting proportionately could require taking small, yet significant steps to handle an issue. Trying to tackle a large issue all at once can overwhelm the person.

Protection

Service users who are in greatest need of support and protection

Support and representation should be given to individuals who are most in need of help in the case of abuse. These include children and babies, people with physical, mental and/or learning disabilities or people who are socially isolated. Alcohol and drug abusers are also at risk, as are individuals who are isolated or weak and old. Regardless of background or circumstances, anyone should have access to the same advice and support. Organisations must ensure that they know:
▶ what to do if there are concerns
▶ how to stop the abuse
▶ how to offer help and support for people who are at risk.

Partnership

Working with a range of professionals, groups and communities to prevent, detect and report neglect or abuse

Safeguarding is a responsibility that is shared across organisations. Community groups, local authorities, healthcare organisations and schools should all understand their role and work together to offer support. Working together in partnership can offer the individual a wider base of support than working as an individual organisation. Sensitive information must only be shared with authorised people (e.g. safeguarding officers) and only when necessary; on a need-to-know basis. Note that the General Data Protection Regulation (GDPR) 2018 (see page 93) does not mean that information cannot be shared in a safeguarding situation. This means that individuals' consent is not needed if a person's welfare and safety is compromised. For example, if a teacher is concerned that a child has been seriously abused, they do not have to contact the parents for consent before they approach safeguarding authorities.

Case study

Winterbourne View

Read this news report from *The Guardian*: 'Winterbourne View care home staff jailed for abusing residents': www.theguardian.com/society/2012/oct/26/winterbourne-view-care-staff-jailed

As a group, discuss the behaviour of the staff at Winterbourne View in relation to safeguarding. What were your impressions of the way the residents were handled?

Accountability

Healthcare professionals need to be accountable for any activities in relation to safeguarding

Safeguarding is everybody's business. Healthcare workers must accept that they are accountable as individuals, services and as organisations. Everyone working in an organisation should be aware and know their safeguarding responsibility and their ability to watch out and raise concerns. At a hospital, for example, it is not just doctors and nurses who are responsible. Doctors, nurses, physiotherapists, porters, volunteers, support staff and hospital cooks, etc. should all know the signs of abuse to look out for and what to do in a variety of situations. All healthcare professionals should look out for signs of abuse.

Why safeguarding is important

Important for protection from harm, abuse and neglect

Safeguarding means protecting children and vulnerable adults from harm, abuse and neglect – there need to be strict safeguarding policies in place. All staff should be trained in safeguarding and be able to protect individuals from abuse. There are many different types of abuse, the most common of which are discussed later in this chapter, and abuse can affect the individual for the rest of their lives. Abuse can happen anywhere, not just in residential care and health settings but also in the home at the hands of family or friends. It is hidden and sometimes difficult to spot, especially if the individual who is being abused fears the abuser and does not want to tell anyone about what is happening to them. They may also feel ashamed and feel that they are somehow to blame for the situation.

To identify signs of abuse, anyone working in healthcare will need to use skills such as observation and communication with other colleagues to capture the full picture. Individuals who are being abused sometimes change their behaviour and show emotional signs, such as retreating into themselves or being bad tempered and lashing out at others. This is particularly the case if the abused individual does not have the vocabulary to describe the abuse, so they feel frustrated. However, this is not always the case, and some individuals may show no external sign of the abuse, instead keeping it locked up inside.

There is legislation and government guidance in place to ensure safeguarding is carried out properly, such as the Disclosure and Barring Service (DBS). All organisations such as schools, hospitals, faith groups, sports clubs, etc. that work with children or vulnerable adults must have safeguarding policies and procedures in place. However, this is only effective in terms of preventing reoffending of known abusers with police records – it alone cannot solve the problem of abuse.

A11.2 How to safeguard individuals in relation to legislation, policies and procedures

Mental Capacity Act (2005) plus Amendment (2019)

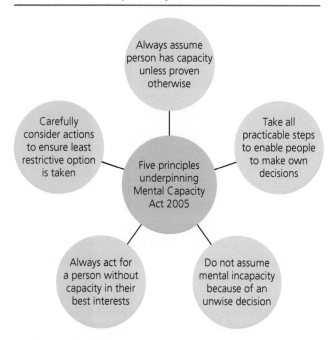

▲ Figure 11.2 Five principles underpinning the Mental Capacity Act 2005

The default for all individuals over the age of 18 is that consent is required for any decisions about health or care and the individual's right to give or withdraw this is paramount. Nonetheless, some adults may be judged to **lack capacity** to do this, for example, individuals with learning disabilities, but this may affect anyone at some time in their life in the form of dementia and/or severe mental health issues. An individual's capacity could also be affected by a stroke or a serious brain injury. The Mental Capacity Act 2005 was introduced in response to widespread concerns about the limited account taken of the voices and rights of such adults to make decisions about their care and treatment. This particularly applies to decisions about people in long-term care. The Mental Capacity Act strengthens and protects the rights of people who wish to plan for their future in the event of becoming incapacitated, as well as the rights of those who currently lack capacity. It also clarifies the rights

and duties of the carers and professionals who assist such individuals (see Figure 11.2).

Other relevant individuals – a health or care professional, other professional, relative or carer – might need to decide whether the individual has the capacity to make a particular decision. In many everyday cases that decision will be the responsibility of the family or carers. Where the decision to be made is more complex, the more formal the assessment of the individual's capacity may need to be, and this may involve doctors or other professionals. For example, where consent is needed for medical treatment or examination, a doctor or healthcare professional will decide if individuals have capacity to consent. The Mental Capacity Act states that before anyone acts on behalf of someone who lacks capacity, they must have a 'reasonable belief' that the person lacks capacity. If the individual is indeed judged to lack capacity, actions can be taken or decisions can be made on their behalf if those actions are in their best interests.

The Act was amended in 2019 after a parliamentary committee examined the Act and found that the rules ordering individuals to be looked after were not being followed properly because staff found the rules too complicated. In addition, many individuals who were unable to make decisions for themselves were ordered to be looked after so their rights were eroded as their wishes and feelings were not being taken into consideration. Under the Amendment, rules should be easier to understand as it changes who decides for people who lack capacity. If the individual is in hospital, the hospital makes the decision. If they are in a care home or their own home or supported accommodation, the local council decides. In other situations, the decision is taken by the NHS **Clinical Commissioning Group (CCG)**.

> ### Key terms
>
> **Lack capacity:** unable to use and understand information to make a decision. This is a term with a specific meaning in law and should not be applied without meeting certain criteria.
>
> **Clinical Commissioning Group (CCG):** most of the NHS commissioning budget is now managed by 209 CCGs. These are groups of general practices which come together in each area to commission the best services for their patients and the local population.

However, the Amendment has made it clear that an individual cannot be ordered to be looked after before talking to:
► the individual
► someone who can make decisions for the individual by law
► an independent mental capacity advocate
► anyone the individual has said can help make a decision for them
► people who care for the individual, for example, a family member or carer.

Care Act (2014)

The Care Act underlines the importance of protecting the most vulnerable in society from harm, abuse and neglect.

It provides the legal framework for how local authorities should protect adults in danger from abuse, harm and neglect. The Act makes it clear that local authorities must put the individual's wellbeing first in everything they do. Local authorities should:
► establish adult safeguarding boards
► lead a multi-agency local adult safeguarding system that prevents abuse, harm and neglect
► investigate when they suspect a vulnerable adult may be at risk of abuse, harm or neglect
► carry out safeguarding adults' reviews when someone dies as a result of neglect, harm or abuse
► arrange for an independent advocate to represent and support an individual who is the subject of a safeguarding inquiry or review.

Just as the Amendment to the Mental Capacity Act above emphasises that any decisions must involve the person concerned, and their wishes, feelings and views must be considered, so too does the Care Act. Any actions taken to support and protect the individual should have minimum effect on their rights and freedom.

Health and Social Care Act (2012)

Improving quality of care was at the heart of the Health and Social Care Act 2012. Although there are many other features of the Health and Social Care Act, this piece of legislation primarily had the effect of bringing personalisation to the NHS. It enables patients to be able to choose services which best meet their needs, including from charity or independent sector providers, provided they meet NHS costs.

This Act therefore intended to empower patients to make choices. If patients were due to have an operation but they did not want to go to their local hospital, they could choose to have their treatment in a hospital of their choice. The Act also established new **Healthwatch** patient organisations locally and nationally to drive patient involvement across the NHS, giving patients a voice. **Monitor** was established as a specialist regulator to protect patients' interests. Although predominantly related to health, the Act did reinforce personalisation in social care. However, in April 2016, Monitor and the NHS Trust Development Authority merged to become part of the **NHS Improvement**.

Key terms

Healthwatch: the national consumer champion in health and care. It has significant statutory powers to ensure the voice of the consumer is strengthened and heard by those who commission, deliver and regulate health and care services.

Monitor: the sector regulator for health services in England. Monitor's job is to make the health sector work better for patients by continually improving the service and getting good value for money.

NHS Improvement: works with the NHS to help improve care for patients and provides leadership and support for the NHS.

Safeguarding Vulnerable Groups Act (2006)

The Safeguarding Vulnerable Groups Act 2006 provided the legislative framework for the Disclosure and Barring Scheme (DBS). This scheme works closely with the police and helps to safeguard both adults and children from harm and abuse by preventing unsuitable people from working with vulnerable adults and children.

This involves:
► processing requests for criminal record checks by searching police records and barred list information
► deciding whether it is appropriate for a person to be placed on or removed from a barred list
► placing people on the DBS children's barred list and adults' barred list for England, Wales and Northern Ireland.

An employer will request a DBS check for roles that may involve working or volunteering in health, social care and childcare settings, or any role involving interaction with children and vulnerable adults.

NICE guidance and quality standards

This is one of many types of guides produced by NICE on healthcare, public health and social care topics. The idea behind these guides is to offer advice to agencies to help improve the quality of care provided. In 'Domestic violence and abuse: multi-agency working', NICE provides clear written guidance for agencies to deliver to healthcare staff on how to recognise and deal with patients who are being abused or subject to domestic violence. The guide aims to reduce abuse and suggests that working together with agencies in a multi-agency partnership is the best solution. NICE gives advice on training and suggests that ongoing support from within an organisation is also needed for individual practitioners. Without training in identifying domestic violence and abuse and responding appropriately after disclosure, healthcare professionals may fail to recognise its contribution to a person's condition and to provide effective and safe support.

The quality standard is expected to contribute to improvements in the following outcomes:
- harm from domestic violence and abuse
- mortality from domestic violence and abuse
- emergency attendances for domestic violence and abuse
- quality of life
- personal safety
- duration of domestic violence and abuse
- re-occurrence of domestic violence and abuse.

Research

Ask your workplace supervisor about multi-agency working. How many outside agencies do they work with? Which agencies do they work with regularly? What do they feel are the benefits to this way of working? Are there any negatives (from the workplace's perspective) from working this way?

Share findings on return to school/college. You may wish to produce bar charts, graphs, etc. of the agencies they work with if there are enough of them to do so.

What conclusions can you draw from this evidence? Is multi-agency working common across the sectors your class worked in?

NHS England guide

NHS England produce a pocket guide called *Safeguarding Adults* designed to help healthcare professionals working with adults to recognise signs of abuse which they may see in their patients who are receiving care. Although only 40 pages in length, the guide covers a diverse range of topics related to abuse. The guide provides advice and guidance for healthcare staff on the steps to take if they suspect harm and abuse. Topics covered include:
- the Care Act in relation to safeguarding
- healthcare staffs' responsibilities
- the role of the member of staff raising the abuse alarm
- information sharing
- the Mental Capacity Act 2005
- assessing capacity chart
- domestic violence and abuse
- female genital mutilation (FGM)
- human trafficking
- modern slavery.

Research

Research NHS England pocket guide: *Safeguarding Adults*. Go to: **www.england.nhs.uk/wp-content/uploads/2017/02/adult-pocket-guide.pdf**

Read this condensed guide to safeguarding, including signs of abuse. Do you find it easy to understand? Why? If not, explain how you would improve the guide. If you were a healthcare worker, do you think you would find this guide useful if you had a suspected case of abuse? Explain your answer.

Test yourself

1. Explain the meaning of safeguarding.
2. What is the role of the Disclosure and Barring Scheme checks?
3. List three principles that underpin the Mental Capacity Act 2005.
4. The Care Act 2014 makes it clear that local authorities must put the individual's wellbeing first in everything. Describe two ways in which this can be achieved.
5. Explain why the Mental Capacity Act (2005) was amended in 2019.

A11.3 Factors that may contribute to an individual being vulnerable to harm or abuse and the vulnerable groups that require protection

Factors that can contribute to abuse

While anyone can be a victim of abuse, members of certain groups are more vulnerable to it:

- women
- people from Black, Asian and minority ethnic (BAME) backgrounds
- children
- young people
- elderly people
- pregnant women and those with young children

- people with mental and/or physical disabilities
- people who speak English as an additional language
- people affected by substance misuse
- LGBTQ individuals
- people with poor literacy skills.

Abuse sometimes happens because people like to have power over others. Abusers usually prey on victims who they see as being weaker or more vulnerable than themselves. People who are being abused often feel ashamed because the abuser may make them feel or tell them that the abuse is their fault. This is one reason why victims often do not report the abuse, i.e. shame and embarrassment. They may also experience self-doubt, especially if the abuser tells them that they are blowing it out of proportion, or they may feel that their family and friends will blame them for their own abuse (victim blaming). They may also feel it is safer to stay as they have nowhere to go.

Factors that contribute to abuse	Vulnerable groups where this factor is most relevant
Age Age can be a factor in abuse as young children, babies and older people do not have the ability, understanding or physical strength to challenge any individual who abuses them. The abuser may often be in a position of trust such as a healthcare professional, relative or neighbour.	• Children/young people/elderly people
Individuals with health issues/being physically dependent on others Health issues can result in individuals being dependent on those who care for them, whether they are family or healthcare professionals. Sometimes the individual is too ill or too frail to report the abuse. If they are physically dependent on others, they may worry that their care could be withdrawn if they make a fuss or complain.	• Adults receiving care in their home • Individuals with physical, mental or sensory impairments • Individuals with learning disabilities
Lack of mental capacity This can be an issue as the individual being abused does not have sufficient understanding of what is happening to them or may forget. They may feel as if it is their own fault and they are ashamed.	• Individuals with learning disabilities • Older people with dementia
History of abuse Individuals who have been abused over a long period of time may think that this abuse is part of everyday life which happens to everyone, particularly if their abuser reinforces this. They may believe that no one has the power to stop the abuse.	• Adults receiving care in their home • Individuals with physical, mental or sensory impairments • Individuals with learning disabilities

Factors that contribute to abuse	Vulnerable groups where this factor is most relevant
Social isolation Social isolation is often used to gain control over someone for an abusive purpose. The person being abused has no one to talk to apart from the abuser. Isolation reduces the opportunity of the abused person to escape from the abuse, making the abused person more dependent on the abuser.	• Adults receiving care in their home • Individuals with physical, mental or sensory impairments • Individuals with learning disabilities • People who do not live near other friends and family
Drug/alcohol abuse NICE lists alcohol or drug use as a risk factor for abuse, in other words, abusers are more likely to have problems with addiction or misuse of these substances. This is also a risk factor in terms of when an individual is drunk or under the use of drugs, it is easier for someone to take advantage of them, as their reactions will be affected. However, it is important to understand that the use of drugs or alcohol does not implicate the victim or excuse the abuser.	• Young people
Finance Individuals can be abused for their money. Someone caring for an older person may target them for their possessions or money, particularly if they seem to have something the carer does not. Some cases have occurred where a healthcare worker has been dependent on the older person for their wages or accommodation and felt resentful. Some individuals may be financially dependent on their abusers, for instance if they do not earn and their family/partner does, or their partner collects benefits on their behalf. They may fear they will not be able to afford to live alone, and those who have children or dependants may be afraid that they will struggle to look after them or risk them being taken away if they leave the abuser. Young people may still be in full-time education and may be dependent on the abuser for food, clothing, etc.	• Older people, especially those who require healthcare • Unemployed individuals or low-paid workers • People financially dependent on others, e.g. their partner and family

Vulnerable groups

People from Black, Asian and minority ethnic (BAME) backgrounds suffer from the same types of abuse as the rest of the community. However, members of certain social, cultural or religious groups may be more at risk of **honour-based violence** (HBV – see page 210). Also, data from the Office for National Statistics (ONS) shows that in the year 2018–19, the rates of domestic abuse among people from BAME communities were higher than their white counterparts, and were highest amongst those of mixed ethnicity (**www.ethnicity-facts-figures.service.gov.uk/crime-justice-and-the-law/crime-and-reoffending/domestic-abuse/latest**).

People from BAME backgrounds are less likely to report incidents of abuse and crime in general, due to higher levels of distrust of the police and criminal justice system, on top of victims' reluctance and difficulties in reporting abuse.

Women, especially women with children, are more at risk of being abused than men. They may be particularly afraid in case the perpetrator starts on the children as well as herself. Pregnant women, too, may be scared of being physically attacked or of their pregnancy being affected.

The other groups listed as vulnerable are due to a variety of factors. Children and young people are dependent on their families and do not always recognise when they are being abused as they have less life experience. They may think that the abuse they are experiencing happens to everyone. If adults are living in their own home, this can mean that the abuse goes undetected for some time. Individuals with learning disabilities may not understand what is happening to them. They may not have the vocabulary to describe the abuse. The same applies to individuals with physical, mental or sensory impairments who may feel they will not be believed. They may depend on others and feel powerless to prevent the abuse from happening, or may have been threatened by the abuser and feel afraid of the consequences of reporting.

A11.4 A range of different types of abuse and harm

Physical

Female genital mutilation

Female genital mutilation (FGM), also previously known as female circumcision or cutting, is when a female's external genitals are deliberately removed, cut or injured for non-medical reasons. Reasons for this may include expectations in an individual's cultural, social or religious community to do so, where it may be seen as beneficial for female hygiene or making a woman marriageable.

This practice takes place between infancy and 15 years of age and can cause many medical complications and discomfort or pain for the individual. It is usually performed by someone with no medical training and without anaesthetic or antiseptic treatment. It is illegal in many countries including the UK but is still carried out in certain African, Middle Eastern and Asian countries.

Hitting

If someone deliberately hurts another person by hitting or slapping them, this is a form of physical abuse. This type of abuse can start off small but can soon escalate into punching and beating.

Burns

Burns could be non-accidental, which means they were inflicted by someone else. These burns could be caused by bathing or immersing the service user in water that is too hot. The injury could be cigarette burns, easily recognised by their small round shape. Other common household items causing burns are hot pans, boiling kettles, hot irons, radiators and electric fires.

Case study

Dionne

Dionne is two years old and goes to nursery three mornings a week. She has missed the last four weeks as her mother says she was ill with measles. She seems uncomfortable when she sits down. The nursery practitioner is concerned when Dionne wets herself as she appears to have a big round burn on her bottom. When questioned, her mother explained that Dionne had climbed on to the cooker and sat on a hot ring, which caused the burn.

▶ Why could this situation constitute a safeguarding concern?

▶ Explain what action the nursery staff should take.

Modern day slavery

Exploitation of individuals for work using threats and violence

Modern day slavery is the illegal exploitation of people (children included) for personal or commercial gain. Victims are often hidden away, and may be unable to leave their situation, or may not come forward because of fear or shame. They are deceived or coerced into working, having been promised a better life and the opportunity to earn money for themselves and their families. Instead, they end up working for individuals who threaten them and may use violence against them. Some enslaved individuals are immigrants, so they are afraid of going to the authorities about abuse for fear of detention or deportation because of their immigration status.

Figure 11.3 lists the types of modern day slavery.

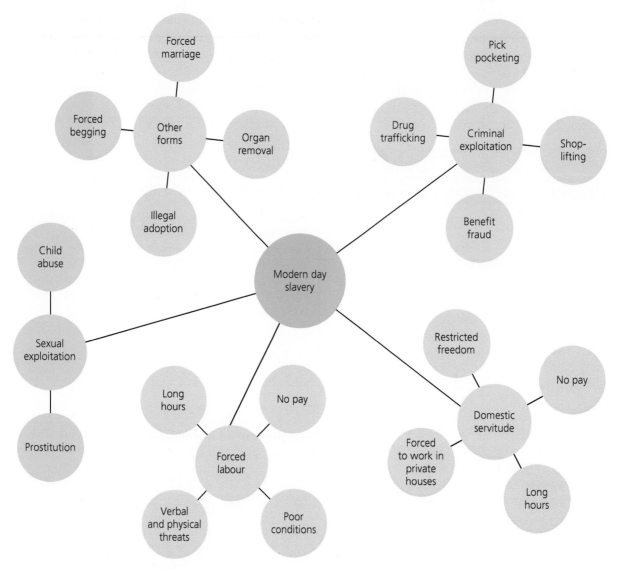

▲ Figure 11.3 Types of modern day slavery

Sexual

Sexual abuse can take place anywhere, for example, a stranger on a crowded train touching a fellow passenger sexually, or at school or university. It can happen to people regardless of their age, gender, ethnicity or sexuality. Generally, the motivation for sexual abuse is about more than just sex and, in common with other forms of abuse, is about the perpetrator trying to exert control or dominance over the person who they are abusing.

Sexual abuse can happen to adults as well as children. Legally speaking, any sexual activity with someone under the age of 16 can be prosecuted as the individual is not considered old enough to give consent. Adult sexual abuse is any sexual activity which takes place without consent, or where consent cannot be given because of lack of understanding of what is happening. It could take the form of rape (non-consensual sexual activity), groping or other inappropriate touch or sexual violence.

Adults who have been sexually abused may feel ashamed to report the assault as they may feel that they have led the perpetrator on. However, it is important to recognise that sexual assault is always the perpetrator's fault never the victim's, regardless of what a victim was wearing, doing or if they were drunk or otherwise incapacitated. Children or young people who are victims of sexual abuse may be scared to tell someone as they think it is their fault or that they will be judged or blamed, or they may not trust adults to protect them or not disclose their allegations.

Forcing someone to take part or watch sexual activities

If it is a young person or child (who, as described in the previous section, under the age of 16 cannot consent to sex) and/or individuals who are tricked into sexual activities, they might not understand what is happening or that it is abuse.

Sexual abuse can be divided into contact and non-contact:

▶ Contact is where the abuser makes physical contact with the individual. This can include:
  – sexual touching of any part of an individual's body, whether they are clothed or not
  – using a body part or object to rape or penetrate an individual
  – forcing an individual to take part in sexual activities
  – making an individual undress or touch someone else.
  Contact abuse can include touching, kissing and oral sex – sexual abuse is not just penetrative.

▶ **Non-contact abuse** is where an individual is abused without being touched by the abuser. This can be in person or online and includes:
  – exposing or flashing
  – showing pornography
  – exposing an individual to sexual acts
  – making them masturbate
  – forcing an individual to make, view or share abuse images or videos
  – making, viewing or distributing abuse images or videos
  – forcing an individual to take part in sexual activities or conversations online or through a smartphone.

Source: www.nspcc.org.uk/what-is-child-abuse/types-of-abuse/child-sexual-abuse/

Emotional

Belittling

Belittling is putting someone down so that they feel small and unimportant. It can be in the form of criticising, judging or humiliating. It can erode an individual's confidence and self-esteem, making them feel worthless. This could happen anywhere, for example, at school where a member of staff makes a child feel small because they cannot follow a maths problem or are struggling to spell a word. In a relationship, this may look like one partner telling their partner they always get everything wrong.
A healthcare worker might notice this when visiting an older patient in their home and they find that when they are explaining the treatment, family members tell the patient it is far too difficult for them to follow.

Bullying

Bullying can take place anywhere – at school, at work, at the gym, on the sports field, etc. There is no legal definition, but it is usually defined as repeated behaviour which is intended to hurt someone either emotionally or physically. It is often aimed at certain individuals because of a perceived difference, which may include their ethnicity, religion, gender, sexual orientation or any other aspect such as appearance or disability.

Verbal abuse

Verbal abuse is a range of words or behaviours used to manipulate, intimidate and maintain power and control over someone. It can include insults, humiliation and ridicule and attempts to scare, isolate and control someone.

Gaslighting

Gaslighting is a form of psychological abuse where a person makes another question their perception of reality, or memories. People experiencing gaslighting are often left feeling confused, anxious, and unable to trust themselves. A victim of gaslighting can be pushed so far that they question their own sanity. The term 'gaslighting' comes from a play and subsequent film called 'Gaslight'. In the movie, the devious husband manipulates and torments his wife to convince her she is going mad.

Coercion/control

Coercion is making an individual do something they do not want to do, usually through force.

Assaults

Assault could be threatening or carrying out physical force or action that makes someone frightened, for example, through physical blows or beatings or using weapons. It could also be sexual assault.

Threats and intimidation

A threat is an expression of intent to injure or hurt someone, often as a consequence of not complying with their request or instructions. Intimidation is making someone scared or fearful, including by making threats towards them or shouting and acting aggressively. Stalking too can be frightening for the victim. This is when someone is following or watching an individual over a period of time, paying them unwanted attention. They may send unwanted gifts or turn up uninvited to the person's home, school or workplace. The person being stalked may be afraid for their safety.

Humiliation

Humiliation means putting down a person and making them feel small or embarrassing them. It means interfering with their pride and dignity to make them feel inferior. Humiliation is a common form of abuse. It may not cause physical harm but is very upsetting. The more shame and embarrassment an individual feels, the less likely they are to share their abuse with anyone, and it makes the victim feel worthless and useless. It is important for medical staff to respect patients and treat them with dignity, giving them space and privacy to get undressed/dressed or during a medical examination.

Organisational/institutional

Regimented mealtimes

Institutional settings sometimes involve rigid routines, such as set mealtimes that do not respect individuals' privacy, comfort and unique needs. People are used to choosing when they eat when they are in their own home, where they can also have a snack or drink whenever they want. Under this regime, if they do not feel like eating in the early evening they have to go hungry until breakfast the next day, which, as well as being harsh and neglectful, can be dangerous, particularly if they have a health condition such as anorexia nervosa. This regimented system happens because the organisation has systems and processes that are designed for the convenience of the staff and not those of the individuals using the service.

Having said that, set mealtimes do not suit everyone, this does not mean that individuals should be left to decide to miss meals. Individuals who have conditions such as diabetes should be encouraged to eat at regular times for optimum management of their condition. The key is to ensure that individuals' needs are met, even where they differ from each other and the solution may not be the most time efficient.

Removing personal choices

This failure to uphold individuals' rights will have a negative effect on their quality of life, as well as affecting their dignity and autonomy. Removing choice about bedtime, what clothes they wear, what food they eat, etc. has a negative effect on their self-esteem because they lose their independence and they may not feel in control of their life. It is very important to allow for individual choice wherever possible so they feel they have been consulted and have made their own decisions about matters that concern them.

Financial

Withholding/taking of money

Many adults are vulnerable to financial abuse, particularly if they have a limited understanding of money matters. Withholding money is a form of control, as individuals should have the freedom to spend how they wish as long as it is in their best interests and unless, where they lack mental capacity, they are in danger of giving away all their money. Information about money should also not be withheld, for example, how much money from benefits is available to an individual who is receiving healthcare. It is important that a healthcare worker is honest and transparent when dealing with any money belonging to an individual in their care. They must always provide receipts for money they have been given to spend on items for the individual.

Neglect

Neglect is the failure to give minimum standards of care to meet an individual's basic needs. It can include nutritional neglect, ignoring medical issues that should be dealt with or providing inadequate heating or clothing. It can manifest itself in both emotional and physical ways.

Self-neglect

Self-neglect covers a wide range of behaviours, such as neglecting personal hygiene or neglecting to eat. It could also involve neglecting one's own health and surroundings and can include behaviour such as hoarding. It is important to consider mental capacity when self-neglect is suspected. Sometimes self-neglect is related to deteriorating health and ability in older age. It can also be a sign of depression or a mental health condition. For example, an individual may become depressed and neglect their own needs after the death of a lifelong partner.

Neglect by others

This includes:

- withholding access to food or the right food for a person: this could be starving the individual or giving them food that they are unable to eat. They may be unable to eat it as they have difficulty chewing or swallowing. This would also include being given food which is not appropriate for their religious or other beliefs, for example, giving a vegetarian a meal containing chicken

- not supporting a person to wash and maintain appropriate personal hygiene and comfort: if the person is unable to wash themselves, they will have to be supported to wash their hair and body and in personal grooming. They will feel dirty, smelly and itchy if they are not helped to keep clean, and will feel neglected and uncomfortable. Their teeth will also need brushing. Being left without support in this area can be very demeaning

- not supporting a person to change soiled or wet clothing: if a person cannot walk to the toilet themselves and a member of staff does not answer their buzzer, they may wet or soil their clothing. They need to be cleaned up as soon as possible. As well as being unhygienic, it will have a detrimental effect on their skin

- not seeking medical assistance when a person needs it: if a person is ill and cannot seek help themselves, it is up to the healthcare assistant to contact their GP, ambulance or other medical professionals, depending on the condition

- withholding access to appropriate medication or treatment for a person: medication that is necessary for the health of the person must be provided as and when necessary. For example, some people have to take medication to reduce blood pressure or to help cognitive functioning.

Reflect

Hannah, aged 75, has recently started to go to day care twice a week because of a visit to her home from social services. Hannah lives with her son, aged 40, who has been responsible for looking after her. However, a neighbour had recently reported that Hannah had been seen in the street looking dishevelled and dirty. When the social worker arrived, she found Hannah sitting in a cold, dirty house. She was dressed in soiled clothes and was not wearing any underwear or anything on her feet.

Hannah has since been diagnosed with dementia. Social services offered Hannah two separate days of day care in a residential home where she could have a bath and a good meal and her clothes would be washed. Hannah did not want to leave her home as she loved it and her son. Social services brought in home help to clean the house and organise the paying of bills, etc.

Was Hannah being abused? If so, what type of abuse was it?

Domestic

Abuse that takes place in the home by a family member

Domestic abuse occurs in the home and is usually committed by a partner or family member. It can include harassment, bullying, physical violence, emotional abuse, stalking, female genital mutilation, forced marriage and 'honour-based' abuse. It can also include trafficking.

73 per cent of the victims of domestic violence incidents reported to police in the year to March 2021 were female.

Source: www.ons.gov.uk/
peoplepopulationandcommunity/crimeandjustice/articles/
domesticabusevictimcharacteristicsenglandandwales/
yearendingmarch2021

Nonetheless, it is important to appreciate that it can happen to men or women. It is also somewhat a hidden crime: many victims do not report it, and abusers may not be prosecuted, both for a variety of reasons. Victims are often afraid to do this as they may depend on the person for money, etc. and may feel that the authorities will not be sympathetic to their situation.

Professional abuse

Abuse by someone in a position of power over the victim or a position of trust

Abuse can be perpetrated by all kinds of people, including any professional healthcare worker who is responsible for providing healthcare. This includes GPs, nurses, physiotherapists, occupational therapists and healthcare assistants. Types of abuse by professionals include physical, financial, sexual, verbal, emotional, psychological, discriminatory abuse or neglect. It is essential that all healthcare workers follow standards of care, including keeping professional boundaries. They must treat individuals with dignity and respect.

Honour-based abuse

Honour-based abuse is any practice used by families to control behaviour in order to protect the reputation of the family. Victims are most likely to be female but it can happen to males as well. If an individual is deemed to have brought shame or dishonour to their family by behaviour such as having relationships with friends or partners who their family do not approve of, members of the immediate family will punish that individual, including with violence. Being in a gay relationship or becoming pregnant outside of a family-approved marriage may also be causes of such disapproval. Sometimes the extended family and even other members of their community become involved, either directly or by collusion or covering up the abuse. Forced marriage is one form of honour-based abuse.

This behaviour is found across countless cultures and communities, including but not limited to faith-based communities, but is often found where there is a heavily male-dominated culture. It is not just adults who can suffer from honour-based abuse – children, too, can be victims if their families dislike behaviour, such as wanting to wear make-up or clothes the family don't approve of. Children with additional needs or SEND may suffer this abuse too.

Violence

Violence can include verbal abuse or threats as well as physical attacks such as punching, grabbing, pushing and slapping. Victims may be overpowered by the abuser. It can also include rape or other forms of sexual abuse.

Cruelty

Cruelty means inflicting mental or physical suffering on an individual who is weaker than themselves. They know the victim has no chance of returning the cruelty. An example could be a person who locks their child or partner in a cupboard because they know they will be terrified.

Forced marriage

According to www.gov.uk/government/publications/what-is-a-forced-marriage, a forced marriage is where one or both people do not (or in cases of people with learning disabilities or reduced capacity, cannot) consent to the marriage as they are pressurised, or abuse is used, to force them to do so. It is recognised in the UK as a form of domestic or child abuse and a serious abuse of human rights.

The pressure put on people to marry against their will may be:

▶ physical, for example, threats, physical violence or sexual violence
▶ emotional and psychological, for example, making someone feel like they are bringing 'shame' on their family
▶ financial abuse, for example, taking someone's wages, may also be a factor.

As you can see, forced marriage is one form of honour-based abuse as it also tries to make an individual feel that their actions cause shame for the family.

> **Reflect**
>
> Visit: www.youtube.com/watch?v=wO6yRKIDKLA
> Alternatively enter the terms "University of Derby forced marriages" into a search engine.
>
> Watch the short film from the University of Derby 'Forced Marriages and Honour Based Abuse' about this type of abuse. It features several survivors of forced marriages telling their story.
> ▶ Which two of the following subcategories of abuse are mentioned? Physical, sexual, psychological, emotional, neglect.
> ▶ Did the information on statistics about the number of reported honour-based abuse cases in the UK surprise you?
> ▶ Has this helped you understand this form of abuse? Explain why/why not.

Child sexual exploitation (sexual, labour or forced criminality)

Child sexual exploitation is abuse by people (usually adults) who have power over young people and use it to sexually abuse them. This can involve a broad range of exploitative activity, from seemingly 'consensual' relationships and informal exchanges of sex through to serious organised crimes.

Victims may receive gifts, such as money, drugs and alcohol, or be given status and affection in exchange for performing sexual activities. Where children and young people are tricked into believing they are in a loving and consensual relationship, this is called **grooming**.

Source: www.nspcc.org.uk/what-is-child-abuse/types-of-abuse/child-sexual-exploitation

Test yourself

1 List three factors that can contribute to abuse.
2 Name three groups of individuals who are more at risk from abuse.
3 Describe what is meant by female genital mutilation (FGM).
4 List four types of modern-day slavery.
5 Explain the meaning of child sexual exploitation.
6 Describe what is meant by bullying.
7 Explain the meaning of honour-based abuse.

A11.5 Some of the possible signs of abuse or harm that may be identified in individuals using healthcare

Physical

Possible signs

Bruising

Trips and falls can result in bruising for anyone. However, if bruises are suspicious and are in well-protected areas, such as inner arms or thighs or abdomen, it is more likely that abuse is involved. Bruises may show fingertip patterns or the shape of items used to inflict the injury (for example, the shape of a belt or belt buckle). There could be symmetrical bruising on both sides of the body. Bruises on the wrists may indicate that the individual has been restrained.

Unexplained bleeding

This could be from the face, head, nose or ears. The explanation of how the bleeding happened does not match the pattern of the injury.

Emotional

Possible signs

Depression

This is often linked to emotional abuse, but depression can also be a reaction to physical or sexual abuse, bullying or family breakdown. This is because emotional abuse can rob an individual of their **self-esteem**. Depression is a common mental health condition, the symptoms of which include low mood, sadness, loss of energy, eating too much or too little, sleeping badly and general lack of interest in everything. There may be increased anger or irritability, and the individual may also have feelings of self-loathing or worthlessness. It can occur in a range of circumstances and may not necessarily indicate abuse, but a change in an individual's mental health should always prompt concern.

Low self-esteem

Individuals who are abused have low self-esteem as they feel worthless. They begin to doubt everything and feel incapable of making any decisions as their self-confidence is eroded. This may be a deliberate tactic on behalf of the abuser to nurture this, as it keeps the victim under their control for longer.

Organisational

Possible signs

Restricted visiting times

If someone is denied access to visit an individual in a residential or nursing home this may be a sign of abuse. The home may try to restrict visits in order to prevent family and friends seeing signs of abuse, e.g. neglect. It also gives the individual limited time to talk to their family about what is happening to them.

Patient complaints

If patients have complained about their care, they are entitled to have their complaint acknowledged and fully investigated. They need to feel confident that their concerns will be looked into and that they will be informed about the findings of the investigation. If their complaint is dismissed, especially if this happens very quickly, this may seem to indicate a cover-up and confidence will be lost in the organisation. In any event, patients or individuals receiving care must be treated with respect and their views taken seriously, and the lack of this should raise concerns.

Financial

Possible signs

Lack of money and/or belongings

For an individual who has an unexplained lack of money or whose belongings mysteriously disappear, this could be a sign of financial abuse. Unexplained disappearance of personal possessions or property, plus a shortage of money despite an adequate income, should ring alarm bells. This could be a sign of fraud, theft or exploitation, or could be family members or friends taking advantage of the individual. Perpetrators could have gambling, drug or alcohol problems and are using the individual's money or selling possessions to fund their lifestyle. Alternatively, family members could be repeatedly asking for sums of money in return for looking after the person; if the individual refuses, the family may stop visiting.

Debt

There may be a non-abuse related reason why an individual is struggling with money, but sudden debts and unpaid bills, with the individual becoming anxious over money and talking about the inability to pay bills, should raise the question of financial abuse. This is particularly relevant if the individual has always managed their money in the past. Another possibility is that the individual could have been forced or misled into signing documents for loans, for example, which the perpetrator then uses for their own purposes, plunging the individual into debt.

Sexual

Possible signs

Unwanted pregnancy

While not always the result of abuse, this could be one sign. Young people often do not talk about sexual abuse because they think it is their fault, that they will be judged or blamed, or they have been convinced by their abuser that it is normal or a 'special secret'. They may also be bribed or threatened by their abuser or told they will not be believed. The young person may not realise that they are pregnant or may hide it as they do not want to get the abuser into trouble.

Sexually transmitted infection

A young person may develop health problems, including soreness in the genital and anal areas or sexually transmitted infections. They may also have:

▶ unusual discharge from the vagina, penis or anus
▶ pain when urinating
▶ lumps or skin growths around the genitals or anus
▶ a rash
▶ unusual vaginal bleeding
▶ itchy genitals or anus
▶ blisters and sores around the genitals or anus.

As well as physical signs, their behaviour may change as they become anxious about their symptoms, so they may spend more time in the bathroom or toilet. They may want to shower more. Their behaviour may change, and they may withdraw from their family and not want hugs or cuddles. Their performance at school may suffer as they find it difficult to concentrate. If the child is very young and in hospital, a healthcare worker may notice some physical signs of sexual abuse when they are helping with personal hygiene.

Even when there are no physical signs of abuse such as those listed above, a young person could behave in a way sexually inappropriate to their age, including showing an obsession with sexual matters.

Sexual promiscuity

This is when an individual has indiscriminate sexual intercourse with multiple sexual partners. Sometimes sexual promiscuity can be a way that the sexually abused individual tries to get control over their feelings relating to their sexual abuse. However, it should be noted that not everyone who has been sexually abused is promiscuous.

Neglect

Possible signs

Unkempt appearance

As a result of neglect, individuals can become hungry, ill, dirty and deprived of their support as they are obviously not being cared for or looked after. A healthcare worker who allows this is not ensuring that the service user is receiving help with their personal care and the individual may be unwashed, with hair unbrushed and untidy, and their appearance generally neglected. Their clothes may also be dirty.

Malnutrition

This sometimes happens where patients are not helped to eat or physically fed or in a residential home where individuals cannot feed themselves. If food is put in front of the patient and they lack the capability to feed themselves, the meal may be taken away untouched. This results in malnutrition (see section A9.3, page 154). The signs of malnutrition involve unintentional weight loss, weakness, lack of interest in eating or drinking and taking a long time to recover from their illness. A healthcare assistant may notice that the individual looks hollow cheeked with thin, pale skin and sunken eyes, and they are complaining of feeling cold all the time. A lack of water causes dehydration and signs of this can be very concentrated urine which looks dark yellow in colour. They may have headaches and difficulty in urinating.

A11.6 What action to take if abuse is suspected or disclosed

Communicate with the individual

Respecting confidentiality balanced with assessing risk

Everyone has the right to confidentiality but abuse changes everything. Confidentiality should be kept as much as possible, but given the seriousness of abuse and the fact it may pose a serious risk to the person, disclosing allegations of abuse to safeguarding are an important exception to this principle and to data protection. Certain situations mean that a healthcare worker must pass on information to the person with responsibility for safeguarding because keeping it to themselves could result in harm to the person who is being supported. The information must only be shared with the named lead person for safeguarding and the information should only be shared on a need-to-know basis, i.e. with no-one else unless they are asked for a statement from the police.

Generally, the involvement of the person who has reported the abuse ends once they have passed on the information to the person in charge of safeguarding. If any disclosures are made to them, the healthcare worker must explain to the individual disclosing abuse that they will have to pass on the information because of the risks posed to that person's health and wellbeing. It is the duty of the healthcare worker not to delay reporting disclosures to ensure the individual is protected from any further risk of abuse. To facilitate this, the healthcare worker must also have received training on safeguarding as this is mandatory in all health settings. Information must also be displayed or shared in workplaces, e.g. on a poster, showing who the lead person(s) for safeguarding is/are and how to contact them.

Ensure a record of any disclosure is recorded word for word (for example, using safeguarding disclosure form/safeguarding incident report form)

Any evidence from disclosures of abuse must be carefully recorded word for word with as much detail

as possible included. Concerns should not be passed on verbally without a written record to support this. The reason for this is that verbal statements can be altered, parts conveyed inaccurately and the meaning changed as they are passed on.

To help with this, each healthcare setting should have a special form for recording disclosures. Everything that has happened must be recorded as the healthcare worker may need to make a formal statement to the police or the investigating team, for which there must be a detailed account of what was said and how.

Reporting

Knowledge of the reporting procedure and report line

Each organisation will have its own reporting procedures for both disclosures of abuse and suspected abuse. It is important that the healthcare worker familiarises themselves with these so that when concerns are reported they are doing so in line with their workplace procedures. This may involve reporting suspicions or disclosures to the named person in the workplace, such as line manager or person in charge of safeguarding or making a referral to the NSPCC, CQC, social services or the police (Figure 11.4). Any healthcare worker who does not report abuse appropriately is failing to carry out their role and responsibilities and this may result in an individual or others being in danger.

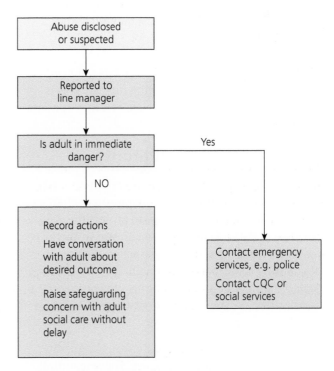

▲ Figure 11.4 Raising a safeguarding concern

Report instance but don't intervene unless immediate or imminent threat to safety

Once the healthcare worker has reported the instance of abuse, their role in the matter is over, until and unless they are called to give evidence in any ensuing legal proceedings. Not all suspected safeguarding issues result in action needing to be taken against anyone, and the safeguarding coordinator may have made an evaluation of the risk and taken steps to ensure the individual is in no immediate danger. It is not the healthcare worker's role to intervene but they should expect the safeguarding coordinator to act if there is an immediate or imminent threat to the individual's safety.

Understand the next point of escalation if suspected abuse is not investigated

In the situation where informing the safeguarding coordinator will involve a delay in a high-risk situation, the healthcare worker should report the concern by telephoning the external agencies such as police or social services immediately. If the healthcare worker has already informed the safeguarding coordinator and no action has been taken, the concerns can be reported to the local authority.

Healthcare providers should clearly record their reasons as to why they did or did not raise a concern and this should be consistent with the Safeguarding Principles, especially proportionality and accountability. For example, if a baby is brought into hospital with an injury consistent with sexual or physical abuse and nothing is done to escalate the matter, the person making this decision (who would be held to account about the decision) has to record their reasons for not doing anything further. This is obviously a serious example of abuse and they should be doing something about it.

Ability to challenge authority

Sadly, sometimes safeguarding is not taken seriously enough by those in authority. If the person in charge of safeguarding fails to take steps to protect the individual at risk, it is up to the healthcare worker who is reporting the abuse to take action. If the safeguarding coordinator is not willing to act, through misplaced loyalty or an unwillingness to confront a difficult situation, the healthcare worker must make a referral to a more senior manager.

Throughout this, the important thing is to safeguard individuals and prevent further abuse. Those reporting disclosures must be prepared to continue going up the managerial chain of command until they are satisfied that they have found the person who is willing to act. If this does not work internally, the healthcare worker must go outside their organisation and refer the case to an outside agency, for example, social services or the police.

Preserving evidence

Documentation of facts

Any evidence that the healthcare worker has of abuse or neglect, be it concerns, hard evidence or allegations, must be carefully documented. This must be fact and not opinion. The evidence should be written down as soon as possible so nothing is forgotten or muddled. There should be an account of what happened, what the healthcare worker saw or were told and how. Anything that is disclosed must be recorded in the words used by the individual.

Observation charts

If there are any physical signs of abuse, such as bruises, cuts or burns, the healthcare worker must make a written, dated and timed note of the facts within 24 hours otherwise they may not be considered reliable as evidence in court. It is a good idea to have another healthcare worker confirm the findings. All staff need to share the same methods of recording and share the responsibility for this. A body map (a basic diagram of a body) could be used to record these physical injuries such as bruises, etc. especially if these could be non-accidental injuries. As well as physical signs of abuse, anxieties and fears should be recorded. Where a child is the alleged victim, they may have started to behave in a different way and this should be recorded. Again, these records should be factual and not have any opinions expressed in them. These observation charts must be kept in a secure place so that only those authorised to investigate the case have access.

Clinical photography

Clinical photography could provide evidence of physical injuries in abuse cases. This could be useful for assessing and evidencing the abused person's condition. Before any clinical photographs are taken, the individual must give their permission and consent. The photographer must ensure confidentiality and security of the photographs as these are medical records which contain sensitive personal information. The photographs must not be used for any other purpose than evidence of physical injuries. Only digital cameras/devices supplied by the health trust should be used. The photographer must ensure that the correct date and time are set. Digital cameras/devices must be carried in a secure bag. Where digital devices such as tablets or smartphones are used, they must be password secure.

Case study

Tabby

Tabby was taken to hospital by ambulance after neighbours rang 999 when they heard screaming and banging. Tabby was unresponsive when the paramedics arrived but has since regained consciousness. She has been severely beaten and has two black eyes, a broken nose and split lips. She also has a large swelling on the back of her head. Her left arm is dislocated and she has several broken ribs. She is covered in bruises, cuts and abrasions.

She tells the nurse on admittance into hospital that her husband was responsible for this. He was angry because she was late home from work and his meal wasn't ready.

▶ Explain what the healthcare professionals need to do to preserve evidence of Tabby's physical attack and why.

▶ Why is this preservation of evidence important?

A11.7 Actions that can be taken by individuals and organisations to reduce the chances of abuse

Raising awareness and educating

Public awareness campaigns can make a big difference in preventing abuse. The public has an important role to play in safeguarding children and adults who they know or encounter by recognising and helping to prevent abuse. It is the responsibility of all agencies and organisations to ensure that there is a lot of public awareness and understanding of child and adult abuse. Public awareness campaigns are designed to inform and educate the public on what is meant by abuse and the signs and symptoms to look out for. They should also inform people about where to get help and advice.

Staff training

Staff in any setting, working with children and vulnerable adults, should undertake up-to-date training courses on safeguarding vulnerable adults. This ensures their knowledge and skills remain current and effective. At the time of writing, government guidance states that safeguarding training must be undertaken by staff at least every three years and at least every two years for designated officers. It must be appropriate to the job role (i.e. relevant to the situations they encounter and the scope of their job role) and include an understanding of the possible signs and symptoms of vulnerable child/vulnerable adult abuse, how to respond when abuse is disclosed or suspected and the latest safeguarding legislation, national and local policies and procedures.

Whistleblowing procedure

Whistleblowing is when a member of staff speaks up or raises a concern ('makes a disclosure') about working practices which are unethical, dangerous and/or break the law and are in the public interest to disclose. These fall into certain categories and often involve unsafe working practices that may harm individuals in their care. Healthcare professionals may whistleblow if the care is poor or dangerous and the patient may be harmed because of this. This is important because, as discussed, they have a duty to report their concerns. (See section A11.11 for further information.)

Whistleblowing about an abusive situation among colleagues can be difficult because of peer pressure. The person raising the concern may be disliked by their colleagues. They may fear they are mistaken about the situation and could risk missing out on future promotion, but it is essential to recognise that safeguarding must come first and nobody must take the chance of not doing something about suspected or disclosed abuse.

In recognition of this worry about being mistaken, the Public Interest Disclosure Act became law in 1998. This Act protects workers from dismissal if they disclose information about malpractice, including abuse at their current workplace, and provides a legal framework for whistleblowing. The Act protects individuals making disclosures about the following offences:

▶ the breach of a legal obligation
▶ miscarriage(s) of justice
▶ a danger to the health or safety of a person
▶ a criminal offence
▶ damage to the environment
▶ deliberately covering up information of any of the above.

The idea of the Act is that the whistleblower is protected if they believe that one of the above offences has been committed. After investigation, even if they are wrong, if they can show that is what they believed to be true then they are protected by this Act from losing their job because of this or from being passed over for promotion.

Effective complaints procedure

An accessible complaints procedure enables individuals and others who work in and visit healthcare settings to openly raise and discuss any concerns and complaints. To make the policy accessible, it should be in different languages, large print and different formats, ensuring everyone who needs to can make sense of it. This in turn will help to create an environment of mutual trust and respect, where individuals take an active role in making their own decisions about whether they complain or not. Care workers have a responsibility to support individuals in their care if they wish to make a complaint. Responding promptly to complaints and concerns and ensuring complaints procedures are available in formats that are understood and reinforced will mean that individuals will be more likely to raise any concerns in relation to safeguarding vulnerable adults.

Risk management procedure

Safeguarding individuals from abuse involves thinking about any risks that could cause them harm as well as taking actions to prevent that harm from happening. Maintaining safety is paramount in health settings, especially as some of the individuals will be vulnerable due to age, disability or medical condition. Risk assessment must be carried out by law. Significant risks should be the focus, rather than minor risks.

Risk management balances the care needs of the service user against the risk, with emphasis on:
▶ collaboration with the service user, asking them for their opinions on what will and will not work for them (that is what they will be happy or unhappy with)
▶ opinions of others involved in their care, e.g. their family and carers
▶ the importance of recognising and building on the service user's strengths
▶ the organisation's role in risk management alongside the individual practitioner's role
▶ weighing up the potential costs and benefits of choosing one action over another
▶ developing plans and actions that support the positive potentials and priorities stated by the service user, and minimising the risks to the service user or others
▶ being willing to take a decision that involves an element of risk because the potential positive benefits outweigh the risk.

Positive risk management means being aware that risk can never be completely eliminated. Therefore, management plans must have decisions that carry some risk. This should be explicit in the decision-making process and should be discussed openly with the service user.

Safeguarding individuals from abuse involves thinking about risks that may cause them potential harm as well as the actions that may be taken to prevent harm from occurring. This is known as **risk assessment** and is required by law. This is an important part of risk management. Risk assessments involve identifying, managing, recording and reviewing any risks that have the potential to cause harm. In this way abuse can be prevented and its likelihood reduced. Risk assessments also promote vulnerable adults' rights to take risks and are a way of enabling them to identify and manage potential and actual risks to themselves and others.

Risk assessments must be updated regularly and the new information should be recorded as individuals' circumstances change. For example, if an individual admitted to hospital must be lifted by hoist as they have a physical disability, there would have to be a risk assessment for lifting them. Their weight would be recorded as there are different slings for the hoist dependent on the individual's weight. The risk assessment would have to be updated regularly to keep up to date with developments as the circumstances can change. For instance, the patient may lose or gain weight and require a different sling.

Risk assessment for each individual case

Each case must be managed on an individual basis as one size doesn't fit all. What is a suitable solution for one person may be totally unsuitable for another as there will be different factors to consider. For example, a person with learning difficulties may want to go to work on the bus instead of being taken there by car. A risk assessment must be carried out and if it is seen to be safe, the person will be allowed to catch the bus on their own. However, for another person it could be decided that it is too far for them to go on their own as they tend to get off the bus too early and then they do not know where they are, in which case they may use the bus but will have to be accompanied by a care worker. These assessments must be weighed up before a decision is reached.

In addition, there may be different views held by the service user or their carers which will affect the decision. Risks are part of everyday life and individuals are entitled to take risks if they want to, within certain limits, i.e. when not life-threatening. As part of person-centred care, carers need to see some risk taking as positive rather than negative. It is now recognised that this can have positive benefits for an individual, allowing them autonomy and control of their lives.

Working with person-centred values

A person-centred approach is to see the person as an individual, focusing on their personal needs, wants, goals and aspirations. The individual becomes central to the healthcare process. The support the individual needs must be designed in partnership with the individual, their family and/or carers.

Key concepts of a person-centred approach are:
- knowing the person as an individual
- empowerment and power
- respecting the individual's values and preferences
- choice and **autonomy**
- respect and dignity
- **empathy** and compassion.

The likelihood of abuse can be reduced by the healthcare workers following the person-centred concepts listed above as they gain in self-worth. If abuse did occur, the individual should, with the person-centred approach, feel more confident to report it, as they will feel that they will be believed and supported. Empowering vulnerable individuals allows them to make their own decisions and to be responsible for their own safety. This allows them to feel valued and improves their self-esteem, which are extremely important.

> ### Key terms
>
> ***Autonomy:*** In the case of safeguarding an adult, staff must respect the competent decisions made by an individual as they have the right to make these independently. Staff should not act without consulting the adult at risk unless the adult does not have the mental capacity for this.
>
> ***Empathy:*** the ability to understand and share the feelings of an individual.

Multi-agency working

Safeguarding children, young people and adults from abuse and promoting their welfare is everyone's responsibility. Agencies such as schools, social services, health services, youth organisations, charities and the police should work alongside one another to protect children, young people and vulnerable adults from abuse and prevent further harm and abuse. A multi-agency approach can help to:
- ensure all concerns are identified early and reported
- ensure professionals and agencies that may have different insights and experiences of individuals and their families come together and appropriately share the information they have
- provide a better insight into the needs and views of children, young people and adults
- ensure professionals and agencies work in consistent ways that focus on building trust, respect and providing support to children, young people and adults.

To ensure that a multi-agency approach is effective, all agencies involved must understand the role they have to play in safeguarding as well as the roles others have. All professionals must be committed to working alongside other professionals who may work in different agencies and have different roles.

A11.8 The meaning of patient safety and clinical effectiveness, including why they're important

Patient safety

The avoidance of accidental or unintended injury or harm during a period of receiving healthcare

Hospitals and many other healthcare settings are security conscious as they do not want any harm to come to their patients while they are in hospital. For example, most hospital sites will have 24-hour 7-days-a-week security with closed circuit cameras to help prevent intruders. All staff will have name badges and all wards will have security doors with intercom buzzers so no unauthorised person can gain access. Hospital staff will carry out regular risk assessment and staff will be encouraged to report safety hazards. Staff should follow policies and procedures related to

key legislation promoting health, safety and security. For example, all staff will be aware of fire evacuation policy and the procedures for the storage of medicines and hazardous substances. Staff should also ensure they pass on all information relevant to patients' progress, safety and any concerns they may have during the handover period to the new staff who are taking over the shift.

In addition to security, the NHS Patient Safety Strategy of July 2019, subtitled 'Safer culture, safer systems, safer patients', set out objectives to be achieved in terms of patient safety. This strategy sits alongside the NHS Long Term Plan (LTP). According to the NHS Patient Safety Strategy, 1000 extra lives could be saved by safer working practices as well as £100 million in care costs by 2023/24. Through this, the NHS aims to achieve its safety vision, i.e. to continuously improve patient safety. Good record keeping and equipping everyone involved with the skills they need are of central importance to this, as is clinical effectiveness (see below), including research into further good practice.

Clinical effectiveness

The application of healthcare, taking into consideration the individual's wishes, healthcare professional's experience, and evidence-based research in the approach

Clinical effectiveness is a key factor of patient safety. It means that information collected from national and international validated and reliable research is used to identify which practices are safe, effective and efficient. In other words, which treatments work and have evidence to verify their success. Drawing all the information together helps healthcare professionals and their patients make decisions about what is best for the patient. The promotion of clinical effectiveness in the NHS has been stated as a key priority of the current government. Clinical effectiveness aims to ensure that healthcare practice is based on the best available data. It is a key component for improving patient safety and quality health service delivery. Evidence-based practice, as the name suggests, means that when a healthcare professional makes a treatment decision with their patient, it is based on their clinical expertise, sound research (see page 371) and the patient's preferences.

> **Key term**
>
> **Clinical:** related to the observation and treatment of patients.

Why patient safety and clinical effectiveness are important

Raises the standard of care, improving the patient's experience and quality

The patient must be at the centre of any treatment and should be treated as an individual. They must be provided with safe and clinically excellent care. The patient must feel a valued and equal partner in any discussion about their care; they need to feel in control and should be treated with honesty, respect and dignity. Patient experience is improved when they can make informed choices about their care because they have been given high-quality information to help guide their decision making. Patients who take part in shared decision making are more likely to follow advice given by the healthcare professional when they are discharged from hospital. Generally, patients who have better experiences have better health outcomes, for example, they are discharged more quickly from hospital because they have recovered faster from their procedure.

Avoids negative outcomes for the provision of care

Poor outcomes from healthcare could mean that the patient needs to stay in hospital longer, therefore they are more likely to pick up superbugs such as MRSA (see Chapter A10, page 194). This could delay their recovery and they may be ill for a longer period than they should be. If patients are treated as a set of symptoms without considering their wider emotional, social or practical needs, this will have an impact on their recovery time as they will not feel or be truly cared for. To avoid a negative outcome, it helps for the healthcare professional to spend more time with the patient to explain all the options available to them. Although this may take more time at the beginning of the treatment, for the healthcare professional it will be worthwhile by having an informed patient who is much happier and more likely to have positive outcomes. This will make them feel involved in their clinical journey and their self-esteem will be boosted. This will have a positive effect on them which should aid their recovery.

Getting It Right First Time (GIRFT) is a national programme designed to improve patient outcomes through reviewing and examining how things are done in NHS hospitals and how they can be improved. Data-driven evidence is reviewed by senior clinicians who then advise or make decisions on the best way to improve outcomes for patients.

Test yourself

1 Explain what is meant by clinical effectiveness.
2 Explain how raising the standard of care improves the patient's experience.
3 Describe how the healthcare professional can help to avoid negative outcomes for the provision of care.

A11.9 What is meant by radicalisation, identifying signs of radicalisation and the purpose of the Prevent strategy (2011)

Meaning of radicalisation

The action or process of someone to adopt or support terrorism, or radical extremist beliefs connected with terrorism or terrorist groups

Radicalisation occurs when individuals believe and support extreme ideas or doctrine around political, religious or social ideals, especially with regard to the use of violence. It is a form of exploitation involving individuals being influenced and coerced into extremism. There are many different reasons why people become radicalised. They may feel lonely or unhappy about themselves or feel they do not fit into their peer group. They may be bullied or harassed or feel discriminated against and are looking for a place to belong and where they feel valued. They may be dreaming of glory and feel they could save the world if they join a terrorist or extremist group. Figure 11.5 suggests some other ideas that may contribute to radicalisation but there are many more.

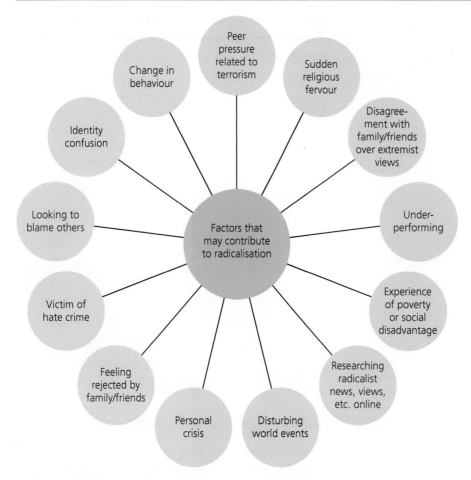

▲ Figure 11.5 Factors that may contribute to radicalisation

Identifying signs of radicalisation

Detachment from family and friends

People who are being radicalised may start to withdraw from family and friends as they do not want them to realise that they no longer have the same views and ideals. They do not respect the values they formerly held or were brought up with as they feel they no longer apply to them. They are also afraid that their family or friends will realise what is happening and try to change their mind. Adolescence in particular is a time of huge physical and emotional change and so it can be very difficult for parents to differentiate between normal adolescent behaviour and attitude that indicates the child may have been exposed to radicalising influence.

Raised levels of anger

Adolescents may have raised levels of anger as their hormones fluctuate, making it difficult for them to keep their emotions under control. This is normal and can lead to mood swings. They may go from sad to happy within a short period of time. Disagreeing with parents and other adults such as teachers is normal behaviour as they are testing the boundaries and questioning authority. Raised levels of anger could be displayed by the adolescent becoming increasingly argumentative and refusing to listen to different points of view. It is difficult to reach a decision about radicalisation on one aspect of behaviour.

Failure or avoidance in discussing own views

Failure to discuss their views is normal for adolescents as they may feel it is a waste of time talking to their parents as 'they don't understand me'. However, it is a good idea for the family to encourage their teenagers to talk about their views. If they are not willing to do so, perhaps they may discuss them with a similar-aged sibling if they have one. If they are unwilling to discuss their views despite the parents' best efforts, the parents cannot force them, but if something relevant appears on the news, this may be a good starting point to lead into a discussion.

Increased interest in privacy or secretive behaviours

Privacy and secretive behaviour are other traits of the adolescent years, as the young person grows up and 'finds themselves'. This alone cannot be indicative of radicalised behaviour as this is normal behaviour for adolescents. They naturally want to be on their own to explore grown-up matters at their own pace.

Case study

Safaa

Examine the factors in Figure 11.5 that may contribute to radicalisation. Read Safaa's story on: www.bbc.co.uk/news/uk-44359958

What do you think helped to radicalise Safaa?

The purpose of the Prevent strategy

To work with communities to support vulnerable people at risk of becoming radicalised

Prevent is a community safeguarding programme about identifying individuals including children and young people before they become radicalised. It is about early intervention. Prevent was set up in 2006 but reviewed in 2011. It originally included promoting integration as well as confronting and preventing terrorism. The government published the Prevent strategy as part of the wider counter-terrorism strategy CONTEST.

CONTEST was published in June 2018 and was the government's response to the terrorist attacks in Manchester and London. Its aim was to reduce terrorist risk to the UK so people could live their lives in safety – see Figure 11.6.

In 2015 the Counterterrorism and Security Act was changed so that organisations funded by the government and working in the public sector, such as education, health, criminal justice, local councils, government departments and social services have a duty in supporting vulnerable individuals and are obliged to prevent them developing extremist or radicalised views. Third-sector organisations as well as faith institutions are also involved in supporting Prevent. Frontline staff are provided with training so that they can recognise and respond to radicalisation. Projects developed by local authorities and community organisations help to reduce the risks of people joining terrorist groups. Prevent provides practical help by giving advice and support on radicalisation to community groups, social enterprise projects, local schools and industry as well as religious organisations.

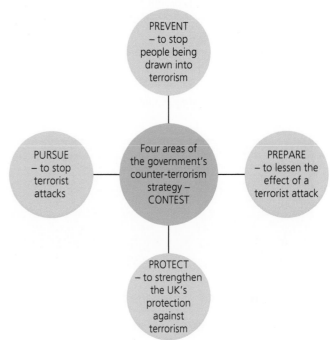

▲ Figure 11.6 The four areas of the government's counter-terrorism strategy CONTEST

If anyone (it could be a professional from any of the above groups or a family member or friend) identifies an individual who may be becoming radicalised, they can make a referral to Channel, a programme designed to provide support for anyone who is drawn to terrorism. Channel is not **compulsory** for individuals who are identified as being in danger of becoming radicalised; they can refuse to go on the programme. It does, however, offer a confidential service as an incentive.

Channel's remit is to provide tailored support for the vulnerable person who may be drawn to terrorism. Each referral will be examined carefully by the Channel panel to see if the referral is genuine and that the individual is at risk. If so, the panel will determine the level of the risk and work out a suitable support plan for the referred individual. Referred individuals are consulted and must give their consent before any support or intervention can go ahead. At no stage is the individual criminalised unless they commit a separate crime such as theft or assault.

Key term

Compulsory: required by law or by other regulations.

A11.10 The importance of positive behaviour, including a range of positive behaviours expected of a health professional

Importance of positive behaviour

Key to safeguarding individuals

The health professional should provide safe person-centred care and services for all individuals. Vulnerable adults and children who have been or are being abused are often left feeling unsafe, fearful and suspicious of others. By building a trusting and professional relationship with individuals, workers can minimise the risk of abuse by:

▶ enabling individuals to confide in them when abuse is happening to them and/or others
▶ building mutual respect so that the individual feels in control of their life
▶ encouraging open discussion and therefore diminishing the risk of abusive relationships.

Failure to comply with behavioural standards could result in noncompliance and deregistration

There are nine statutory health and care regulators (for example, the Nursing and Midwifery Council, General Medical Council, Health & Care Professions Council) who set the standards and code of conduct that healthcare professionals must follow. The target of all nine regulators is to:

▶ protect the public
▶ uphold professional standards
▶ maintain public confidence in the healthcare professions.

They do this by:

▶ setting standards of competence and conduct for healthcare professionals
▶ checking training and education courses are suitable
▶ keeping a register of professionals
▶ following up complaints about registered professionals.

After investigating the complaints, the health and care regulators will decide if a healthcare professional is allowed to continue or whether further training or other criteria must be met before they can continue to practise.

If complaints are upheld, the healthcare professional could be **struck off** (removed from) the register (also known as **deregistration**) either because of their competence or behaviour – this means they will be prevented from working as a registered healthcare professional.

This process is known as **fitness to practise**. Types of behaviour that could cause a healthcare professional to be struck off the register include sexual misconduct, criminal offending for serious crimes such as assault or murder, or for dishonesty. Dishonesty is not just stealing but includes covering up when things go wrong and could or did cause harm to a patient. Examples of incompetence could be inadequately exploring a patient's medical history or misinterpreting baseline observations, such as oxygen saturation or level of consciousness or realising that they are out of their depth but not asking a colleague for help.

Range of positive behaviour expected of a health professional

People first approach (for example, don't make assumptions, acknowledge and accept diversity and choice)

It is important that everyone has the right to be treated fairly and equally; healthcare workers should respect patients' rights, choices and beliefs. Some attitudes towards and assumptions about patients can create barriers, such as stereotyping or lacking respect for cultural and ethnic differences. Unless a healthcare professional communicates with each person as an individual, they are likely to make assumptions about them based on something they have seen or read, for example, that all older people are weak and frail. The judgement or prejudice may be inaccurate but it could affect the interaction with that person.

Diversity recognises and values that everyone is unique. Valuing diversity involves respecting and accepting individual differences such as age, gender, religion, sexual orientation, education, disability, race or beliefs. Several of these are characteristics which are legally protected under the Equality Act 2010 (see page 2).

Individuals may have different views and opinions from the healthcare worker. Choice gives individuals control over their lives and increases their self-esteem because it promotes independence. The role of the healthcare worker is not to judge but to enable individuals to think through what options are available, the advantages and disadvantages of each and then make their choice.

Effective practised clinical competence (for example, communicate effectively, share best practice, work cooperatively)

Effective verbal, non-verbal and written communication between workers, individuals, their families, professionals and agencies is vital in healthcare. This means sharing information, opinions or ideas in a way that others will understand and be able to respond to. In this way the healthcare professional must be competent at passing on information to other professionals in the healthcare team as a patient's health and recovery relies on the clarity of the information passed on. Records that reinforce the verbal information relayed are also vital as a backup.

The idea of sharing good practice is to improve clinical delivery across all areas of the NHS – in other words, treat patients even more effectively. Healthcare professionals must work in **multidisciplinary teams** and co-operate with different disciplines within the hospital if they want the best outcome for their patients. However, sharing good practice is also about sharing successes across different areas of the country, not just within a hospital trust. For example, if operating a seven-day week in northern Lincolnshire and Goole NHS Foundation has allowed patients to have same-day diagnostics and a walk-in clinic so that target waiting

times for patients have been met, this needs to be shared with other hospital trusts nationally so that they can help to reduce their own waiting lists. But sharing good practice should be worldwide, with different countries offering their innovative ideas that work. The aim of this co-operative working is to ensure that good practice is passed on so that everyone reaps the benefits.

Key term

Multidisciplinary team: a team of professionals from different specialisms who work together for the good of the patient, e.g. a physiotherapist working with a dietician and an orthopaedic surgeon after someone has had a traffic accident.

Maintain safety (for example, observe and report on an individual's condition and escalate any issues where necessary, as soon as possible)

Clinical competence is important in healthcare as it could mean the difference between life and death for the patient, or between serious consequences or a good recovery. As stated above in behavioural standards a healthcare professional can be removed from the register if they are incompetent in their clinical decisions. This incompetence can take the form of not passing on any change in a patient's condition or not recognising signs of deteriorating physical condition.

Communicating clearly to other staff members and passing on concerns is vital and this must be done immediately if there is any cause for concern. It is better to be overcautious than wait until it is too late to resolve the situation. This is the reason there is a handover period at the end of a hospital shift so staff can comment on patients' recovery or deterioration to the new duty team so they can act on any concerns. Staff must seek help if they are unsure or feel out of their depth with any patient as there is no shame in asking another practitioner for guidance and support.

Encourage professionalism and trust

When working in healthcare, it is important for all staff to uphold the standards of their profession. They must act with honesty and integrity in all their dealings with patients, the public and other healthcare professionals. They need clear professional boundaries with the people they treat or look after. In this way they can act as role models for students and newly qualified healthcare professionals.

Continuing professional development provides healthcare workers with the opportunities to maintain and enhance their knowledge and skills. This equips them with current knowledge and up-to-date clinical practice and enables them to practise safely and legally. It also gives the professional healthcare worker confidence in their own skills and ability. All these factors encourage trust and confidence from patients as they see the professional behaviour of the healthcare workers.

> ### Test yourself
>
> 1 a There are nine statutory health and care regulators. What are the three targets of all the regulators?
>   b List three ways they do this.
>   c If there is a complaint the regulators will investigate and decide on the 'fitness to practise'. If the professional healthcare worker is struck off the register why might this happen?
> 2 Healthcare professionals are expected to behave with a people first approach. Explain what this means.
> 3 Explain what is meant by clinical competence.

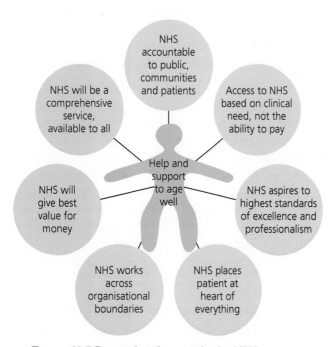

▲ Figure 11.7 Principles that guide the NHS

A11.11 The types of support for managing positive behaviour

Behavioural frameworks (for example, guidance on expected employee behaviour in a trust or workplace)

All NHS workers must follow the NHS Constitution, which has seven principles that guide the NHS, as shown in Figure 11.7. These principles form the basis of all the NHS hopes to achieve.

The six core NHS values support these seven NHS principles and all employees (regardless of their role) are expected to follow:

▶ Working together for patients – this requires all healthcare staff to put patients first. Patients, their families, carers, etc. must be fully involved in the care offered. If staff are unhappy about anything they are expected to speak up.
▶ Respect and dignity – every person is an individual. They should be valued and their needs addressed. They should have a voice, be listened to and taken seriously.
▶ Everyone counts – nobody must be discriminated against or excluded. Available resources must be used wisely for the benefit of the whole community.
▶ Commitment to quality – patients must have quality of care; their treatment should be effective and safe. Feedback from patients should be encouraged and acted on to improve the care.
▶ Compassion – anxiety, pain and distress must be met with kindness, care and compassion. Staff must provide comfort and support to help relieve any patient from suffering.
▶ Improving lives – people's health and wellbeing can be improved by clinical excellence, professionalism, innovative practice and service improvements.

Each NHS trust will use the six core values for its own behavioural framework. They may alter or change the words but the principles behind their policies will remain the same. These values will be used in staff appraisal discussions/performance management as well as forming the basis of any feedback or discussion on everyday practice. Students applying for university courses in healthcare are tested on these values.

Workplace policies (for example, whistleblowing and social media policies setting out what employees should/shouldn't do)

Any organisation will have workplace policies in place covering areas such as health and safety, attendance, bullying and harassment, safeguarding and grievance. As a large organisation, the NHS has an external whistleblowing policy in place, although hospital trusts will also have their own individual whistleblowing policy showing what to do step by step. This policy is for NHS healthcare workers who need to contact an external agency about a concern they have, in cases where they have already reported the concern internally and nothing has happened.

Figure 11.8 shows a number of reasons why an individual might whistleblow in the NHS. There is a list of agencies that the whistleblower may wish to contact besides NHS England. The external whistleblowing policy offers confidentiality and anonymity if that is what the healthcare worker wants. There is an NHS Whistleblowing Helpline that will give them independent advice. Every NHS trust has a Freedom to Speak Up Guardian who will offer advice and support for staff who speak up. Guardians work across the NHS trusts to encourage transparency and openness. This role was created as a result of an investigation in 2013 into a Mid Staffordshire NHS Foundation Trust.

Social media policies give staff clear guidance on what is acceptable and unacceptable usage of social media. Staff are asked not to access social media sites during working hours but only on break times. Obviously, hospital trusts ask that staff do not post photographs of patients or other staff in their workplace or give out confidential information as this would breach data protection legislation and violate patient confidentiality. In addition to this, posts must not contain information that is offensive, threatening, embarrassing, bullying, etc. They must not discuss work-related issues or complaints or anything that may bring the organisation into disrepute. Failure to comply with any of the rules would result in a disciplinary hearing which may lead to dismissal.

> **Research**
>
> Ask your supervisor if they have a social media policy in your placement and if you could have a copy. Alternatively, see if you can find a social media policy online for an NHS trust.
>
> In a group, share the policies you have been able to collect and compare them for the message they give to staff. Are they all very similar? How do they differ?

Performance management (for example, performance improvement plans to support employees to succeed)

Performance management should be an ongoing process between a healthcare worker and their manager. This process involves meetings and observations over time to provide feedback on performance and identify targets for improvement where necessary. These meetings and observations will then contribute to the six- or twelve-monthly (depending on the organisation) appraisal but supervision or management would usually be monthly, especially for someone new to the job. The manager's role is to supervise, support and advise the healthcare worker. They must ensure that the worker has a job description and understands what is expected from them in their role. If there are any concerns or issues, the manager should not wait until the annual appraisal to raise the concern but should raise it when it happens. Managers should consider the possible causes of the concern which may be:

▶ inadequate training
▶ the health and wellbeing of the worker

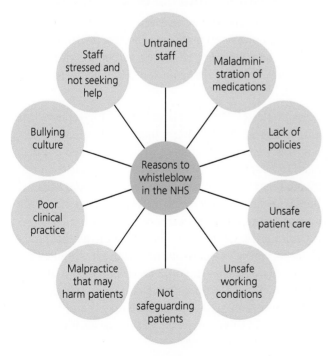

▲ Figure 11.8 Possible reasons to whistleblow in the NHS

- a lack of supervision or support
- broken or damaged equipment, missing materials
- poor systems, policies and procedure.

The healthcare worker must be given the chance to improve so the manager may consider the following help for the worker:

- a coach/mentor
- reviewing systems, policies and procedures
- arranging repairs for faulty/broken equipment, ordering missing materials
- clarifying the job role
- reviewing their workload
- supervision and support
- additional training
- an occupational health referral.

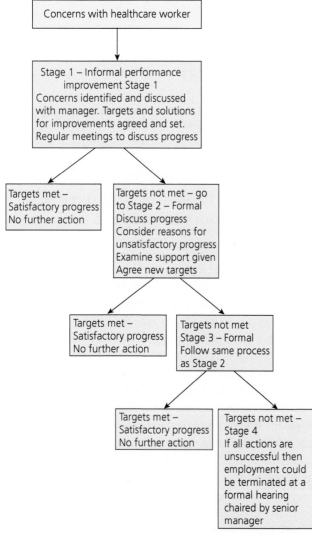

▲ Figure 11.9 The typical stages in an unsatisfactory performance management review

Figure 11.9 shows the typical four stages of an unsatisfactory performance review. This is an option available to managers but it must be stressed that the worker has every opportunity to improve their performance. The target set for them to achieve is jointly agreed between the worker and the manager; the manager will provide support for the worker to meet the targets as far as they can. If the worker is still not meeting the standard by Stage 3 of the review they may be advised to apply for other vacancies within the organisation. These vacancies may be at a lower grade but they will be guaranteed an interview if they meet the minimum requirements. Throughout this unsatisfactory performance management process, the worker will have written confirmation of targets, etc. that have been agreed so they will know exactly what they have to do for their work to be considered satisfactory.

A11.12 What is meant by a conflict of interest and how to deal with those while practising healthcare

What is meant by a conflict of interest

A situation where a person of trust, or an organisation's own interests, are in direct conflict with the interest of the patient

A conflict of interest is where a professional finds themselves unable to make an objective decision as they will be affected by the result, either positively or negatively. This should be declared (see below for more details).

For example, a GP may be discussing a hip replacement with a patient. The GP might mention that there is a long waiting list for the operation to be carried out in an NHS hospital. The patient is willing to pay for a private hospital to carry out the procedure and asks the GP for his opinion of the different private hospitals offering hip replacement procedures. It would be difficult for the GP to recommend the private hospital where he works as a consultant because it would be a conflict of interest as he could make money out of the operation. The GP would have to inform the patient that he is not impartial as he also works there. The patient would then have the facts before deciding which hospital to choose.

Another example of a conflict of interest could be if a close relative, for example, son or daughter, works for a company supplying PPE to the hospital where an individual works. This should be declared, particularly if they have decision-making responsibilities in the company.

If an individual working in the healthcare sector is unsure about whether to declare a conflict of interest, they should fill in the declaration of interests form on the NHS website and return it. If in doubt, they should declare it anyway.

How to deal with conflicts of interest

Be open and honest, acting with integrity

A person acting with integrity is honest and truthful and always follows moral principles. For example, a consultant may be offered free accommodation in a holiday villa as a gift by a patient on the understanding that they will be moved up the waiting list for an operation. If they accept, and the patient is moved up, the consultant would not be honest and open or be acting with integrity. To act openly, the consultant would be expected to turn down the gift. As a public employee, they must be as open as possible about all their decisions and actions. They must also declare any private interests which may relate to their duties as a healthcare worker.

Follow workplace guidelines

The appropriate way to manage any conflict of interest is to follow the guidelines that apply to your role and organisation. The workplace guidelines will give the healthcare worker a framework for how to report conflicts of interest; it will also say which person has

the responsibility for conflicts of interest. It is likely that most healthcare professionals will not have to declare a conflict of interest as they will not benefit from a patient as this would usually be someone who deals with finance or is high up in the management structure. Under current guidelines, healthcare staff working in the NHS can accept small gifts up to the value of £50 from patients without declaring them, for example, a box of chocolates or a bottle of wine; however, gifts of money or vouchers must always be declined. Note that policies and procedures vary according to different health settings and staff should follow their own workplace guidelines.

Declare any personal conflicts (for example, that you have a personal relationship with the individual)

If a hospital manager works in a department that is recruiting new staff members and a good friend of the manager has applied, they would declare an interest as soon as they realise the situation so the organisation can debate on the right level of involvement for the person in the recruitment/management process. The manager would have to fill in a form describing the relationship and the organisation would make a decision based on the information they have received. If the manager does not declare the relationship they could be accused of favouritism or giving preferential treatment to one of the candidates, or potentially they could lose their job.

There must be transparency in the recruitment process as it is essential in avoiding real or perceived favouritism of friends or relations, and that decisions are based on facts and not on relationships or connections with the people involved.

Project practice

In section A11.2 you examined the NHS England guide on abuse. Working alone using your ideas on how to improve the guide, produce your own ideas for a condensed guide that you could give to a student who is just starting out to train as a healthcare worker. Present your guide to the group in a short slideshow presentation. You do not have to produce the whole guide but you should produce a written handout with more detail than your presentation.

1 Read through the guide and choose at least three topics that interest you.

2 Decide what you like and/or dislike about the way these topics are presented. Give reasons why you think they are satisfactory or unsatisfactory.

3 Design your own interpretation of the topics, remembering they are going to be used by a trainee healthcare worker.

4 Turn your ideas into a slideshow presentation to present to your group. Remember not to put too much information on each slide.

5 Produce a more detailed handout, covering only the three topics.

Assessment practice

1 The NHS Constitution has six principles that form the basis of safeguarding in the health sector. List **three** of these principles.

2 a Janine has an 'unsatisfactory' on her observations for her performance management. Name two possible 'causes of concern' her manager should consider.

   b What help may Janine need to improve her performance?

   c Despite getting help, Janine has not met her targets and has failed Stage 3 of her performance review. Explain what happens now.

3 a Describe what is meant by a conflict of interest.

   b Explain the appropriate way to deal with a conflict of interest.

4 Describe how a staff member can ensure they record disclosures of abuse appropriately.

5 Discuss how clinical photography can help to preserve evidence in cases of abuse.

6 Explain the meaning of proportionality in the context of safeguarding.

7 Describe what is meant by empowering individuals.

8 Explain what is meant by an effective complaints procedure.

9 Explain what is meant by clinical effectiveness.

10 a The NHS has six core values that all employees must follow. Describe **four** of these core values.

   b Explain how NHS Trusts will use these core values in everyday practice.

B1.1–B1.32: Core science concepts: Biology

Introduction

Biology is the study of living organisms, which makes it an enormous subject! In this chapter we will cover some important basics, such as the structure of cells and the way in which they are organised. We cannot really understand how organisms work without understanding cells, and we cannot understand how cells work without learning about the main types of biological molecules: proteins, carbohydrates and lipids. Exchange and transport mechanisms – the ways in which substances enter or leave – are essential for the working of individual cells and multicellular organisms. Genetics helps us understand how characteristics are inherited and introduces the fourth main type of biological molecules – the nucleic acids – as well as providing a basis for our understanding of evolution. Microbiology is not just the study of very small organisms; it helps us to understand infectious diseases. Finally, immunology helps to explain how our bodies protect themselves against infection.

Learning outcomes

The core knowledge outcomes that you must understand and learn:

Cells and tissues
B1.1 the 3 principles of cell theory
B1.2 the different types of cells that make up living organisms
B1.3 the structure and function of the organelles found within eukaryotic cells
B1.4 the similarities and differences between plant and animal cells in relation to the presence of specific organelles and their function
B1.5 how eukaryotic cells become specialised in complex multi-cellular organisms
B1.6 how prokaryotic cells differ from eukaryotic cells

Proteins, Carbohydrates and Lipids
B1.7 the relationship between the structure, properties and functions of proteins
B1.8 the relationship between the structure, properties and functions of carbohydrates
B1.9 the relationship between the structure, properties and functions of lipids

Exchange and transport mechanisms
B1.10 how the surface area to volume ratio affects the process of exchange and gives rise to specialised systems
B1.11 the principles of cellular exchange and the transport mechanisms which exist to facilitate this exchange
B1.12 the advantages of having specialised cells in relation to the rate of transport across internal and external membranes

Genetics
B1.13 the purpose of deoxyribonucleic acid (DNA) and ribonucleic acid (RNA) as the carrying molecules of genetic information and the role they play in the mechanism of inheritance
B1.14 the relationship between the structure of DNA and RNA and their role in the mechanism of inheritance
B1.15 the function of complementary base pairing in forming the helical structure of DNA
B1.16 the process and stages of semi-conservative replication of DNA
B1.17 how this semi-conservative replication process ensures genetic continuity between generations of cells
B1.18 the link between the semi-conservative replication process and variation
B1.19 the difference between genetics and genomics

Microbiology
B1.20 the classification and characteristics (size of cell, type of cell, presence of organelles) of the following micro-organisms
B1.21 the benefits of using light and electron microscopes when investigating micro-organisms.
B1.22 how to calculate magnification from the size of the image and the size of the object
B1.23 the uses of differential staining techniques

Immunology
B1.24 the nature of infection
B1.25 causative agents of infection and examples of resulting diseases

B1.26 the different ways in which causative agents may enter the body
B1.27 how infectious diseases can spread among populations and communities
B1.28 the definition of an antigen and an antibody
B1.29 the link between antigens and the initiation of the body's response to invasion by a foreign substance
B1.30 the stages and cells involved in the body's response to an antigen
B1.31 the differences between cell-mediated immunity and antibody-mediated immunity
B1.32 the role of T and B memory cells in the secondary immune response.

Cells and tissues

We can study and understand biology at different levels of organisation. Starting with the whole **organism**, we can move upwards to study the ways in which organisms interact in populations and ecosystems. Alternatively, we can look at the way in which organisms work in increasing levels of detail. The cell is the basic unit of all organisms. We need to learn the structure and organisation of the cell to get a proper understanding of how cells work together and also understand the environment in which the chemical reactions of the cell take place.

Key terms

Membrane: all membranes consist of a **phospholipid** bilayer together with proteins and other components. They are selectively permeable (meaning they let some things through and not others) and can control movement of substances across the membrane as well as being the sites of many important processes in the cell.

Phospholipid: a large molecule formed from a glycerol molecule covalently bound to two fatty acid molecules and a phosphate group. It has a **hydrophilic** (can interact with water) head group (because of the phosphate) and a **hydrophobic** (repels water) tail (because of the fatty acids).

Cytoplasm: is the fluid component of the cell, enclosed by the cell membrane and surrounding the organelles.

Organelles: specialised structures within plant and animal cells that have specific functions. Some types of organelle are also found within bacterial cells.

Organism: an individual plant, animal or single-celled lifeform.

B1.1 The 3 principles of cell theory

Robert Hooke (1635–1703) was the first person to recognise cells, although the 'cells' in cork that he saw using his microscope were the empty spaces between the cell walls of the cork. Hooke laid the foundations for what we now know as the three principles of cell theory. This states that:

▶ All living things are made up of one or more cells. This means that living things can be **unicellular** (single cells) or **multicellular** (made up of more than one cell).
▶ Cells are the most basic unit of structure and function in all living things. Cells contain many components (nuclei, mitochondria, etc.) but these cannot exist or reproduce on their own.
▶ All cells are created by pre-existing cells, i.e. cells cannot just appear from nowhere. New cells are created from pre-existing cells in the process of **mitosis** (cell division).

B1.2 The different types of cells that make up living organisms

There are two types of cell: **prokaryotic** cells and **eukaryotic** cells. Eukaryotic cells are complex and include all animal and plant cells as well as yeasts, other fungi and algae. Prokaryotic cells are simpler and smaller and include the bacteria. Both types of cell have **membranes**, **cytoplasm** and DNA. However, eukaryotic cells have membrane-bound **organelles**, such as mitochondria or chloroplasts. Also, the DNA is contained within the nucleus. The DNA is bound to proteins known as histones and together they form a complex known as chromatin (see below). In prokaryotic cells, the DNA just floats freely in the cytoplasm, or is found as small circular molecules known as plasmids, and is not associated with proteins.

B1.3 The structure and function of the organelles found within eukaryotic cells

Plasma membrane

Also called the **cell surface membrane**, this is found around the outside of the cell and consists of a **phospholipid bilayer** together with proteins and other components. The **plasma membrane** controls entry and exit of substances into and out of the cell.

Key terms

Phospholipid bilayer: a double layer of phospholipids with the hydrophobic tails arranged towards the middle and the hydrophilic head groups on the outside. It forms the basis of all biological membranes.

Plasma membrane: sometimes called the cell-surface membrane, it is the membrane that surrounds all types of cell; animal, plant and bacterial. Like all membranes, the plasma membrane consists of a phospholipid bilayer together with proteins and other components.

Nucleus (containing chromosomes)

The nucleus is the largest organelle and is surrounded by the **nuclear envelope.** This is a double membrane that has many gaps or **pores**.

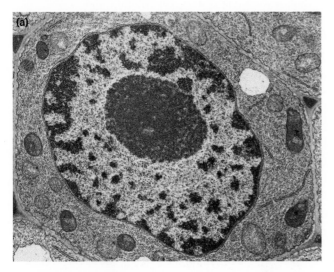

▲ Figure 12.1a An electron micrograph (x 25 000) showing a nucleus

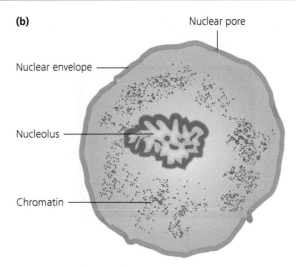

▲ Figure 12.1b A diagram showing the structure of the nucleus

The nucleus contains the genetic information, in the form of DNA. The DNA is combined with proteins known as histones; this forms the complex known as **chromatin**. The chromatin is coiled and super-coiled to form the chromosomes.

Mitochondria

Mitochondria (the singular is mitochondrion) are the site of **aerobic respiration** and therefore the site of adenosine triphosphate (ATP) production. Aerobic respiration is the process where glucose is reacted with oxygen to produce carbon dioxide and water. As this reaction is exothermic, the energy transferred from this reaction is used to produce ATP, the 'energy currency' of the cell. Almost all processes in the cell that require energy obtain it from ATP.

Like nuclei and chloroplasts, mitochondria are enclosed by a double membrane (envelope). The inner membrane is folded into structures called **cristae**.

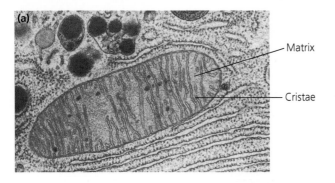

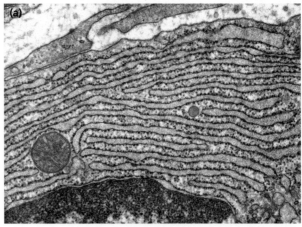

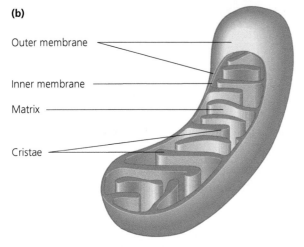

▲ Figure 12.2 A mitochondrion: (a) an electron micrograph (x 1100) and (b) a diagram

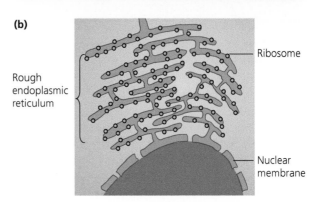

▲ Figure 12.3 Rough endoplasmic reticulum: (a) an electron micrograph (x 18 000) and (b) a diagram

Ribosomes

Ribosomes are the smallest of the organelles and are the site of protein synthesis. Some float free in the cytoplasm and make the proteins needed within the cell, whereas others are attached to the rough endoplasmic reticulum. Ribosomes use the information coded in an mRNA molecule to assemble the correct order of amino acids in the protein.

Rough and smooth endoplasmic reticulum

The **endoplasmic reticulum (ER)** is a system of membrane-bound flattened sacs that fills a large part of the cytoplasm. The **rough ER (RER)** has ribosomes attached to its outer surface. Proteins that will be released from the cell or incorporated into the plasma membrane are made on these attached ribosomes and then folded and transported in the RER to the Golgi apparatus.

The **smooth ER** does not have attached ribosomes and is responsible for synthesising, storing and transporting lipids and some carbohydrates.

Golgi apparatus and Golgi vesicles

The Golgi apparatus is a stack of flattened sacs, known as cisternae (singular is cisterna). Each cisterna is surrounded by a single membrane and filled with fluid. The Golgi modifies proteins that have been transported from the RER, for example by adding carbohydrates to them. These modified proteins are then transported by **Golgi vesicles** that form when the ends of the cisternae are pinched off. These vesicles can form **lysosomes** (see below). Others, called **secretory vesicles**, carry their contents to the plasma membrane where they can be released to the outside of the cell.

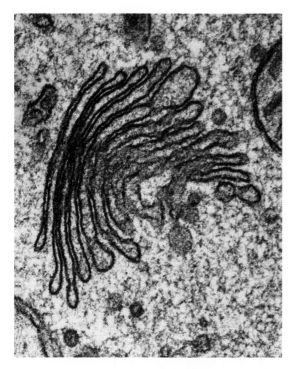

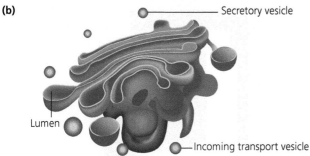

(b)

Secretory vesicle

Lumen

Incoming transport vesicle

▲ Figure 12.4 The Golgi apparatus: (a) an electron micrograph (x 50 000) and (b) a diagram showing the Golgi vesicles and secretory vesicles

Lysosomes

These are the cell's recycling facility. When proteins and other cell components get worn out, they are moved into lysosomes. Digestive enzymes break these down into their constituents, e.g. amino acids that can be re-used to make new proteins. It is important that these enzymes are kept separate from the rest of the cytoplasm because of the damage they could do. Lysosomes are also involved in digestion of invading **pathogens** (bacteria and viruses) that are taken into the cell by the process of **phagocytosis** (see page 256 later in this chapter).

Centrioles

Centrioles are structures made of a tubular protein called tubulin. They are involved in the formation of the spindle in **mitosis** as well as formation of **cilia** and **flagella**. They are not present in many types of plant cells.

Key terms

Pathogen: a micro-organism that causes illness or disease by damaging host tissues and/or by producing toxins.

Cilia: (singular **cilium**) are hair-like structures found on the plasma membrane of some types of cell, particularly in the lungs.

Flagella: (singular **flagellum**) are similar in structure to cilia but are much longer and are involved in propulsion of the cell.

Chloroplasts (in plants)

Like mitochondria, chloroplasts are enclosed by an **envelope** (double membrane) and contain membranes called **thylakoids** arranged in stacks called **grana** (singular is **granum**). The chloroplast is the site of photosynthesis, the process whereby plants and algae use light energy to make complex organic molecules from carbon dioxide and water. There are two stages to photosynthesis. The first stage occurs in the thylakoid membranes which contain chlorophyll and other pigments that absorb light energy as well as proteins involved in the production of ATP. The rest of the chloroplast consists of a fluid called the **stroma**, which is where the second stage of photosynthesis take place.

(a)

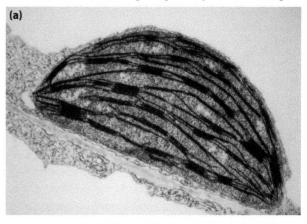

(b)

Inner membrane   Stroma

Outer membrane

Thylakoid

Granum

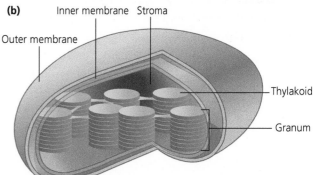

▲ Figure 12.5 A chloroplast: (a) an electron micrograph (x 13 750) and (b) a diagram

Cell wall (in plants)

Plant cell walls consist mainly of the carbohydrate **cellulose.** Cell walls provide strength and rigidity for protection and support. If animal cells take up too much water they burst, whereas in plants the cell wall prevents this.

Cell vacuole (in plants)

Cell vacuoles are fluid-filled sacs surrounded by a single membrane. Their size varies; in some cells the vacuole almost fills the cell. The fluid is a dilute solution of molecules and ions. The vacuole can be used to store mineral salts, amino acids, sugars and waste products. Vacuoles are also involved in maintaining the water balance of the cell.

B1.4 The similarities and differences between plant and animal cells in relation to the presence of specific organelles and their function

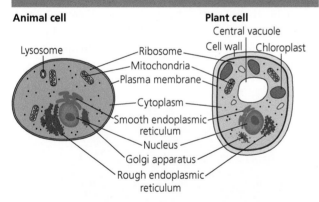

▲ Figure 12.6 Components of plant and animal cells

If you compare the animal and plant cells shown in Figure 12.6 you will see that there are many similarities. In fact, the main difference between the two types is that plant cells have structures such as the cell wall, chloroplasts and vacuoles that are not found in animal cells.

The cell wall provides support to plant cells and helps to keep them rigid. This also means that they have similar shapes. There are some types of highly specialised plant cells, but there is a much greater variety of types of animal cells. Animal cells also have a larger variety of shapes as they do not have a cell wall to keep them rigid and hence the need for skeletons in larger organisms.

B1.5 How eukaryotic cells become specialised in complex multi-cellular organisms

In multicellular organisms, different cells are specialised to fulfil different functions. This is controlled by which genes are expressed (i.e. genes that are switched on and therefore have an effect). Every **somatic** cell (i.e. all cells excluding gametes) contains in its nucleus the whole **genome** (all the genes) of the organism. How the cell functions is determined by which of the many genes are expressed and which are not.

The process by which a cell changes from one cell type to another is known as **cell differentiation.** To understand this, consider how a **zygote** (fertilised egg cell) develops into an embryo and how one single cell gives rise to not just many cells, but many different types of cell.

Stem cells can differentiate to form specialised cells. The human embryo contains stem cells that can give rise to the more than 200 cell types of the adult human body. By the time a baby is born, most cells have already differentiated. This is why the term 'adult cells' applies to cells in babies and children as well as in adults. However, adult stem cells persist and are responsible for cell turnover, e.g. production of red blood cells from bone marrow cells (see Figure 12.7). These bone marrow cells also differentiate to form the various types of lymphocytes involved in the immune response (see section B1.30). Most epithelial cells (see section B1.12) need to be replaced throughout the life of an organism. Examples include cells in the skin, lungs, cornea and intestine. In each case, stem cells are responsible for replacement of worn-out cells.

Key term

Stem cells: undifferentiated (non-specialised) cells that can give rise to one or more types of differentiated (specialised) cell.

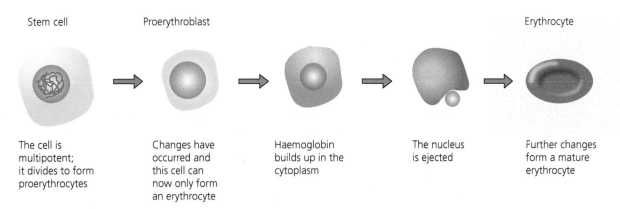

Stem cell   Proerythroblast   Erythrocyte

The cell is multipotent; it divides to form proerythrocytes

Changes have occurred and this cell can now only form an erythrocyte

Haemoglobin builds up in the cytoplasm

The nucleus is ejected

Further changes form a mature erythrocyte

▲ Figure 12.7 Differentiation of red blood cells (erythrocytes)

B1.6 How prokaryotic cells differ from eukaryotic cells

You need to be able to distinguish between prokaryotic and eukaryotic cells based on drawings. Differences can also be identified on electron micrographs.

Figure 12.8 shows a diagram of a typical prokaryotic cell. The table summarises the differences between prokaryotic and eukaryotic cells.

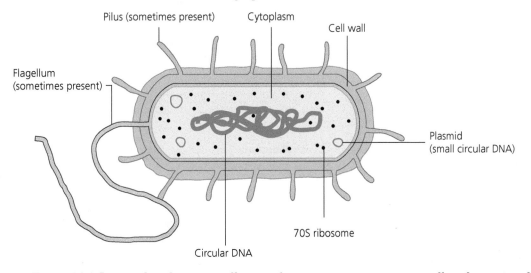

▲ Figure 12.8 A typical prokaryotic cell: some features are not present in all prokaryotic cells.

Prokaryotic cells	Eukaryotic cells
They have cytoplasm that lacks membrane-bound organelles.	They have cytoplasm containing membrane-bound organelles.
They have smaller ribosomes.	They have larger ribosomes.
They have no nucleus; instead, they have a single circular DNA molecule that is free in the cytoplasm and is not associated with proteins.	Chromosomes are linear and contained within the nucleus. The DNA is associated with proteins called histones.
They have a cell wall that contains murein/peptidoglycan, a glycoprotein.	Plant cells have a cellulose cell wall while fungi have a cell wall made of chitin.
They may have one or more plasmids.	There are no plasmids.
They may have a capsule surrounding the cell.	There is no capsule, even in plant cells. Some fungal cells can form a carbohydrate capsule.
They may have one or more simple flagella.	Flagella, where present, are more complex.

1   What are the three principles of cell theory?
2   State two differences between prokaryotic and eukaryotic cells.
3   State two differences between plant and animal cells.

Proteins, carbohydrates and lipids

Proteins, carbohydrates and lipids are three of the main classes of large biological molecules. We will encounter the fourth class in section B1.14 (page 244).

B1.7 The relationship between the structure, properties and functions of proteins

Dipeptides are formed by joining two **amino acids** in a **condensation reaction** (Figure 12.10). **Polypeptides** are formed by the condensation of many amino acids, joined by **peptide bonds**.

Key terms

Peptide: a compound containing two or more amino acids joined together by **peptide bonds**. A **dipeptide** contains two amino acids bonded together.

Amino acid: a molecule with both an amino group and a carboxyl group. Amino acids are the small molecules (monomers) from which all **proteins** are made. There are 20 naturally occurring amino acids found in proteins and all have the amino and carboxyl groups attached to the same carbon. This carbon also has a hydrogen and another substituent – the side chain, or R-group – which is different in each different amino acid; see Figure 12.9. Amino acids are the monomers from which all proteins are made.

Protein: a **polypeptide** with a recognisable three-dimensional structure. It may contain more than one polypeptide chain.

Condensation reaction: a reaction between two small molecules to produce a larger molecule and water; most large biological molecules are formed by condensation reactions.

Polypeptide: a **polymer** of amino acids joined together by peptide bonds.

Polymer: a long molecule made from many small molecules called **monomers**.

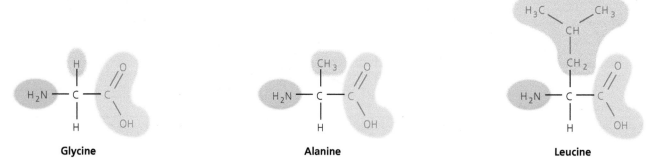

The 20 different amino acids that make up proteins in cells and organisms differ in their side chains (R groups). Below are three examples.

Glycine   Alanine   Leucine

▲ Figure 12.9 The basic structure of an amino acid and three examples of different amino acids.

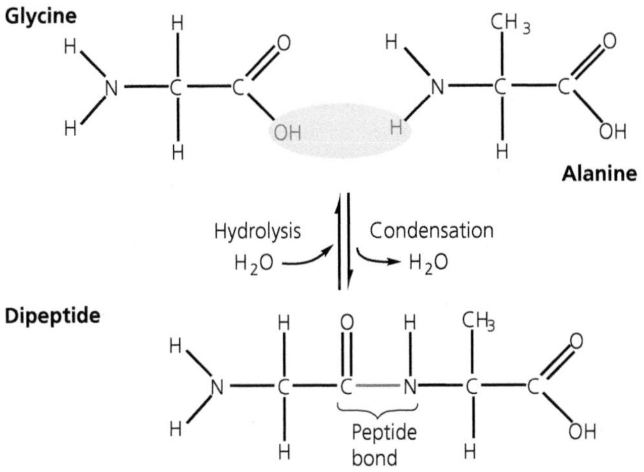

Glycine

Alanine

Hydrolysis
H_2O →

Condensation
→ H_2O

Dipeptide

Peptide
bond

▲ Figure 12.10 The formation of a peptide bond between two amino acids in a condensation reaction produces a dipeptide. The reverse reaction is a hydrolysis.

Functional proteins, such as fibrous proteins or globular proteins, contain one or more polypeptide chains. The sequence of amino acids is different in each different protein. It is the amino acid sequence which will determine how the polypeptide chain folds up. This, in turn, determines the three-dimensional shape of the protein.

B1.8 The relationship between the structure, properties and functions of carbohydrates

Carbohydrates are important energy sources, for example, sucrose ('sugar', refined from sugar cane), lactose (found in milk) or maltose (used as an energy source for yeast in the brewing industry). Polysaccharides are polymers formed by condensation reactions of many monosaccharide molecules (monomers). As they are such large molecules, they are usually insoluble. This makes them suitable to carry out storage functions (glycogen and starch) and support functions (cellulose).

Type of carbohydrate	Examples	Notes
Monosaccharides	Glucose 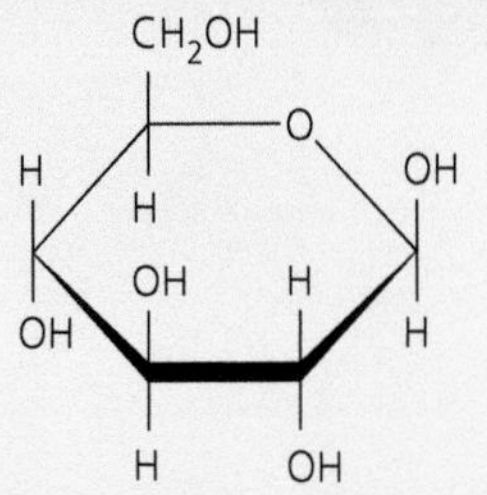	Monosaccharides contain just one sugar molecule and include glucose, fructose and galactose.
Disaccharides	Maltose 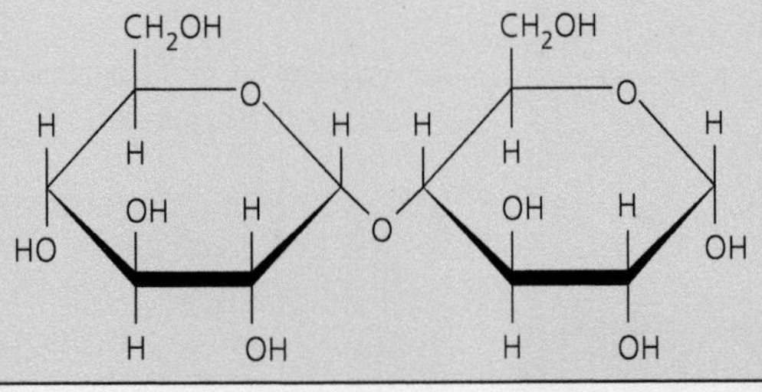	Disaccharides are formed by condensation reactions between two monosaccharides – the bond formed is known as a glycosidic bond. Common disaccharides include maltose (containing two glucose molecules), sucrose (containing glucose and fructose) and lactose (containing glucose and galactose).
Polysaccharides	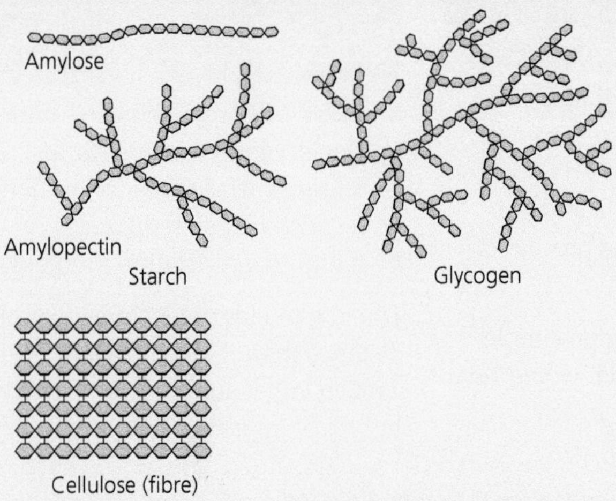 Amylose, Amylopectin, Starch, Glycogen, Cellulose (fibre)	Polysaccharides are polymers of monosaccharide monomers. The most common are starch (straight chain amylose or branched chain amylopectin), glycogen and cellulose, all of which are polymers of glucose.

Key term

Diffusion: is the movement of a substance from a high concentration to a low concentration. For instance, if you drop a crystal of copper sulfate into a beaker of water and watch the blue colour spread then you can see diffusion occur.

B1.9 The relationship between the structure, properties and functions of lipids

Lipids are the only group of large biological molecules that are not polymers. They all contain carbon, hydrogen and oxygen and are usually insoluble in water. More complex lipids can also contain phosphorous and nitrogen.

Lipids consist of two or three fatty acids, which are joined to a molecule of glycerol in condensation reactions. The fatty acids have long hydrocarbon chains, which explains why lipids are generally insoluble.

The main groups of lipids are:
▶ **triglycerides** (for example, fats and oils). These are used mostly as energy stores as well as for insulation (under the skin) and protection (around delicate organs such as the kidneys)
▶ **phospholipids**. These are found in plasma membranes and provide flexibility and help control what can move into and out of cells.

The role of phospholipids in membranes was covered in section B1.2.

Exchange and transport mechanisms

All organisms exchange substances with their surroundings. Single-cell organisms that respire aerobically need to absorb oxygen and get rid of carbon dioxide. They also need to absorb nutrients and get rid of waste products. This happens by the process of simple **diffusion**.

Large multicellular organisms cannot rely on simple diffusion. The distances are too great and it would take too long, as illustrated in Figure 12.11.

Single-celled organism (*Paramecium caudatum*)
Maximum distance for diffusion = 50 μm
Time taken = 8 seconds

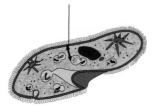

Maximum distance for diffusion = 15 cm
Time taken = 7 hours

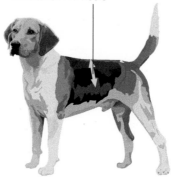

▲ Figure 12.11 The problem of increasing size on the rate of diffusion.

B1.10 How the surface area to volume ratio affects the process of exchange and gives rise to specialised systems

Efficient exchange (of gases, nutrients or waste products) requires three things:
▶ a large surface area for exchange
▶ a short diffusion distance
▶ a high concentration gradient.

The dog in Figure 12.11 has a much longer diffusion distance than the *Paramecium*, although it does have a much larger surface area. However, for efficient exchange the surface area must be large in comparison to the volume. We describe this as having a large surface area to volume ratio. This is illustrated in Figure 12.12. To make it simpler we have used a cube, but the principle is the same for animals with more complex shapes.

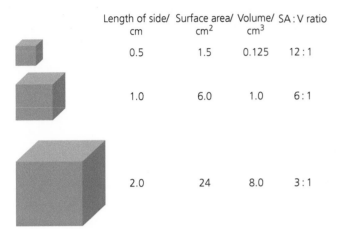

Length of side/ cm	Surface area/ cm^2	Volume/ cm^3	SA : V ratio
0.5	1.5	0.125	12 : 1
1.0	6.0	1.0	6 : 1
2.0	24	8.0	3 : 1

▲ **Figure 12.12 Decrease of surface area: volume ratio in cubes of increasing size**

Where the surface area is small compared to the volume (i.e. a low surface area to volume ratio), organisms cannot rely on simple diffusion across the whole body area like in *Paramecium*. Specialised exchange and transport mechanisms are required to maximise the rate of diffusion, such as lungs or gills and the heart and circulatory system.

Gills and lungs are adapted to make the diffusion distance as short as possible; between the air or water and the blood. For example, the walls of the alveoli in the lungs are only a single cell thick. There are also mechanisms, such as breathing, that maintain a high concentration gradient. Breathing brings air into the lungs that has a higher concentration of oxygen than within the blood. This ensures that oxygen diffuses into the blood.

Reflect

Temperature and the rate of the chemical reactions needed to support life (**metabolic rate**) also play a part. The heart rate of a mouse is about 500–600 beats per minute, whereas an elephant's heart rate is about 25–30 beats per minute. Why is this?

Think about the following:
▶ Heat loss also depends on surface area to volume ratio.
▶ Mammals, such as mice and elephants, generate body heat from respiration.

More active animals have a higher metabolic rate and therefore require more substances such as glucose for aerobic respiration. This increases their need for specialised exchange and transport mechanisms. In terms of heat loss, the mouse has a larger surface area to volume ratio and therefore has an increased rate of heat loss. Because of this, they need to generate more heat from respiration, increasing their need for glucose and oxygen within their cells, explaining their higher heart rate.

B1.11 The principles of cellular exchange and the transport mechanisms which exist to facilitate this exchange

The lipid component of cell membranes consists of a double layer known as the phospholipid bilayer. As discussed in section B1.2, phospholipids consist of a **hydrophilic** head group and a **hydrophobic** tail. This is shown in Figure 12.13 and is a very stable structure. Either side of the membrane is in an aqueous medium (meaning the main solvent is water). This means the tails arrange themselves on the centre, due to being hydrophobic. As a result, the hydrophilic heads arrange themselves on the outside, creating the phospholipid bilayer.

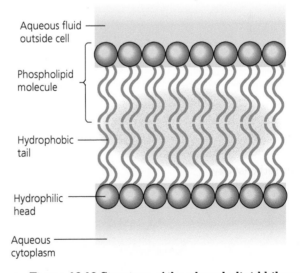

▲ **Figure 12.13 Structure of the phospholipid bilayer**

The phospholipid bilayer acts as a barrier to diffusion of many substances and only allows small, non-polar molecules through. Polar substances (see section B1.42, page 271) such as water, glucose, amino acids or inorganic ions (e.g. Na+, K+ or Cl-) cannot diffuse through the hydrophobic core of the bilayer.

This means that they require specialised transport systems involving proteins and glycoproteins (proteins with sugar molecules attached) embedded in the phospholipid bilayer. We can see an example of an adaptation to increase the efficiency of exchange if we look at the small intestine. The intestine is effectively a tube, and the central space (where digestion occurs) is called the lumen. The epithelial cells that line the small intestine are specialised cells; the plasma membrane facing the lumen is folded into many tiny finger-like projections called microvilli. This greatly increases the surface area for absorption of the products of digestion. Figure 12.14 illustrates the **fluid mosaic model** of the plasma membrane.

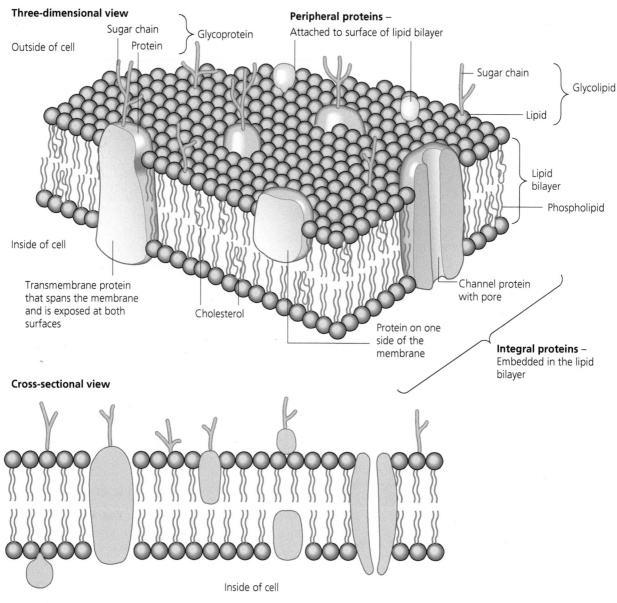

▲ Figure 12.14 The fluid mosaic model of the eukaryotic plasma membrane

Mechanisms: passive, active and co-transport

Simple diffusion, facilitated diffusion and osmosis are all passive processes, meaning that they do not require energy. Therefore, movement is always from high concentration to low concentration, sometimes described as down a diffusion gradient.

Simple diffusion

The phospholipid bilayer with its hydrophobic core can be a barrier to diffusion of polar substances; we say that it is *partially permeable*. So, small, non-polar molecules (e.g. carbon dioxide, oxygen, steroid hormones, lipids or fat-soluble vitamins) can move into the phospholipid bilayer and diffuse across the membrane.

Facilitated diffusion

Polar molecules, such as water, glucose and ions such as Na^+ or Cl^- cannot diffuse across the membrane,

so they rely on **facilitated diffusion**. This is where diffusion is assisted by proteins in the membrane. Ions and small polar molecules (including water) are transported by **channel proteins** (Figure 12.15) that act like pores in the membrane. Some of these can open and close, and these are called **gated channels**. Ion channels are usually specific for particular ions such as Na^+ or Ca^{2+}.

Larger polar molecules, such as glucose or amino acids, use **carrier proteins** (Figure 12.16). They are specific to the substance being transported which binds to the carrier protein in a similar way to a substrate binding to an enzyme (see section B2.5, page 321). The carrier protein then changes shape, which transfers the substance to the other side of the membrane.

The rules of diffusion still apply to both channel proteins and carrier proteins. Substances move only from a high concentration to low concentration.

Channel proteins help the diffusion of ions. Some ion channels have gates that open and close.

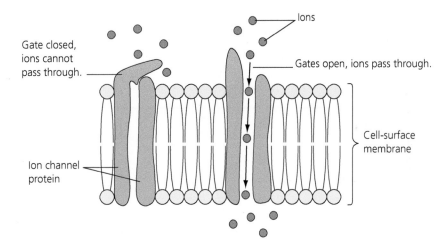

▲ Figure 12.15 Facilitated diffusion through a channel protein. The ones shown here are gated (they can open and close) while others are open all the time

Diffusing molecules bind to a carrier protein. The protein changes shape and takes the molecules through the membrane.

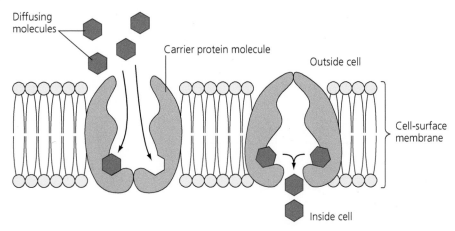

▲ Figure 12.16 Facilitated diffusion by a carrier protein

Osmosis

This is a particular type of facilitated diffusion where water moves across a partially permeable membrane from a high concentration of water molecules to a low concentration of water molecules. Do not be confused by this – a dilute solution (or pure water) will have a high concentration of water molecules, whereas a concentrated solution (e.g. a high concentration of glucose) will have a low concentration of water molecules. Therefore, water moves by osmosis from pure water or a dilute solution to a more concentrated solution.

Active transport

Substances do not move by themselves from low to high concentration (i.e. up a concentration gradient). However, **active transport** is a process that uses energy to move substances against a concentration gradient. This involves carrier proteins that use ATP as a source of energy. The mechanism is like that shown in Figure 12.16 with the addition of ATP as an energy source. These types of active transport proteins are often called pumps.

Co-transport mechanisms

The absorption of glucose from the gut is an example of a co-transport mechanism. Epithelial cells lining the small intestine have carrier proteins that only transport a glucose molecule together with a sodium ion. A sodium ion pump in the plasma membrane pumps sodium ions out of the epithelial cells into the blood capillaries which lowers the concentration of sodium ions inside the epithelial cells. This creates a sodium ion concentration gradient from the inside of the small intestine into the epithelial cells. It is this concentration gradient that causes sodium ions to diffuse into epithelial cells via a co-transport protein which brings with them glucose molecules. This helps ensure all the glucose is absorbed from the small intestine and is known as co-transport. Once inside the epithelial cell, the glucose diffuses down a concentration gradient into the blood. However, as glucose is a polar molecule, this requires a carrier protein too. The process is illustrated in Figure 12.17.

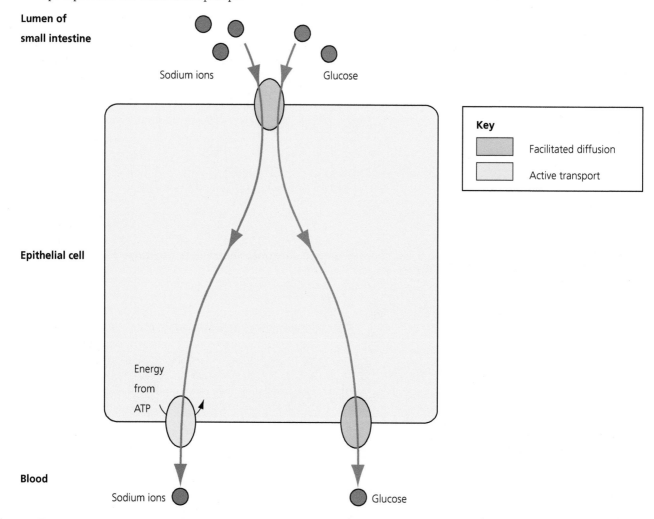

▲ Figure 12.17 Co-transport of glucose and sodium ions in the gut

B1.12 The advantages of having specialised cells in relation to the rate of transport across internal and external membranes

We saw in section B1.10 that multicellular organisms above a certain size can no longer rely on diffusion for exchange of substances with their environments. This usually means that specialised exchange organs have evolved, such as:

▶ gills or lungs for gas exchange
▶ the gut for absorption of nutrients
▶ kidneys for excretion of nitrogenous waste (urea).

Each of these organs have specialised cells adapted to maximise the efficiency of transfer of specific substances. Many of these cells are described as **epithelial** or **endothelial** and they are well adapted to their function.

Reflect

Epithelial and endothelial tissues are usually single layers of cells that line or coat organs. The easiest way to decide whether a particular cell or tissue is epithelial or endothelial is to consider if it is in contact with the outside world. Of course, the place where it interacts with the 'outside world' can be contained within the body – just think about the gut, which is really just a long tube from mouth to anus.

Think about the following and decide whether they are examples of epithelial or endothelial:
▶ skin cells
▶ cells lining the mouth
▶ cells lining the trachea and lungs
▶ cells lining the gut
▶ cells lining the kidney tubules and bladder
▶ cells lining blood vessels (arteries, veins and capillaries).

Hint: only one of these is an example of endothelial cells!

Research

Choose an organ from the following list and research ways in which specialised cells in that organ are adapted to maximise the rate of transport across membranes:
▶ blood vessels
▶ lungs
▶ gut.

Test yourself

1 Explain why large multicellular organisms require specialised exchange and transport mechanisms.
2 What are the three features of a good exchange surface?
3 Describe the fluid mosaic model of cell membranes.
4 Explain why polar molecules require special transport mechanisms to cross cell membranes.
5 State two differences between active transport and facilitated diffusion.

Genetics

Genetics is the study of inheritance. We resemble our parents, but do not look exactly like either of them. **Genes** are passed from parent to offspring and these interactions control the appearance of those offspring.

The laws of genetics were worked out in the nineteenth century by Gregor Mendel. However, the role of DNA as the genetic material was only established for certain in the middle of the twentieth century.

We can study genetics using Mendel's laws that have been built on by subsequent researchers. We can work out the rules and how to apply them, and in this way, genetics is a type of logic puzzle. More recent approaches involve trying to work out what is happening at the molecular level. That requires an understanding of DNA, RNA and the synthesis of proteins. This section will help you gain a good understanding of this modern approach to genetics.

Key term

Gene: a sequence of bases in DNA that codes for (contains the information to make) a polypeptide, or, in some cases, functional RNA (this is involved in regulating how genes are expressed).

B1.13 The purpose of DNA and RNA as the carrying molecules of genetic information and the role they play in the mechanism of inheritance

Our understanding of genetics is based on some key points. We now know:
- Genes consist of **DNA** (deoxyribonucleic acid) and so we can say that DNA holds the genetic information.
- Genes control production of proteins by transferring the genetic information from DNA via **RNA** (ribonucleic acid) to the ribosomes where proteins are synthesised.
- Proteins are what determine the characteristics of an organism.

To fully understand genetics, we need to understand:
- how DNA stores the genetic information
- how DNA is replicated to pass on that genetic information to future generations
- how DNA and RNA are involved in the production of proteins.

B1.14 The relationship between the structure of DNA and RNA and their role in the mechanism of inheritance

As with all biological molecules, there is a strong relationship between the structure of nucleic acids (DNA and RNA) and their function. Both molecules are polynucleotides – that is polymers of nucleotides – in the same way that a polypeptide is a polymer of amino acids.

Each nucleotide contains a **pentose** (5-carbon sugar), a nitrogen-containing **organic base** and a phosphate group.
- In RNA (ribonucleic acid) the pentose is ribose, in DNA (deoxyribonucleic acid) the pentose is deoxyribose.
- In RNA the organic bases are adenine (A), cytosine (C), guanine (G) or uracil (U), while in DNA the organic bases are adenine (A), cytosine (C), guanine (G) or thymine (T).

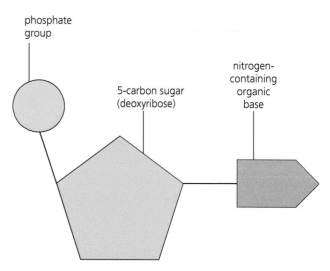

▲ Figure 12.18 General structure of a DNA nucleotide

The nucleotides are joined together in long chains by phosphodiester bonds between the pentose sugars; this is often described as a **sugar-phosphate** backbone. Phosphodiester bonds are formed in a condensation reaction like the one that forms peptide bonds (see Figure 12.10 in section B1.7).

The DNA molecule is a double helix where two very long polynucleotide chains are wound around each other and held together by hydrogen bonds between **complementary** base pairs: A pairs with T and C pairs with G. Complementary base pairing is central to how DNA stores and passes on genetic information, as well as to how genes control the synthesis of proteins.

RNA is a much shorter single-stranded polynucleotide chain.

The structure of DNA and RNA is shown in Figure 12.19.

The sequence of bases (sometimes called the **base sequence**) of DNA is how the genetic information is stored and passed on to future generations.

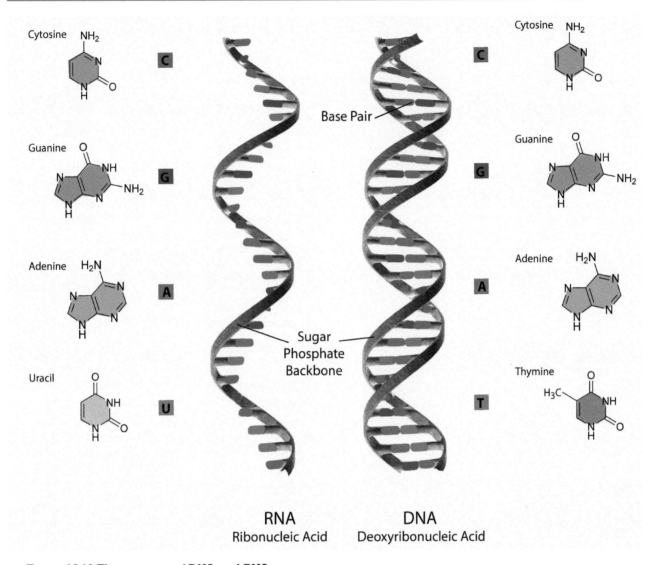

Cytosine

Guanine

Adenine

Uracil

Cytosine

Guanine

Adenine

Thymine

Base Pair

Sugar
Phosphate
Backbone

RNA
Ribonucleic Acid

DNA
Deoxyribonucleic Acid

▲ Figure 12.19 The structure of DNA and RNA

B1.15 The function of complementary base pairing in forming the helical structure of DNA

Complementary base pairing holds the two strands of DNA together in the double helix structure. This makes the DNA molecule very stable, which is important for the molecule that contains and passes on the genetic information. Complementary base pairing is also the basis for how DNA is replicated.

B1.16 The process and stages of semi-conservative replication of DNA

The stages of DNA replication are as follows:
▶ The DNA double helix is progressively unwound. This involves an enzyme (**helicase**) that breaks the hydrogen bonds between the bases, allowing the strands to separate.
▶ Each strand now has unpaired bases.
▶ The strands each act as templates to assemble new strands. DNA nucleotides bind to the unpaired bases through complementary base-pairing.
▶ The enzyme **DNA polymerase** catalyses (speeds up) the formation of the phosphodiester bonds between the nucleotides.

This process is shown in Figure 12.20.

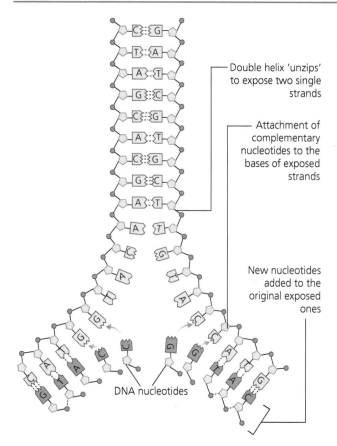

Double helix 'unzips' to expose two single strands

Attachment of complementary nucleotides to the bases of exposed strands

New nucleotides added to the original exposed ones

DNA nucleotides

▲ Figure 12.20 Semi-conservative replication of DNA

Key terms

Semi-conservative replication: when DNA replicates two new double helix molecules are formed, but each one consists of one of the original strands and one newly synthesised strand.

Mutation: a change in the sequence of bases in DNA. This can occur in a number of ways. When a mutation occurs within a coding region of DNA a new **allele** can be formed.

Allele: a variant of a gene.

Genetics: the study of how single genes, or a small group of genes, function and how they affect the appearance and functioning of the organism.

Genomics: the study of how all the genes in an organism interact, as well as the role of non-coding sequences of DNA.

Genome: the entire genetic material of an organism. This includes DNA that does not code for proteins as well as the coding DNA (genes).

B1.17 How this semi-conservative replication process ensures genetic continuity between generations of cells

The product of **semi-conservative replication** of DNA is two molecules of DNA, both identical to the original. This is how the genetic information, contained in the DNA, can be passed from one generation of cells to the next. Because the two new molecules are identical to each other and to the original, the new generation of cells will be identical to the previous generation.

B1.18 The link between the semi-conservative replication process and variation

We saw in section B1.17 how semi-conservative replication ensures genetic continuity between generations of cells. However, the process is not always 100 per cent accurate. Sometimes the 'wrong' base is inserted by DNA polymerase. This random event is one source of **mutation**. A mutation is a change in the sequence of bases in DNA, although this very rarely results in the formation of new **alleles**, partly because a lot of the DNA does not code for proteins. However, when a mutation occurs within the coding region of a gene, a new allele can sometimes be formed leading to the formation of a new characteristic. This is the source of genetic variation.

Genetic variation is the reason that we do not all look the same and is the basis of natural selection and evolution.

B1.19 The difference between genetics and genomics

We saw at the start of this section how the laws of **genetics** were worked out by a nineteenth-century monk working with pea plants. In contrast, **genomics** requires a great deal of technology to analyse and understand the **genomes**, particularly DNA sequencing and bioinformatics.

Both genetics and genomics are important in medicine. Genetics allows us to understand how inherited disorders like haemophilia, sickle cell anaemia or Huntingdon's disease are passed on. This understanding helps us assess the risk of children inheriting such conditions from their parents. Genomics is being used to investigate the link between all the genes we carry and the development of a wide range of diseases and conditions, from obesity and diabetes to heart disease and cancer.

> ### Practice points
>
> The terms 'genetics' and 'genomics' are similar and easily confused. Use of precise language is essential in science, so it is a good idea to develop good practice at an early stage that will stand you in good stead throughout your career.

> ### Test yourself
>
> 1 What is a gene?
> 2 State two differences between DNA and RNA.
> 3 What is meant by 'complementary base pairing'?
> 4 Give the names of two enzymes involved in DNA replication.

Microbiology

B1.20 The classification and characteristics (size of cell, type of cell, presence of organelles) of the following micro-organisms

Micro-organisms are often thought of simply as pathogens. This may be because that is how we see them having the greatest impact on our lives. However, that is only part of the story.

> ### Reflect
>
> Think of all the ways in which micro-organisms are of benefit or even essential. You could include:
> ▶ foods and food production
> ▶ production of medicines, such as antibiotics
> ▶ agriculture
> ▶ production of chemicals and clean-up of chemical contamination.

> ### Practice points
>
> See sections B1.62 and B1.63 (pages 295 and 296) for more about SI units and conversion between units. These are two units that you will encounter when studying micro-organisms.
>
> **Micrometre** (μm) is the most commonly used measure of size when studying micro-organisms and is 10^{-6} m (one millionth of a metre) or 10^{-3} mm (one thousandth of a millimetre).
>
> **Nanometre** (nm) is 10^{-9} m (one billionth of a metre), 10^{-6} mm (one millionth of a millimetre) or $10^{-3}\mu$m (one thousandth of a micrometre).

Bacteria

Bacteria are typically 1–2μm (micrometres) long (i.e. about 1/1000 to 2/1000 of a millimetre) and usually roughly cylindrical, although other shapes, such as rods and spirals, do occur. They do not have membrane-bound organelles (see sections B1.3 and B1.6) and so are prokaryotes. See Figure 12.8 for a diagram of a typical bacterium.

Fungi

As well as the more familiar mushrooms and toadstools, many fungi are microscopic – the yeasts, including those used in fermentation to produce ethanol, are single cell organisms. Yeast cells are bigger than bacteria – in the range of 4–12μm.

Fungi are eukaryotes, meaning they have chromosomes contained within a nucleus and other membrane-bound organelles. Multicellular fungi are composed of microscopic threads or hyphae that grow over or through their food source. Figure 12.21 shows a diagram of the mould fungus, *Penicillium chrysogenum* (the original source of the antibiotic penicillin.

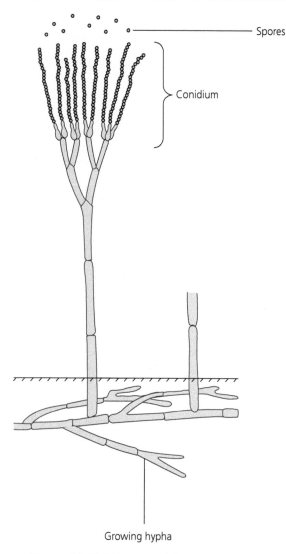

Spores

Conidium

Growing hypha

▲ Figure 12.21 Structure of the mould fungus, *Penicillium chrysogenum*

A honey fungus measuring 2.4 miles (3.8 km) across in the Blue Mountains in Oregon, USA is thought to be the largest living organism on Earth. That is certainly not microscopic! The structures that we recognise as mushrooms or toadstools are actually fruiting bodies, formed from very compact hyphae, that release spores.

Parasites

A parasite is an organism that lives on or in another organism at the expense of that organism. This includes multicellular organisms such as parasitic plants (e.g. mistletoe) and flatworms (e.g. tapeworms). Microscopic parasites are single-celled eukaryotic organisms such as *Plasmodium* (Figure 12.22), the parasite that causes malaria, or *Phytophthora infestans*, a parasite of plants that causes potato blight. Microscopic parasites can be different sizes, but usually in the range 1–10 µm.

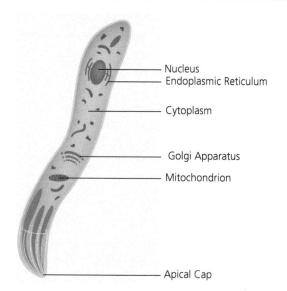

Nucleus
Endoplasmic Reticulum

Cytoplasm

Golgi Apparatus

Mitochondrion

Apical Cap

▲ Figure 12.22 Diagram of *Plasmodium*, a microscopic eukaryotic parasite

Viruses

As we saw in section B1.1, viruses are acellular (they are not made of cells) and do not contain organelles in the way that prokaryotes and eukaryotes do. They consist of genetic material (DNA or RNA) surrounded by a protein coat. Sometimes, the protein coat is itself surrounded by an envelope of lipid bilayer and glycoproteins that originated from the cell in which the virus replicated. Most viruses are very small – in the range 20–200 nm, although some giant viruses are as large as 1 µm – about the size of a bacterium and come in many shapes as well as sizes (Figure 12.23).

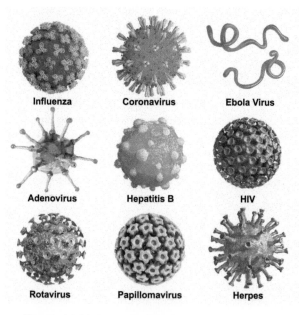

Influenza   Coronavirus   Ebola Virus

Adenovirus   Hepatitis B   HIV

Rotavirus   Papillomavirus   Herpes

▲ Figure 12.23 A small selection of different virus structures

Are viruses alive? It is a question that has been asked many times and there is no simple answer. What we *can* say is that viruses are **acellular** – they are not made up of cells – and need to infect other cells to reproduce. Think about whether the first principle of cell theory (section B1.1) means that viruses cannot be classed as living organisms. If we consider viruses as alive, is the first principle wrong? Nothing in biology is ever simple!

B1.21 The benefits of using light and electron microscopes when investigating micro-organisms

As the name suggests, micro-organisms cannot be seen with the naked eye. Therefore, we need to use some form of microscope to view and study them. The type of microscope used will depend on the size of the micro-organism we want to study – and, as some microscopes are more expensive, what we have access to.

Key terms

Magnification: how much bigger the image is than the actual object we are viewing. It should not be confused with **resolution**.

Resolution: the ability of a microscope to distinguish between two adjacent points. The resolution of a microscope is the smallest distance between two points that can be seen as separate. A high-resolution microscope can show a clearer image.

You have probably encountered resolution when using a camera phone. An old phone will probably have quite a low resolution. If you take a photo you may be able to enlarge the image to the same size as one taken with the latest high-resolution camera phone, but the modern phone will give a much clearer, sharper image.

(a)

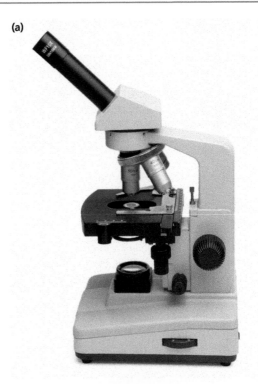

(b)

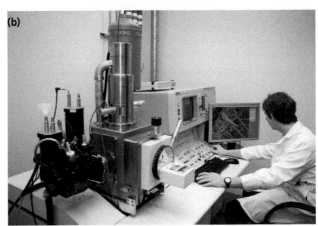

▲ Figure 12.24 (a) A light microscope and (b) an electron microscope

The principle of light and electron microscopes is the same: lenses are used to magnify the image. The difference is that, unlike light microscopes, electron microscopes use a beam of electrons to obtain an image. Whereas light microscopes use glass lenses for **magnification**, electron microscopes use magnets as lenses.

Light microscopes

The good news about light microscopes is that they are relatively inexpensive. They are also relatively easy to use, although they must be used with care to avoid damage. Thin sections of plant and animal tissues are usually prepared, but light microscopes can also be used to examine living micro-organisms as long as they are not too small, like most viruses. Electron microscopes cannot use living material as they have to operate in a vacuum.

> ### Health and safety
>
> Modern light microscopes usually contain a built-in light source. Halogen bulbs are likely to become very hot during use, so make sure you do not touch the bulb or try to disassemble the microscope.
>
> When using a high power objective lens it is easy to drive the lens through the slide as you focus. This is likely to damage the lens as well as creating a hazard from the broken glass of the microscope slide. To avoid this, always lower the stage when changing lens. Ensure the stage is lowered and raised carefully when using the highest power lens. Once in view, only adjust the focus using the fine focus knob to prevent damage to the lens or slide.

Scanning electron microscopes

In a **scanning electron microscope** (**SEM**), the beam of electrons is scanned across the surface of the sample. The electrons bounce off the surface and a computer is used to build up a 3D image of the surface of the sample, showing more surface detail than is possible with a light microscope.

Transmission electron microscopes

In a **transmission electron microscope** (**TEM**), the electrons pass through the sample in the same way as light rays pass through a sample in the light microscope. This means a TEM shows a 2D image of the sample. Very thin sections are required as electrons cannot penetrate materials very deeply. This allows a TEM to reveal details of virus particles or cell organelles that would not be visible with the light microscope. A series of thin sections can be used to take multiple 2D images that can be assembled into a 3D image.

The table compares the approximate magnification and **resolution** of these three types of microscope.

Instrument	Maximum magnification	Maximum resolution
Light microscope	× 1500	200 nm
SEM	× 100 000	10 nm
TEM	× 500 000–1 000 000	0.2 nm

Figure 12.25 illustrates what can be seen with the human eye, a good quality light microscope and a transmission electron microscope.

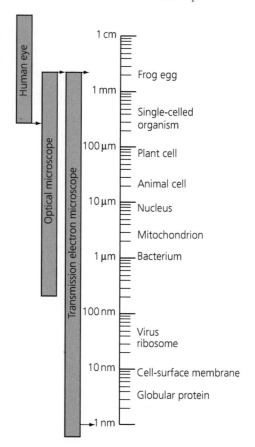

▲ Figure 12.25 A scale from 1 nm to 1 cm showing what can be seen with the naked eye, a light microscope and a transmission electron microscope. A log scale has been used because of the large range of measurements

> ### Practice points
>
> #### Units
> The following units are commonly used in microscopy:
>
> μm (micrometre) = 10^{-6} m
>
> nm (nanometre) = 10^{-9} m

B1.22 How to calculate magnification from the size of the image and the size of the object

Magnification is simply how much bigger the image is than the object. We can express that mathematically as:

$$magnification = \frac{size\ of\ image}{size\ of\ object}$$

It looks simple – and it is – but it can cause confusion. When calculating magnification, make sure you use the same units for the size of the image and the size of the object. We would normally measure the size of an image (e.g. a photomicrograph) in cm or mm, but microscopic objects are usually measured in μm. It is better to measure the size of the image in mm. When you calculate the magnification, make sure both sizes are expressed in the same units – either mm or μm, as shown in the example. There is more about converting between units in section B1.63.

A photomicrograph of a cell shows a mitochondrion that you know to be 1.5 μm long. You measure the image of the mitochondrion and find that it is 112.5 mm long. What is the magnification?

Method 1: convert the measurement of the image from mm to μm = 112 500 μm by multiplying by 1000 so 112.5 mm.

Now divide the size of the image by the size of the object to calculate the magnification:

$$magnification = \frac{112\,500}{1.5} = \times\,75\,000$$

Method 2: convert the size of the object from μm to mm by dividing by 1000 so 1.5 μm = 0.0015 mm

Now, divide the size of the image by the size of the object to calculate the magnification:

$$magnification = \frac{112.5}{0.0015} = \times\,75\,000$$

As you see, both methods give the same result. Remember that magnification should be quite a large number and always greater than 1. If your answer is not, then you have made a mistake!

B1.23 The uses of differential staining techniques

Staining uses dyes to help make objects clearer under the light microscope by increasing contrast and making it easier to see cells. Unstained cells are almost transparent, which makes it very difficult to see them. Staining makes micro-organisms stand out against the background.

Differential staining adds another dimension by allowing us to distinguish different cell types, including specific types of bacteria or even parasites. There are a number of common ways this is done.

> **Health and safety**
>
> If you are involved in preparing stained sections, make sure that you are aware of any hazards associated with the chemicals used.

Gram staining

The **Gram stain** differentiates bacteria by detecting the peptidoglycan present in the cell wall of Gram-positive bacteria. Crystal violet is used to stain the peptidoglycan and then iodine is added to fix the stain permanently to the peptidoglycan molecules. Stained bacteria appear dark blue or violet. Gram-negative bacteria only have a very thin peptidoglycan layer – they have an outer membrane of lipopolysaccharides – and so the stain can be washed out of the cells. A counterstain of fuchsin or safranin is then used to stain all bacteria red/pink. As Gram-positive bacteria have already been stained dark blue/violet, only the Gram-negative bacteria appear red/pink.

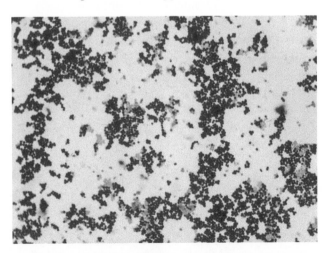

▲ Figure 12.26 Gram staining showing Gram positive (purple) and Gram negative (pink) bacteria

Giemsa staining

The Giemsa stain contains a mixture of Azure B, methylene blue and eosin stains. The methylene blue stains the chromosomes and nucleus dark purple while Azure B and eosin stain the cytoplasm pale blue or pink.

Giemsa stain can be used for:
▶ identification of specific bacteria such as *Chlamydia trachomatis*; these are stained blue-mauve to dark purple
▶ identification of *Plasmodium vivax* and *Plasmodium falciparum*, the malarial parasites; these are stained with a red or pink nucleus and blue cytoplasm
▶ identification of blood diseases such as anaemia and leukaemia; the different blood cells stain differently with Giemsa stain and any abnormalities can be identified (Figure 12.27).

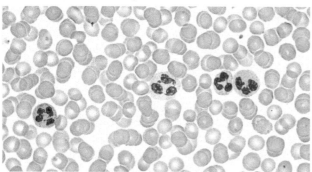

▲ Figure 12.27 A peripheral blood smear stained with Giemsa stain. Red blood cells do not have nuclei and so are stained pink, while the white blood cells have prominent nuclei that stain purple. This allows the different types of blood cell to be identified

Haematoxylin and eosin staining

Also known as H&E staining, this is the most widely used stain in medical diagnosis. The haematoxylin stains cell nuclei blue while the eosin stains the cytoplasm pink.

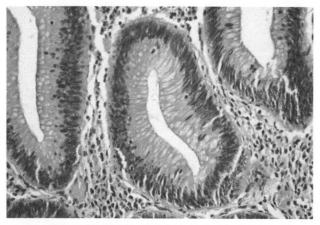

▲ Figure 12.28 Human breast cancer tissue section stained with H&E

Immunology

Immunology is the study of the immune system, which is an important part of the body's response to infection. We will see in section B1.30 that the immune system is just one way in which the body defends itself against disease. First, we need to consider the causes of infectious diseases.

B1.24 The nature of infection

Infection describes an organism replicating inside the body, resulting in disease. Some organisms, including all viruses, some bacteria and some parasites, infect body cells. Others replicate in organs such as the gut, in the blood or the spaces between cells.

B1.25 Causative agents of infection and examples of resulting diseases

Pathogen	Example of disease	Notes
Bacteria	• chlamydia • gonorrhoea • tuberculosis	Bacterial infections are treated by antibiotics, but bacteria are becoming increasingly resistant to antibiotics.
Viruses	• common cold • mumps • measles	SARS-CoV-2, the coronavirus that causes COVID-19, has recently become the best-known virus.
Fungi	• yeast infection (thrush)	Other fungal skin infections include toenail fungus and athlete's foot.
Prions	• Creutzfeldt-Jakob disease (CJD)	Prions are non-living pathogenic proteins. The mutant form of prion protein, when ingested, can cause normal prion proteins to change shape. This causes damage to the nervous system and eventual death.
Protoctists	• malaria	Don't confuse the pathogen (*Plasmodium*, a protoctist) with the *Anopheles* mosquito that transmits the pathogen.
Parasites	• toxoplasmosis	Toxoplasmosis is caused by *Toxoplasma gondii*, a parasitic protoctist. Many multicellular parasites can also cause infections, particularly in developing countries.

You may notice that there is an overlap between protoctists and parasites; malaria and toxoplasmosis are both caused by parasitic protoctists. However, some parasite diseases are due to infection by multicellular parasites, such as tapeworms.

B1.26 The different ways in which causative agents may enter the body

During the COVID-19 pandemic everyone paid much greater attention to hand hygiene, mask wearing, social distancing and improved ventilation of indoor spaces. Although many people died from COVID-19, one effect of these precautions was that there were far fewer deaths from seasonal flu. This illustrates the importance of understanding the ways in which infections are transmitted.

Direct transmission

▶ Physical contact with an infected person (for example, skin-to-skin contact) or contaminated surface (for example, door handles and other hard surfaces).
▶ Sharing of needles can result in transmission of blood-borne pathogens.
▶ Pathogens such as HIV or hepatitis C virus can be spread by transfusion with contaminated blood or blood products. Unprotected sexual contact can lead to **STIs**.

Key term

STI or **sexually transmitted infection:** caused by a pathogen that is passed from person to person during sexual contact.

Airborne transmission

The pathogen is carried by dust or droplets in the air. Some droplets (aerosols) can exist in the air for many hours and inhaling infected droplets can lead to infection. COVID-19 and tuberculosis are spread in this way.

Indirect transmission

Vehicle transmission occurs when infected food or water are ingested (eaten or drunk). Faecal-oral transmission is the result of poor hand hygiene and is a significant cause of food poisoning. Another example of vehicle transmission is from infected blood on inanimate objects such as clothing or bedding.

Another form of indirect transmission is being bitten by an infected **vector** (the organism that transfers the pathogen from host to host). Insect bites can introduce pathogens into the body. The best-known example is the malaria protoctist (*Plasmodium*), for which the vector is the *Anopheles* mosquito. There are many others, including Lyme disease (caused by a bacterium) and Zika fever (caused by a virus).

B1.27 How infectious diseases can spread among populations and communities

Understanding how infection spreads from person to person helps our understanding of how infectious diseases spread among populations. Once we understand that, we can consider ways in which the spread can be prevented, or at least minimised.

Inadequate sanitation includes:

▶ a lack of access to clean water for washing. Clean water is also unlikely to carry water-borne diseases

▶ inadequate sewage disposal, which increases the risk of faecal-oral transmission of a wide range of pathogens, including parasites that have evolved alongside human populations.

Dense populations lead to overcrowding in households as well as a lack of social distancing outside the home. These will both increase the rate of transmission by direct, airborne and indirect routes.

Inadequate healthcare infrastructure, such as inadequate hospitals or clinics, or a lack of doctors or nurses, increases the risk of disease spreading unnoticed as well as making it harder to treat and prevent further spread.

Ignorance can be deadly. Lack of accessible health promotion information means that people are less likely to take necessary precautions to prevent spread of infection. They may also be more resistant to prevention measures, such as vaccination.

It is worth noting that while all these factors are more prevalent in countries with developing economies, they are associated with areas of deprivation worldwide.

Case study

Between 1846 and 1860, a worldwide pandemic of cholera was responsible for over a million deaths worldwide. Cholera was thought to be caused by particles of decaying matter in the air ('miasma'). During 1854 there was a severe outbreak near Broad Street in the Soho district of London. A physician, John Snow, had been studying cholera for several years by this time. He mapped all the outbreaks of cholera in the district and showed that they were concentrated around a public water pump on Broad Street. Snow did not understand that cholera was caused by a bacterium, but the evidence he collected showed that in this outbreak it was transmitted by infected water from the Broad Street pump and not miasma. The authorities were unwilling to accept the results of Snow's work, although the pump handle was temporarily removed to prevent its use.

Snow also investigated the quality of water provided by different water companies. Individual houses in the same area received their water supply from different companies. Snow showed that there was a higher incidence of cholera in those households receiving their water from two large companies who extracted it directly from the River Thames. At that time, the river was heavily contaminated with raw sewage. Other households obtained their water from smaller companies who provided cleaner, better filtered water. These households had much lower incidence of cholera.

John Snow's work was a good example of the scientific method, including his use of statistical analysis. His work led, eventually, to great improvement in sanitation through the installation of more efficient sewage handling and provision of clean water.

▶ Think about the nineteenth-century cholera outbreak. Can you see any parallels with the COVID-19 pandemic?

▶ John Snow investigated a range of different factors in order to see a pattern. Can you think of factors that should be considered when studying the COVID-19 pandemic?

▶ Do you think that we have learned the lessons of John Snow's work?

B1.28 The definition of an antigen and an antibody

Key terms

Antigen: a substance that is recognised by the immune system as self (the body's own cells) or non-self (foreign cells and pathogens) and stimulates an immune response. Antigens are found on pathogens but also on the surfaces of all body cells.

Antibody: a blood protein that is produced in response to a specific antigen. An antibody binds specifically to an antigen in a similar way to an enzyme binding specifically to its substrate.

B1.29 The link between antigens and the initiation of the body's response to invasion by a foreign substance

We can think of **antigens** as chemical markers rather like ID cards. They are usually proteins or **glycoproteins** (proteins with sugar molecules attached) on the surface of pathogens or body cells.

Some antigens on the surface of body cells allow the immune system to distinguish between the body's own cells ('self' antigens) and foreign cells, including pathogens ('non-self' antigens).

The response to invasion by a foreign substance involves several stages that we can think of as defence mechanisms. The immune response is part of that process but is not the only part.

B1.30 The stages and cells involved in the body's response to an antigen

The stages of defence against non-self antigens, for example, on pathogens, is shown in Figure 12.29.

Physical and chemical barriers

The first line of defence is to keep pathogens out. The skin plays a significant part as an external barrier. Mucous membranes are also important. These line the gut, airways and reproductive system. Goblet cells produce thick, sticky mucous that helps to trap bacteria and other pathogens. Antimicrobial proteins and peptides also help to destroy pathogens and can also be involved in stimulation of the immune system.

Lysozyme is an enzyme that hydrolyses bonds in the cell wall components of some bacteria. This weakens the cell walls, meaning that the bacteria swell and burst. Lysozyme is present in tears, helping to protect the surface of the eyes, as well as in breast milk providing protection to infants while their immune systems are developing.

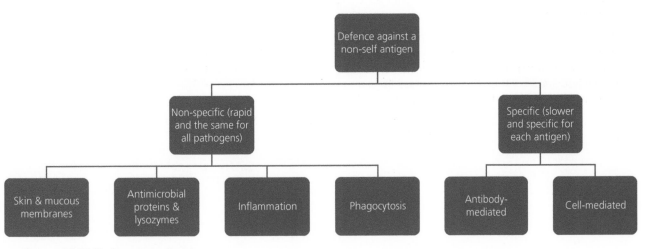

▲ Figure 12.29 Defence mechanisms

Inflammation

Inflammation is a response to injury or infection where the area becomes hot, red and swollen as a result of increased blood flow. Mast cells respond to tissue damage (caused by injury or infection) by secreting histamine. This **cell-signalling** compound stimulates a range of responses, including:

▶ increased blood flow in capillaries;
▶ capillaries begin to leak more, allowing fluid to enter the tissues resulting in swelling;
▶ **phagocytes** leave the blood and enter the tissues where they can engulf foreign material.

Histamine also stimulates cells to release cytokines, including interleukins that lead to more inflammation. Cytokines also lead to the promotion of **phagocytosis**.

Key terms

Innate immunity: the non-specific mechanisms, present from birth, that protect against a wide range of pathogens. These mechanisms, including inflammation, phagocytosis and antimicrobial proteins, work quickly, but are not always very effective.

Inflammation: a local response to injury and infection.

Cell-signalling: the process by which cells communicate with each other, usually by release of chemicals such as histamine, cytokines and interleukins.

Phagocytes: produced in the bone marrow and circulate in the blood. Some leave the blood and are present in the tissues.

Phagocytosis: the process of a phagocyte engulfing a pathogen or other foreign material.

Lymphocytes: small white blood cells. B lymphocytes, or B cells, are responsible for antibody production. Different types of T lymphocytes, or T cells, play different roles in the immune response.

Phagocytosis

Chemicals released by pathogens into the blood attract phagocytes. Receptors on the surface of phagocytes bind to antigens that are present on the surface of most pathogens, and this leads to the phagocyte engulfing and digesting the pathogen (Figure 12.30).

Some types of phagocyte known as macrophages do not completely digest the pathogen. Instead, antigens from the partially digested pathogen are processed and then appear on the plasma membrane of the macrophage. These are then known as antigen-presenting cells (APCs), as they 'present' the antigens to **lymphocytes** (T cells). This process of antigen presentation initiates the immune response. This is the slower, more specific and more effective stage of defence against infection.

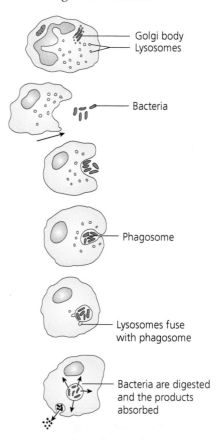

Golgi body
Lysosomes

Bacteria

Phagosome

Lysosomes fuse with phagosome

Bacteria are digested and the products absorbed

▲ Figure 12.30 The stages in phagocytosis

The role of T cells

The two main groups of T cells are T helper cells (T_H cells) and cytotoxic T cells (T_C cells) also known as T killer cells (T_K cells).

T_H cells have a type of cell-surface receptor known as CD4. There are many different shapes of CD4 receptor corresponding to the millions of antigen shapes that we might encounter. When a T_H cell encounters an APC, the CD4 receptors on the T_H cell may be complementary to the antigen, i.e. the shapes match. If so, the following events happen:

▶ The T_H cell binds, via its CD4 receptor, to the APC.
▶ This activates the T_H cell.
▶ The activated T_H cells divide by mitosis to form a clone of active T_H cells and memory cells.
▶ Activated T_H cells are then able to activate T_w and B cells.

This is shown in Figure 12.31.

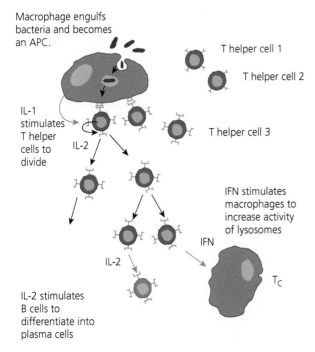

▲ Figure 12.31 The activation of T_H cells in the immune response. Three different T_H cells are shown, but only T_H cell 3 has a CD4 receptor complementary to the antigens on the APC

When body cells are infected by pathogens such as viruses, they also process pathogen antigens and present them on their cell surfaces, becoming APCs. T_C cells also have cell-surface receptors known as TCRs. Like CD4 receptors on T_H cells, there are many different shapes of TCR, complementary to different antigens. If a T_C cell encounters an APC with complementary antigens the following series of events occurs:

▶ The T_C cell becomes activated. This process also involves T_H cells.
▶ Once activated, the T_C cells will divide by mitosis to form a clone of activated T_C cells and memory cells.
▶ The T_C cells will bind to the surface of other infected cells and destroy them.

It might seem drastic to destroy the body's own cells, but infected cells will usually end up dead anyway and the action of T_C cells prevents pathogens such as viruses replicating inside the infected cells. This process is shown in Figure 12.32.

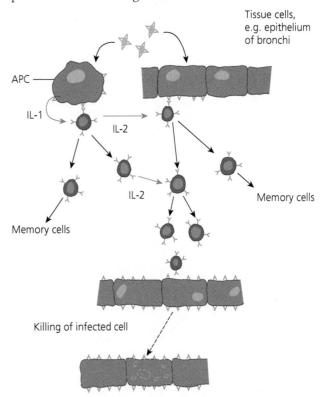

▲ Figure 12.32 Activation of T_C cells by infected host cells leads to killing of other infected cells

The role of B cells

B cells also have cell surface receptors, the B cell receptor or BCR. Again, there are many different shapes of BCR. When a B cell encounters antigens complementary to (i.e. which match) its BCR, the following events take place:

▶ The antigen binds to the BCR.
▶ B cell takes in the BCR and antigen.
▶ The B cell processes the antigen and so becomes an APC.

At this stage, activated T$_H$ cells become involved.
- Any activated T$_H$ cells with complementary CD4 receptors will then bind to the antigens on the APC.
- The T$_H$ cell then secretes cytokines (such as IL-1 and IL-2).
- The cytokines activate the B cell.
- The activated B cell divides to form a clone of activated B cells and memory cells.
- The activated B cells differentiate to form plasma cells that produce large quantities of antibodies.

This process is shown in Figure 12.33.

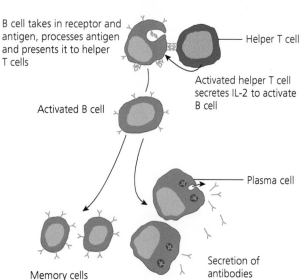

▲ Figure 12.33 Selection and activation of B cells with a BCR complementary to pathogen antigens

Antibodies bind to antigens on the surface of pathogens. Antibodies protect against pathogens in several ways, including:
- binding to toxins produced by bacteria and making them harmless;
- cross-linking pathogens so that they are too large to spread or infect cells;
- signalling to phagocytes to engulf the pathogens;
- binding to pathogen proteins that the pathogens use to enter body cells, for example, the spike protein on the surface of the SARS-CoV-2 virus.

B1.31 The differences between cell-mediated immunity and antibody-mediated immunity

In the previous section, we looked at the parts that T cells and B cells play in the immune response. It is useful to separate the two parts of the immune response. T$_H$ cells play a key role in both of these parts, but there are important differences between the way in which the immune system protects the body from pathogens.

In the **cell-mediated response**, T cells destroy pathogens by destroying infected body cells. This means the pathogens cannot replicate and infect more body cells. Antibodies are not involved in the cell-mediated immune response.

In the **antibody-mediated** response, B cells produce antibodies, and it is the antibodies that lead to destruction of pathogens. Some antibodies are known as antitoxins, because they bind to and neutralise toxins produced by pathogens.

B1.32 The role of T and B memory cells in the secondary immune response

If we are infected by a pathogen, it takes the body about 10–17 days to produce antibodies. This process, known as the primary response, was described in section B1.31 and explains why we get ill with an infection. Once antibodies (and active T$_C$ cells) are produced, the pathogen is removed and we get better. Plasma cells do not live long in the blood and the antibodies they produce are gradually broken down.

If, after some time, we are infected with the same pathogen, then antibodies are produced more rapidly and in much larger quantities. This is known as the **secondary immune response** and is illustrated in Figure 12.34.

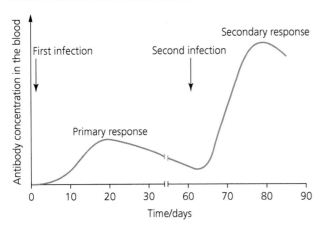

▲ Figure 12.34 The change in the concentration of antibodies during the primary and secondary immune responses

We saw how memory T cells and memory B cells were produced during the primary immune response. These remain in the body for a long time. When they encounter the pathogen for a second time, they multiply much more rapidly to form clones of plasma cells and T_C cells. The plasma cells produce high concentrations of antibodies in just a few days. In this way, the secondary immune response can clear pathogens from the body before we even show symptoms of the disease.

The secondary immune response is the basis of how vaccines work. A vaccine will stimulate the primary immune response without needing exposure to the pathogen, so the body is ready when it is exposed to the same pathogen later.

Test yourself

1 Give two examples of diseases caused by each of the following types of pathogen:
   a Bacteria   b Viruses
2 Explain the difference between a pathogen and a vector.
3 Give two examples of each of the following methods of disease transmission:
   a Direct   b Airborne   c Indirect
4 Describe two factors that cause infections to spread within populations.
5 What is an antigen?
6 Give two differences between the specific and non-specific immune responses.
7 What is meant by an antigen presenting cell (APC)?
8 Give two differences between the primary and secondary immune responses.

Project practice

You are working in a lab that analyses ingredients for use in food manufacture. It is important that these meet required standards of identity, purity and safety. Choose one of the following areas.
▶ DNA analysis of meat to confirm species (lamb, beef, pork, etc.)
▶ Microbiological analysis of ingredients for contamination with pathogens.
▶ Immunological techniques for confirming identity and purity of ingredients.

You then need to carry out the following:
1 Research a strategy.
   a Carry out a literature review.
   b Justify why you have chosen specific sources and not others.
2 Plan a project using the sources that you selected in your literature review.
   a Set out the techniques you would use in your chosen form of analysis.
   b Include all appropriate risk assessments.
   c Identify the data that you would need to collect and how you would record the data.

3 Analyse the data.
   a You will normally be presented with the data you need, as there will not be time to actually carry out the investigation.
   b Produce a report of your analysis; think about what statistical tests you might need to apply.
4 Present your outcomes and conclusions in the form of a scientific poster showing:
   a the techniques being used
   b the strengths and weaknesses of your chosen technique
   c your conclusions about the technique you have chosen.
5 Group discussion covering topics such as:
   a the need for food analysis
   b the practicality of different techniques
   c do these techniques help to reassure consumers?
6 Reflection – write a reflective evaluation of your work.

Assessment practice

1 For each of the following organelles, state whether they are found in eukaryotes, prokaryotes, or both:

  a Nuclei

  b Plasma membrane

  c Ribosomes

  d DNA associated with proteins

  e Plasmids

2 Which of the following statements is true?

  A Lipids are polymers of fatty acids and glycerol.

  B Polysaccharides are highly soluble molecules which makes them suitable as energy stores.

  C Proteins are used as a form of storage molecule.

  D Proteins, polysaccharides and lipids are all formed by condensation reactions.

3 A short section of DNA has the following base sequence.

  A G C T T A G C T

  Give the base sequence of the complementary strand of DNA.

4 Explain how semi-conservative replication ensures genetic continuity from one generation of cells to the next.

5 A student was using a light microscope to study a stained section of animal tissue.

  a Explain what type of stain is likely to have been used in preparing the section.

  b The student made a labelled drawing of part of the section. Explain why the student was told to label the position of the plasma membrane but not the plasma membrane itself.

6 A class was studying micrographs of animal cells.

  a One micrograph showed a mitochondrion that was labelled as being 1.5 μm long. A student measured the micrograph and found that the image of the mitochondrion was 11.3 cm long. Calculate the magnification of the microscope.

  b Another micrograph was labelled 'x 500 000'. The student measured the thickness of the plasma membrane on the micrograph and found it was 2 mm wide. Calculate the actual width of the plasma membrane in nm.

  c Explain what type of microscope will have been used to create the micrographs.

7 Antibiotics can be used to treat bacterial infections because they do not harm eukaryotic cells.

  a Explain why antibiotics cannot be used to treat malaria.

  b Explain why malaria can be controlled using insecticides.

8 During the COVID-19 pandemic, the UK government's advice was built around the slogan 'Hands, face, space'. This was later amended, adding 'fresh air'. Evaluate the use of this slogan.

9 Which of the following are involved in antibody-mediated immunity?

  A B cells, T helper cells, plasma cells, phagocytes

  B B cells, T killer cells, plasma cells

  C Phagocytes, T killer cells, plasma cells

  D Phagocytes, T killer cells, T helper cells

10 During the early stages of development of a COVID-19 vaccine, the concentration of antibodies in the blood of volunteers was measured in the weeks after vaccination. One vaccine produced significantly more antibodies than another type of vaccine. However, both were found to be similarly effective in preventing COVID-19 infection. Suggest an explanation for this finding.

B1.33–B1.44: Core science concepts: Chemistry

Introduction

Chemistry is the study of substances, their properties and how they combine to make other substances. All substances are made up of atoms, so we need to understand the structure of atoms and the arrangement of electrons within atoms. This is important because electrons are responsible for the bonds between atoms and chemical reactions involve making and breaking bonds.

This chapter also covers basic concepts of acids and bases, the factors that affect the rates of chemical reactions and some methods we can use to analyse substances.

Learning outcomes

The core knowledge outcomes that you must understand and learn:

Materials and chemical properties

B1.33 the relationship between the atomic structure and physical and chemical properties of metals

B1.34 how the arrangement of electrons is linked to the way in which elements are situated within groups in the periodic table

B1.35 the correct names for sub-atomic particles and their position in an atom – protons, electrons and neutrons

Acids/bases and chemical change

B1.36 the physical properties of acids

B1.37 the concept of strong and weak acids (as distinct from dilute and concentrated solutions)

B1.38 how to determine the name of the salt produced in acid-base reactions

Rates of reaction and energy changes

B1.39 the principles of collision theory

B1.40 the effect of temperature on rates of reaction

B1.41 the definition of a catalyst and the role of catalysts in a reaction

Chemical analysis of substances

B1.42 the principles of tests and techniques that are used to separate, detect and identify chemical composition

B1.43 the tests that could be used to quantify components in a mixture

B1.44 the principle of titration.

Practice point

Standard form

Throughout the coming chapters, and elsewhere in this book, you will see numbers written in what is known as **standard form**.

For example, the number 3200 can be written as 3.2×10^3.

10^3 is one thousand ($10 \times 10 \times 10$; try it on your calculator). So we are writing a number which we might say as three thousand two hundred as 3.2 thousands, hence 3.2×10^3.

3200 is not a very large number, so you might ask, 'why bother?' But what about the following number?

3 200 000 000 000 000 000 000

That takes too much space to write. But it also has the complication of working out millions, billions and so on. It is much easier to write it as 3.2×10^{21}.

The same is true of very small numbers:

5.5×10^{-11} is much easier to work with than 0.000000000055. Can you be sure to keep track of all those zeroes?

Numbers in standard form always have two parts. The number before the '×' sign is always greater than or equal to 1 but less than 10. The number after the '×' sign is always a power of 10. Here are some examples:

$1.25 \times 10^3 = 1250$

$3.5 \times 10^{-4} = 0.00035$

You can count decimal places to convert between standard form and 'ordinary' numbers.

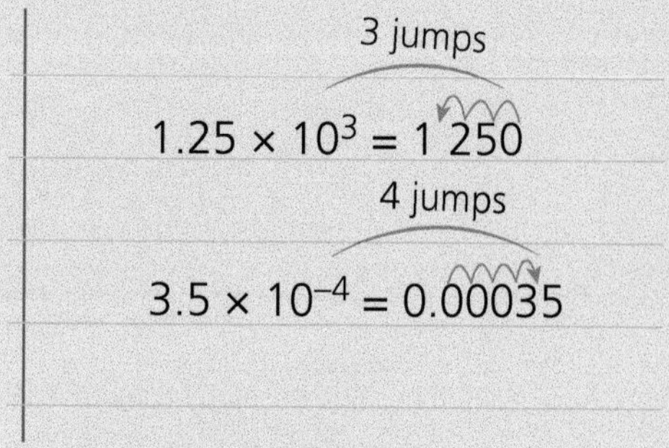

▲ Figure 13.1 Converting between standard form and 'ordinary' numbers

There are two ways to work out if the power of 10 is positive or negative:
▶ If the decimal point jumps to the left, it is a positive power of 10. If it jumps to the right, it is a negative power of 10.
▶ If the number is greater than 10, then the power is positive. If the number is less than 1, the power is negative.

You will find more detail about this topic with further examples in section B1.64.

Materials and chemical properties

Materials science is the study of the properties of solid materials and how they are determined by the chemical and physical composition of the material. Materials science is of great importance in the modern world. It inhabits the space between chemistry, physics, biology and engineering. Therefore, in chemistry, we must study both the physical and chemical properties of substances and understand how they are related to get a full understanding of the substances we are studying.

B1.33 The relationship between the atomic structure and physical and chemical properties of metals

Key terms

Ions: atoms that have lost electrons (positive ions) or gained electrons (negative ions).

Delocalised electrons: 'free' electrons that are not associated with any single atom.

Physical properties

Metals are usually solids at room temperature (mercury is the only metal that is liquid at room temperature), with particles packed closely together in a repeating three-dimensional grid arrangement called a lattice. The atoms in the lattice have lost their outer shell electrons, so the structure consists of metal **ions** and a sea or cloud of **delocalised electrons**. The attraction between the positive ions and the negative electrons holds the particles together in the lattice. This is known as **metallic bonding** and is shown in Figure 13.2. Metallic bonding explains the physical properties of metals.

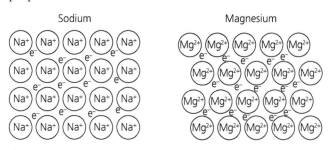

▲ Figure 13.2 A two-dimensional diagram of metallic bonding in sodium and magnesium

Conductivity (electrical and thermal)

The delocalised electrons are free to move throughout the lattice. This means that they can carry an electric current (a flow of charge), so metals are good electrical conductors.

The delocalised electrons can move and vibrate and so transfer thermal energy from one to another through the metal, making metals good conductors of heat.

Malleability/ductility

Metals are **malleable** (they can be hammered into shape) and **ductile** (they can be drawn into wires). This is because of the layered structure. As you can see in Figure 13.3, if a force is applied to a metal, the layers can slide without disrupting the bonding.

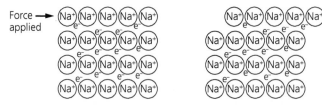

▲ Figure 13.3 Applying a force to part of a metal causes the layers to slide over each other without disrupting the bonding

Strength

The close packing of the particles in a metal explains their high density. You can see from Figure 13.3 that the Mg^{2+} ions have twice the charge of the Na^+ ions and there are also twice as many delocalised electrons. This is because magnesium has 2 electrons in its outer shell, so forms 2+ ions, whereas sodium has only 1 electron in its outer shell, so forms 1+ ions (see section B1.34). This means that magnesium has 2+ ions and twice as many delocalised electrons compared with the 1+ ions and fewer delocalised electrons in sodium. Therefore, there is a greater electrostatic attraction between the positive ions and delocalised electrons in magnesium. As a result, more energy is needed to overcome these forces in magnesium and so magnesium is stronger and has a higher melting point than sodium. The transition metals have even more delocalised electrons, which explains their greater strength and density – for instance, iron or tungsten. These are very hard compared with sodium which is soft enough to be cut with a knife and spread with a spatula.

Chemical properties

See section B1.34 for more information about how elements are divided into groups and blocks.

Group 1

Group 1 metals are all highly reactive. They react with water to form hydrogen gas and the metal hydroxide, for example, sodium:

$$2Na(s) + 2H_2O(l) \rightarrow 2NaOH(aq) + H_2(g)$$

They react with oxygen to form solid white oxides, for example:

$$4Na(s) + O_2 \rightarrow 2Na_2O(s)$$

Group 1 metals all have a single electron in their outer shells and so they form ionic compounds containing 1+ ions (Na^+, K^+, etc.). The outer electrons are further from the nucleus as you move down the group, from lithium to rubidium. This means there is a weaker force of attraction between the negative outer shell electron and the positive nucleus (because of the increased distance and increased shielding from the other electron shells). That means the outer electron is lost more easily in rubidium, making it more reactive.

The reactivity of group 1 metals increases down the group from lithium (least reactive) to rubidium (most reactive).

Transition metals

Transition metals are much less reactive with oxygen and acids compared with either group 1 or group 2 metals. Iron will rust (in other words, form iron oxide), but only when in contact with air containing water vapour – there is no reaction with dry air or oxygen-free water. Other transition metals react even more slowly, which makes them resistant to **corrosion**.

> ### Key term
>
> **Corrosion:** the process where metals react with substances in the air to form oxides, carbonates, hydroxides or other compounds.

The reaction of transition metals with acids is variable – it depends on the metal and the acid.

For example, iron will react with hydrochloric acid to produce iron chloride and with sulfuric acid to produce iron sulfate. In both cases hydrogen is also produced and the iron forms Fe^{2+} ions.

The reaction with nitric acid is a little different because concentrated nitric acid is a stronger oxidising agent than either sulfuric, hydrochloric, or dilute nitric acids. This means that the Fe is oxidised to Fe^{3+} rather than Fe^{2+}. Also, the nitrate (NO_3^-) in nitric acid is reduced to nitrogen monoxide (NO).

Copper is one of the least reactive transition metals and does not react with dilute hydrochloric or sulfuric acids. However, nitric acid and concentrated sulfuric acids are strong oxidising agents, and will both react with copper:

Dilute nitric acid reacts to form copper nitrate and nitrogen monoxide.

Concentrated sulfuric acid reacts to form copper sulfate and sulfur dioxide.

Notice that hydrogen is not produced in either case.

The table compares some properties of transition metals with group 1 metals.

Property	Group 1 metals	Transition metals
Melting points	Low	High
Density	Low – lithium, sodium and potassium are less dense than water	High
Hardness and strength	Soft and weak (can be cut with a knife)	Hard and strong
Reactivity with:		
Oxygen	High to very high (need to be stored under a protective layer of oil)	Slow to very slow
Chlorine	React vigorously to produce solid metal chlorides	Less reactive. Iron wool heated strongly will react with chlorine to produce iron (II) chloride
Water	Vigorous to very vigorous	Relatively unreactive

> ### Reflect
>
> Think about metallic bonding – positive ions surrounded by a sea of delocalised electrons.
>
> Can you use this to explain the difference in physical properties between the group 1 metals and the transition metals?

The relationship between the structure and properties of the following materials

Composite materials

As the name suggests, composite materials are made from two or more materials that have different properties. Reinforcing fibres or particles are embedded in a softer matrix that helps to bind the material together. Some common examples include:

- Concrete, used since Roman times, consists of small stones embedded in a matrix of sand and cement.
- Fibreglass has the strength of glass but is not brittle. Relatively rigid glass fibres act as reinforcement in a flexible resin matrix. Fibreglass can be created in a mould to produce a strong but lightweight material.
- Carbon fibre consists of carbon nanotubes embedded in a polymer matrix. It can combine great strength in a lightweight material. Although it is more expensive than metals such as iron and steel, carbon fibre is used increasingly in engineering applications (automotive and aircraft), sports equipment (golf clubs and tennis racquets) and many others.

Ceramics

Ceramics are made from materials such as clay, sand and other minerals that are moulded and then baked to form strong bonds between the atoms in the structure. This makes them hard, strong under compression and chemically unreactive.

- Clay ceramics have been made for thousands of years by moulding clay and heating in a furnace to produce decorative items and tableware.
- Glass is made from sand (a silicate) with either sodium carbonate and limestone to make soda-lime glass or with boron trioxide to make the stronger, heat-resistant borosilicate glass.

Polymers

Polymers are long chain molecules made from repeating monomer units. For example, poly(ethene) is a polymer with many thousands of repeating units based on ethene.

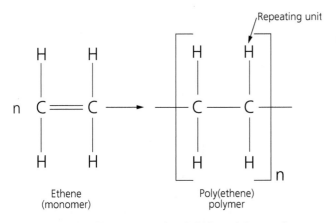

Ethene (monomer)   Poly(ethene) polymer

Repeating unit

▲ Figure 13.4 Formation of poly(ethene) from ethene. The square brackets with n indicates that the repeating unit is repeated n times (i.e. many times)

Some polymers have weak forces between the chains – this makes them softer and more flexible – while others have strong bonds holding the chains in a stronger and more rigid structure.

Polymers are chemically unreactive and electrical insulators (as they do not have any delocalised electrons to carry a current). This makes them very useful for storing and packaging items to keep them from changing.

Poly(ethene) is known commonly as **polythene**. Low density poly(ethene) (LDPE) and high density poly(ethene) (HDPE) are examples of **thermosoftening** polymers. Weak forces between the molecules allow the chains to slide over each other. This means they can be heated to soften them, allowing them to be moulded and reformed. Recycling thermosoftening polymers is therefore relatively easy and it is used in various consumer products to take advantage of this fact.

- HDPE is stronger and more rigid because it has a higher density. This is because it contains unbranched chains that can pack together more tightly. HDPE is used for bottles and other containers.
- LDPE is weaker and more flexible because it has a low density. This is because the chains are branched and therefore cannot pack together as easily. LDPE is used for bags, sheets and films.

Thermosetting polymers use heat to create cross-links between the chains. This makes the polymer stronger and less flexible. However, thermosetting polymers cannot be heated and reformed, which means they are less easily recycled.

> ### Research
>
> Make a list of the different types of material covered in this section. Choose at least one of each type.
>
> Then make a list of the different uses of the materials. For each example, try to show how the properties are related to the use.

B1.34 How the arrangement of electrons is linked to the way in which elements are situated within groups in the periodic table

The simplest definition of an **atom** is a **nucleus** surrounded by a cloud of **electrons**. The atom is more complex than this, but this model of the atom can be useful in some circumstances.

The **nucleus** is at the centre of the atom. It consists of **protons** and **neutrons** and contains most of the mass.

Elements consist of only one type of atom. **Compounds** consist of two or more types of atoms.

Electrons do not orbit the nucleus like planets orbiting the sun. Instead, they are located in **shells**, numbered from 1 to 7. Each shell is higher energy than the previous.

We can think of each shell being further from the nucleus than the last, and you will often see shells represented like this in diagrams. However, this can be misleading, making it look as if the electrons really are orbiting the nucleus. It is better to think of these 7 shells as being the 7 principal energy levels.

Electrons within each shell are located in various orbitals – s, p, d and f. The **orbitals** are found in different shells as follows:

▶ Each shell has only one s orbital.
▶ In shell 2 and above, there are also p orbitals.
▶ In shell 3, there are also d orbitals.
▶ In the highest shells, there are also f orbitals.

The modern periodic table is arranged in increasing order of **atomic number**, but the elements are also arranged according to their electronic structure into the s, p, d and f blocks (Figure 13.5).

The periodic table is also organised into **groups** – the columns in the table. Elements in the same group have similar chemical properties. This is because they have the same number of electrons in the outer shell.

The periodic table can be divided into blocks depending on which type of orbital the outer electrons are located in (Figure 13.6):

▶ Group 1 (the 'alkali metals') have one electron in the outer shell. It is in an s orbital, so these are all in the s block.
▶ Group 2 (the 'alkaline earths') have two electrons in the outer shell, both in the s sub-shell, so these are also in the s block.
▶ Groups 3 through 0 have from three to eight electrons in the outer shell. These are all in p orbitals, so these are in the p block.
▶ The d block includes the transition metals.

Key terms

Atomic number: refers to the number of protons in the nucleus.

Group: refers to the columns in the periodic table. Elements in each group have the same number of outer shell electrons. Period refers to the rows in the periodic table. Elements in each period have the same number of shells.

Orbitals: are where electrons are located. Each orbital can be empty or can contain one or two electrons.

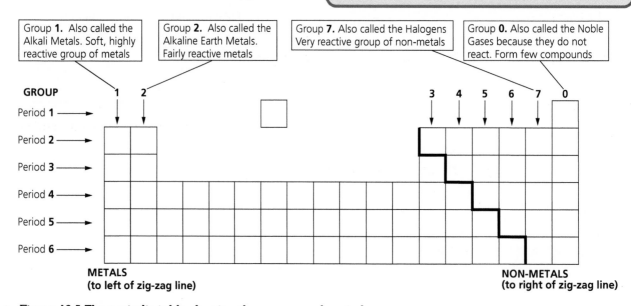

Group **1**. Also called the Alkali Metals. Soft, highly reactive group of metals

Group **2**. Also called the Alkaline Earth Metals. Fairly reactive metals

Group 7. Also called the Halogens Very reactive group of non-metals

Group 0. Also called the Noble Gases because they do not react. Form few compounds

METALS (to left of zig-zag line)

NON-METALS (to right of zig-zag line)

▲ Figure 13.5 The periodic table showing the groups and periods

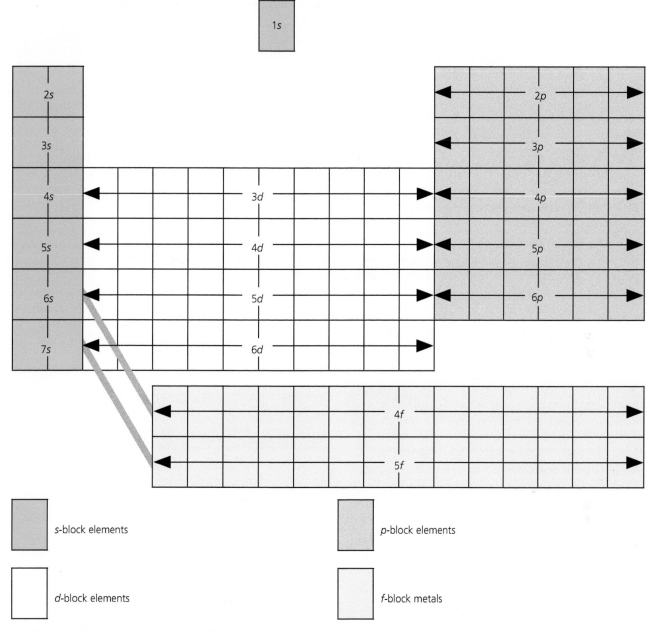

▲ Figure 13.6 The periodic table divided into blocks according to electronic structure

B1.35 Sub-atomic particles – protons, electrons and neutrons

An atom was originally thought of as being the smallest particle that an element could be broken down into. We now know that is not the case. Nuclear physics studies the many types of sub-atomic particle, but in chemistry we are only concerned with three types:

▶ Protons are found in the nucleus and have a charge of +1 and a relative mass of 1.

▶ Neutrons are also found in the nucleus. They have no charge but also have a relative mass of 1.

▶ Electrons are found in orbitals around the nucleus and have a charge of −1. The relative mass of electrons is approximately 1/2000th that of a proton or neutron.

From this, you can see that the majority of the mass of an atom is in the nucleus.

1 Explain the terms 'malleable' and 'ductile'.
2 Explain how the structure of metals means that they are good conductors of electricity.
3 Explain, with examples, the difference between a composite and a ceramic.
4 State what is meant by the following:
   a an atom
   b an element
   c a compound.
5 Explain the difference between a shell and an orbital.
6 Complete the following table:

Particle	Location	Charge	Relative mass
Proton			
	Nucleus	0	
			approx. 1/2000

Acids/bases and chemical change

pH is a measure of the hydrogen ion concentration. It is a **logarithmic scale**, usually from 0 to 14, although pH values can go above or below this range. Because it is a logarithmic scale, a change of one pH unit means the hydrogen ion concentration changes by a factor of 10. At room temperature, pure water has a pH of 7, which is considered the neutral point. Below pH 7 the solution is **acidic** and above pH 7 the solution is **alkaline**. **Neutralisation** occurs when acid and **base** react to form water and a salt.

Acid-base reactions are particularly important in chemistry. As well as being used to determine concentrations in titration (see section B1.44), they are used for preparation of a wide range of salts.

Acid: a proton (H^+ ion) donor. An **acidic** solution contains H^+ ions.

Alkali: a water-soluble base, such as sodium hydroxide. An **alkaline** solution contains hydroxide (OH^-) ions.

Base: a proton (H^+ ion) acceptor. Examples include hydroxides as well as ammonia and amines. (See B1.38.)

B1.36 The physical properties of acids

Acids release hydrogen (H^+) ions – we say that they are H^+ **donors**. This explains the properties of acids:
▶ They are an irritant (cause inflammation of the skin) and often corrosive.
▶ They react with bases in a neutralisation reaction to produce a salt and water (see section B1.38).
▶ They react with most metals to form hydrogen gas (H_2).
▶ Because they have a high concentration of H^+ ions, they have a pH value less than 7.

B1.37 The concept of strong and weak acids

It will be useful to look at sections B1.62 and B1.63 on units before going further if you are at all unsure about use of the different units used for concentration in this section. Anyone who has tried drinking orange squash without diluting it will be familiar with the idea of concentrated and dilute solutions. To use a more chemical example, if we prepare a solution containing 0.1 mol hydrochloric acid in 1 dm^3 water, the hydrochloric acid will dissociate completely into its ions:

$$HCl(aq) \rightarrow H^+(aq) + Cl^-(aq)$$

In this equation, '(aq)' means **aqueous**, a solution in water. The concentration of H^+ will be 0.1 mol/dm^3 and the solution will have a pH = 1.00. This process is usually described as **dissociation** of the acid (into its constituent ions), but you will also come across the term **ionisation** to describe the same thing.

We can do the same with nitric acid or sulfuric acid:

$$HNO_3(aq) \rightarrow H^+(aq) + NO_3^-(aq)$$

$$H_2SO_4(aq) \rightarrow 2H^+(aq) + SO_4^{2-}(aq)$$

The only difference with sulfuric acid is that the concentration of H^+ will be 2 mol/dm^3 because 1 mol of sulfuric acid releases 2 mol of H^+.

In contrast, if we have a 1 mol/dm^3 solution of ethanoic acid and measure the pH, it will be 2.88 because the H^+ concentration is only 0.0013 mol/dm^3. This is because ethanoic acid is a weak acid, which means that it only partially **dissociates** in aqueous solution. We can represent this as the following reversible reaction:

$$CH_3COOH(aq) \leftrightharpoons H^+(aq) + CH_3COO^-(aq)$$

A **reversible reaction**, also known as an equilibrium reaction, is represented by the double arrow $\leftrightharpoons$ and can move in either direction. In any **equilibrium**, there will be a mixture of all the components (reactants and products) in varying proportions. In the case of weak acids, such as ethanoic acid, the position of the equilibrium lies well to the left, i.e. only a small amount will dissociate – most will remain as CH_3COOH.

Once we understand the difference between strong/weak and concentrated/dilute, it should be clear that we can have a dilute solution of a strong acid and a concentrated solution of a weak acid.

You will also see from the above that when we have solutions of the same concentration, e.g. 0.1 mol/dm^3, the pH of the strong acid (pH = 1.00) will be lower than that of the weak acid (pH = 2.88). If you consider the H^+ concentration you will see that ethanoic acid (the weak acid) has a H^+ concentration almost one thousand times lower than the hydrochloric acid.

This illustrates another important feature of pH. For each one unit decrease in pH, the H^+ concentration increases by a factor of 10.

B1.38 How to determine the name of the salt produced in acid-base reactions

Bases, such as sodium or potassium hydroxide, react with acids, such as hydrochloric acid, in a neutralisation reaction to produce a salt plus water. For example, with hydrochloric acid and sodium hydroxide:

$$NaOH(aq) + HCl(aq) \rightarrow NaCl(aq) + H_2O(l)$$

Group 2 hydroxides (hydroxides of Group 2 elements) react in the same way. The salt formed always takes the name of the metal (positive ion) together with the name corresponding to the acid used. Ammonia solution (ammonium hydroxide) reacts in the same way to form ammonium salts.

The table shows the names of salts formed from some common acids.

Practice point

The table shows the modern (systematic) names of the chemicals. You will probably encounter older, non-systematic names as well, such as 'acetate' for 'ethanoate'. There are many other examples, although we will not be covering those chemicals here.

Test yourself

1 What is meant by:
   a an acid   b a base?
2 Explain the difference between a concentrated solution of a weak acid and a dilute solution of a concentrated acid.
3 Name the salts produced in the following acid-base reactions:
   a Potassium hydroxide and nitric acid.
   b Calcium hydroxide and phosphoric acid.
   c Ammonia solution and sulfuric acid.

Acid	Formula of acid	Type of salt formed	Formula of anion	Example
Hydrochloric	HCl	Chlorides	Cl$^-$	Sodium chloride, NaCl
Sulfuric	H$_2$SO$_4$	Sulfates	SO$_4^{2-}$	Sodium sulfate, Na$_2$SO$_4$
Nitric	HNO3	Nitrates	NO$_3^-$	Sodium nitrate, NaNO$_3$
Phosphoric	H$_3$PO$_4$	Phosphates	PO$_4^{3-}$	Sodium phosphate, Na$_3$PO$_4$
Ethanoic	CH$_3$COOH	Ethanoates	CH$_3$COO$^-$	Sodium ethanoate, CH$_3$COONa

Rates of reaction and energy changes

We need to understand the factors that affect the rate of chemical reactions. That understanding is important if we are running a chemical factory producing ammonia for use in artificial fertiliser or preparing a sample of a medicine such as aspirin in the laboratory.

B1.39 The principles of collision theory

Our understanding of rates of reaction and energy change in chemical reactions is based on **collision theory**. This was originally worked out for reactions between gases, but the principles also apply to reactions in solution. We can summarise this theory in three statements:

1 Molecules must collide in order to react.
2 Molecules must have sufficient energy when they collide. Chemical reactions involve breaking chemical bonds (which requires energy) before new bonds are made (which releases energy). The energy required to break bonds is known as the activation energy. If molecules that have less energy than the activation energy collide, they will just bounce off each other without reacting.
3 Molecules must be in the correct spatial orientation when they collide. The bonds being broken and reformed will be in specific positions in space. This means molecules must be aligned correctly when they collide – see Figure 13.7.

B1.40 The effect of temperature on rates of reaction

As temperature increases, the kinetic energy of the molecules increases. This means they move faster. If they move faster, they are more likely to collide. So increasing temperature increases the rate of reaction in two ways:

▶ The probability of collision increases.
▶ The proportion of molecules with sufficient energy to react also increases.

On the other hand, decreasing temperature decreases the kinetic energy of molecules. Therefore, molecules move slower, decreasing the probability of successful collisions and hence decreases the rate of reaction.

B1.41 The definition of a catalyst and the role of catalysts in a reaction

Catalysts increase the rate of chemical reactions. They do this because they provide an alternative reaction pathway that has a lower activation energy. This means that more molecules will have sufficient energy to react and this will increase the rate of reaction. In short, more reactants will exceed the activation energy and so can successfully collide.

Transition metals are often used as catalysts. In some reactions between gases the solid transition metal catalyst provides a surface for the reaction to take place. In other cases, the transition metal takes part in the reaction. Acids are common catalysts in organic chemistry. In both cases, the catalyst will participate in the reaction but will be reformed at the end of the reaction. This means that the catalyst is not **permanently** changed. It is used, but not used up. In all cases, remember the catalyst provides an alternative reaction pathway that has a lower activation energy.

Test yourself

1 What are the three statements of collision theory?
2 Explain why temperature increases the rate of reaction.
3 Explain how a catalyst increases the rate of reaction.

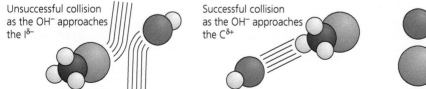
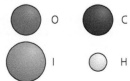

Unsuccessful collision as the OH⁻ approaches the I$^{\delta-}$

Successful collision as the OH⁻ approaches the C$^{\delta+}$

O   C
I   H

▲ Figure 13.7 Effect of orientation on reaction outcome

Chemical analysis of substances

Our knowledge of chemistry is built upon the ability to analyse substances. We need to understand the composition of substances and how this changes when they undergo chemical reactions.

B1.42 The principles of tests and techniques that are used to separate, detect and identify chemical composition

Separation is central to most forms of analysis. As well as separating the components of a mixture, we sometimes need to **quantify** them (work out how much of them there is).

Examples of analysis based on separation of the components of a mixture include:
- detecting additives in foodstuffs
- analysing urine samples to detect use of performance-enhancing drugs in sport (doping)
- determining the purity of pharmaceutical raw materials.

Reflect

List as many types of substance you might need to analyse as you can. For each one, decide whether it would be enough to know what is present (**qualitative analysis**) or whether you would need to know how much of each substance is present (**quantitative analysis**).

Key terms

Chromatography: the separation of the components of a mixture dissolved in a liquid or gas (the mobile phase) carrying it through a structure holding the stationary phase.

Adsorption: when a substance (e.g. a gas, liquid or solute) binds to or attaches to another, usually solid.

Adsorbent: often used to describe the stationary phase in chromatography because substances become adsorbed to it during separation.

In all types of **chromatography**, separation depends on substances in a mixture having a different **affinity** or attraction towards two phases. The **stationary phase** is fixed while the **mobile phase** (a liquid or gas) is able to move. It is important, in this context, that we use the term **adsorption** for the process of binding to a material in the stationary phase. (This is not the same as **absorption**, which is a term sometimes used, incorrectly, in this context. In absorption, one substance is taken in or **absorbed** by another, rather like a sponge absorbing water.)

Thin layer chromatography

Thin layer chromatography (TLC) is used to separate non-volatile mixtures such as amino acids, pharmaceuticals or dyestuffs. These are substances that cannot be easily vaporised. Separation is based on their solubility in the mobile phase (solvent) or affinity for (attraction to) the stationary phase (on a coated plate). The stationary phase is a thin layer of **adsorbent** such as silica gel, alumina or powdered cellulose on a flat, **inert** (non-reactive) support, such as glass or (more usually) plastic.

TLC can be used to detect the number of components in a mixture. The stages are:
1 A pencil line (the **origin**) is drawn about 1 cm from one short edge of the TLC plate.
2 The sample or samples are applied in solution at various points along the origin and left to dry.
3 The plate is placed vertically in a container with a shallow layer of solvent, so that the origin is above the level of the solvent (Figure 13.8).
4 The container is covered or sealed to prevent evaporation. The solvent will be drawn up the paper by **capillary action** (the process where a liquid is drawn into narrow spaces like those between the fibres in filter paper or a kitchen towel).
5 When the solvent reaches the origin, substances in the sample will dissolve and begin to move.
6 Substances with greater affinity for the stationary phase will move more slowly than substances with a greater affinity for the solvent and so the mixture will become separated.
7 After the solvent has moved far enough up the paper (usually almost to the top), the plate is removed from the container.
8 The position that the solvent has reached (the **solvent front**) is marked.

Efficient separation requires choice of solvent (mobile phase) so that the different components of the mixture will have different solubility in the mobile phase. If all components are equally soluble, they will all move the same distance. If they are insoluble, they will remain at the origin. Therefore, different solvents or mixtures of solvents with a range of **polarities** (ability to mix or dissolve) are used depending upon the substances being separated.

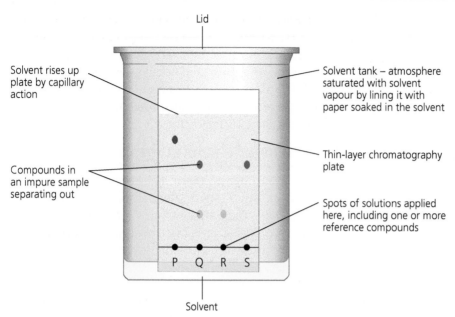

Lid

Solvent rises up plate by capillary action

Solvent tank – atmosphere saturated with solvent vapour by lining it with paper soaked in the solvent

Thin-layer chromatography plate

Compounds in an impure sample separating out

Spots of solutions applied here, including one or more reference compounds

P   Q   R   S

Solvent

▲ Figure 13.8 Apparatus for TLC. Samples for analysis are spotted on the origin at P, Q, R and S

In the same way, the nature of the stationary phase will determine how far a particular substance moves. If a substance has a high affinity for the stationary phase, it will not move far up the plate. If it has a low affinity for the stationary phase, it will move further.

TLC is often used to separate the different coloured dyes in a mixture or to analyse the different coloured pigments in a plant extract. In other cases, the components of the mixture are colourless. This means we need to make the spots visible in some way. A common method is to use a dye that will bind to the chemicals in our mixture:

▶ Ninhydrin will stain amino acids purple. If a TLC plate is used to separate a mixture of amino acids, it can be dried and then sprayed with ninhydrin solution. The amino acids spots are then stained purple.

▶ Iodine vapour will stain many chemicals brown.

Another method to make the spots visible is to use a TLC plate that contains an inert fluorescent dye. After the separation is done and the plate is dried it can be illuminated with UV light. The spots will appear dark on a bright background.

If we analyse a substance by TLC and see just a single spot, it suggests the substance is pure. However, it is possible that two substances move the same distance. To be sure a sample is pure, we need to repeat the analysis in a different system, for example, with a different solvent mixture or different adsorbent.

As well as separating the components of a mixture, paper chromatography and TLC can be used to identify the components. One way is to run pure samples (**standards**) alongside the mixture. The distance travelled by a component of the mixture can then be compared to the distance travelled by one of the standards.

Another method is to calculate the **retention factor** or R_f **value**. R_f values can be used in TLC to identify unknowns based on standard published literature values.

Column chromatography

Column chromatography uses similar stationary phases to TLC but a much wider range is available, particularly those used in the separation of biologicals. In all cases, the sample is applied to the top of the column and **eluted** with a suitable mobile phase, the **eluent**. The stationary phase runs the entire length of the column. The substances then travel down the column based on their affinity for the eluent. Substances with a higher affinity for this mobile phase, will be separated and eluted earlier from the bottom of the column. The advantage of column chromatography is that the **eluate** can be collected in small amounts (**fractions**) as it emerges from the bottom of the column. Different substances will be in the different fractions because they elute from the column at different times. This allows column chromatography to be used for purification of a single chemical compound as well as for analysis.

Key terms

Elution: to wash out. In column chromatography this means 'washing out' a substance that has become adsorbed to the column (stationary phase).

Eluent: the solvent (mobile phase) used to wash substances out of a column.

Eluate: the mobile phase, containing dissolved substances, as it emerges from a column.

Gas chromatography

Gas chromatography (GC) is used to separate and analyse **volatile** compounds (ones that can be vaporised). GC uses an inert carrier gas as the mobile phase. The stationary phase can be a thin layer of high boiling point liquid on an inert solid support packed into a column. Substances that have a higher affinity for the stationary phase, will interact with it more, meaning it will take longer for it to emerge from the column. Substances with a lower affinity for the stationary phase, will then emerge sooner and be detected first. More recently, capillary GC uses a polymer lining a very fine capillary column as the stationary phase. The column will be coiled inside an oven to maintain the relatively high temperature needed (Figure 13.9).

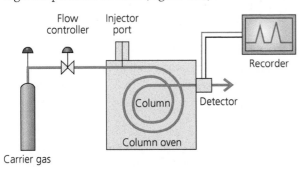

▲ Figure 13.9 Apparatus for GC

The sample is injected into the gas stream and the components of the mixture being separated will interact with the stationary phase to different degrees and so will emerge from the column at different times. The substances emerging from the column are detected, usually by a **flame ionisation detector (FID)** or a **thermal conductivity detector (TCD)**. These work with a wide range of substances, although other detection methods are available for specific applications.

The time taken between injection and detection of a particular component is known as the **retention time**. We saw how R_f values can be used in TLC to identify unknowns based on standard published literature values. The same is true of retention time in GC. However, conditions used for the analysis must be identical to those used when determining the standard values. This includes use of the same column (not just the same stationary phase), mobile phase, temperature, etc.

Another way to confirm the identity of a substance in a mixture is to add a purified sample of that substance (a standard) to the sample when it is injected onto the column (GC or HPLC, see below). If the substance in the mixture **co-elutes** with the standard (i.e. has the same retention time), it is strong evidence of identity.

High performance liquid chromatography

High performance liquid chromatography (HPLC) is a type of column chromatography that uses very small particles and high pressures to achieve better separation. The very fine particles make it difficult to force the solvent through and so HPLC requires powerful pumps and pressure-resistant columns to be fitted. The sample being analysed or purified cannot simply be applied to the top of the column – the system is sealed and under pressure – so the sample needs to be introduced by injection through a valve or port. The advantages of using HPLC for separation are much greater speed and higher resolution (ability to separate two very similar substances). HPLC has become one of the standard methods of separation in analytical laboratories. It can also be scaled up to operate as a purification method on a much larger scale, handling grams or even kilograms of substance.

A more recent development of HPLC, **ultra-high performance liquid chromatography** or **UPLC**, uses capillary columns to separate mixtures before analysis by mass spectrometry.

Mass spectrometry

Mass spectrometry (MS) can identify the amount and type of compound, which makes it very useful in identifying unknown compounds. The sample is ionised by removing electrons. The mass spectrometer then measures the ratio of mass to charge (m/z) of the positive ions produced. This can be done in various ways:
- By measuring how far the ions were deflected by a magnetic field; ions with greater mass are deflected less (Figure 13.10).

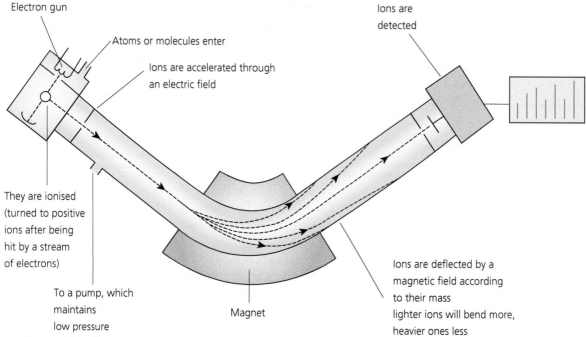

Electron gun

Atoms or molecules enter

Ions are accelerated through an electric field

Ions are detected

They are ionised (turned to positive ions after being hit by a stream of electrons)

To a pump, which maintains low pressure

Magnet

Ions are deflected by a magnetic field according to their mass lighter ions will bend more, heavier ones less

▲ Figure 13.10 Diagram of a mass spectrometer

▶ More recent methods such as **time of flight (TOF)** measure how long it takes for ions to reach the detector; ions with greater mass are slower and take longer.

MS provides the molar mass (M_r) of the compound, but additional information about the structure of the compound can be obtained from the way in which the ion breaks up (fragments) in the mass spectrometer.

By feeding the output of a GC column into a mass spectrometer, it is possible to identify the compounds being separated much more accurately than simply by retention time. This technique, known as GC-MS, is used widely because of the compact nature of the equipment, its speed and relatively low cost. Applications (uses in the real world) include airport screening for drugs and explosives, fire forensics (investigating the causes of a fire) and space exploration. Probes containing miniaturised GC-MS have been sent to Mars, Venus and Titan.

Research

A similar approach to GC-MS can be taken with liquid chromatography. In LC-MS, a very small capillary column is used for separation of complex mixtures such as proteins and peptides. Other applications involve analysis of drug metabolites in pharmacology and anti-doping laboratories. An internet search for 'applications of LC-MS' will help you learn more.

B1.43 The tests that could be used to quantify components in a mixture

GC, HPLC and MS are all powerful analytical techniques that separate the components of a mixture. This means they can be used to determine whether a sample is pure or is contaminated with other substances. To be really useful, we need to be able to calculate the percentage of each component, so that we can work out the percentage purity.

In both GC and HPLC, substances emerging from the column pass through a detector. The output from the detector gives a type of graph called a chromatography trace where the area under the peaks is proportional to the amount of the substance. This data is captured by a computer and analysed to show the percentage of each component.

It is also possible to use a standard of known content to convert the relative values we get from measuring peak area into absolute values, i.e. actual masses, in µg or mg.

In mass spectrometry, the output gives the relative abundance of each component. It is possible to determine the absolute quantity of each component using standards made with heavy isotopes.

B1.44 The principle of titration

Key terms

Mole: an amount of substance. This helps us to work out the reacting proportions in any reaction. We can also use the mole to work out reacting masses or volumes. The abbreviation is **mol**.

Indicator: a substance that changes from one colour to another or from coloured to colourless depending on whether it is in acidic or basic solution.

Analyte: the solution of unknown concentration in a titration.

Standard solution: the solution of known concentration in a titration.

Burette: a long glass tube that has a tap at the bottom and is marked in $0.1cm^3$ divisions. It is used to deliver an accurate volume of liquid (the **titre**) to reach the **end point**.

End point: the point in a titration where the indicator changes colour.

Equivalence point: the point of neutralisation where the number of moles of acid and base are equal. This should ideally be the same as the **end point**.

Titre: the volume of standard solution needed to neutralise the analyte (i.e. to reach the end point of the titration).

Neutralisation occurs when an equal number of **moles** of H^+ (from an acid) and OH^- (from a base) react together to form water. If a strong acid, such as hydrochloric acid, reacts with a strong base, such as sodium hydroxide, in exactly equal proportions, the mixture will be neither acid nor base but neutral (pH7.0). At this point an **indicator** will change colour. We use this in the process of **titration** to calculate the concentration of a solution of acid or base.

In titration we have one unknown – the number of moles in the **analyte**. We titrate this against the **standard solution**. Titration involves adding the standard solution from a **burette** to a known volume of the analyte in a conical flask until we reach the **end point** – when the indicator changes colour. This should

be the **equivalence point**, where we have equal moles of acid and base. Because we know the concentration of the standard solution, we can use the **titre** to calculate how many moles were required to reach the equivalence point. This will tell us the number of moles of analyte in the flask and therefore the concentration of the analyte.

Test yourself

1 Explain the difference between the terms adsorption and absorption.
2 Explain what is meant by the mobile phase in chromatography.
3 Give two examples of a stationary phase.
4 Explain the similarities and differences between column chromatography and HPLC.
5 State the meaning of the following terms:
   a titre
   b end point
   c equivalence point.

Project practice

You have been asked to prepare visuals for a school outreach display that your company is supporting.

Choose one of the following themes and prepare a poster or PowerPoint illustrating how this is relevant to your workplace. Use resources from the internet where necessary.

► 'The right material for the job' – the ways in which different types of material are suited to particular applications in science or healthcare.
► 'Not just a corrosive liquid' – the importance of strong and weak acids in industry, foodstuffs and analysis.
► 'Time is money' – the importance of rates of reaction in industrial processes.
► 'What's in my lunch?' – the use of chemical analysis to test the quality and purity of the food and drink we consume.

Your presentation should include at least one graph, chart or diagram to help illustrate the relevance of your theme to your workplace.

Assessment practice

1 Explain the reasons for the properties and the uses of the following metals:

  a Sodium is soft and low density, but iron is hard and high density.

  b Sodium reacts vigorously with cold water, but iron only reacts very slowly with water.

  c Copper is used to make electric wiring.

  d Copper is used to make pipes in central heating systems.

2 The table shows a range of applications with the corresponding material. For each combination, select the appropriate explanation for why the material is suited to the application.

  A Lightweight, can be formed into wires (ductile) good electrical conductor

  B Lightweight, strong

  C Strong, can be moulded into shape (malleable)

  D Inert, strong and can be moulded into shape

  E Transparent, inert, heat-resistant

  F Strong, inert, very heat resistant

  G Strong, can be formed into shape, non-conductor of electricity

Application	Material	Explanation (letter)
Body panel for budget-priced car	Steel	
Body panel for high performance sportscar	Carbon fibre composite	
Bottle for storage of corrosive liquids	High density polyethene (HDPE)	
Crucible for heating solids at high temperatures	Clay ceramic	
Flask for use in reflux where the contents are heated for a prolonged period	Borosilicate glass	
Insulator for use in high-voltage power lines	Clay ceramic	
Cable for use in high-voltage overhead power lines	Aluminium	

3 Use the periodic table to complete the following table.

Element	Group	Period
Sodium		
Magnesium		
Iron		
Nitrogen		
Neon		

4 Classify the following as to whether they are (i) strong or weak and (ii) concentrated or dilute:

  a a 5 mol/dm^3 solution of ethanoic acid

  b a 0.001 mol/dm^3 solution of hydrochloric acid

  c a 10 mol/dm^3 solution of sulfuric acid.

5 Name the salts that would be produced by mixing each of the following pairs of acid and base:

  a nitric acid and calcium hydroxide

  b sulfuric acid and barium nitrate

  c hydrochloric acid and ammonia

  d ethanoic acid and potassium hydroxide.

6 One method of preparing a salt involves adding an excess of insoluble substance such as a metal, metal oxide, metal hydroxide or metal carbonate to an acid. Suggest how you could prepare a solution of copper sulfate from insoluble copper oxide and sulfuric acid. Explain the advantage of this method over mixing an acid and a soluble base.

7 Collision theory states that particles with sufficient energy must collide in order to react.

  a Explain why increasing the concentration of reactants in solution will increase the rate of reaction.

b Suggest why increasing the temperature has a bigger effect on rate of reaction than increasing the concentration.

8 You have been asked to analyse the amino acids in a food supplement to show that it contains the amino acid lysine.

a Outline how you would use TLC with ninhydrin spray and a pure sample of lysine to do this.

b You find that the food supplement contains two spots. The impurity spot moves a shorter distance than lysine. What can you tell about the properties of this impurity?

c Describe how you could use chromatography to obtain a sample of the impurity for further analysis.

9 You have been asked to analyse a sample of petrol to see if it is contaminated. You are provided with a pure sample of the potential contaminant.

a Explain how you could use GC to show that the contaminant was present in the sample.

b Explain how you could use MS coupled to GC to identify an unknown contaminant in the sample.

10 Describe how you would determine the percentage purity of the following:

a crude pellets of sodium hydroxide

b a volatile compound for use in food flavouring using gas chromatography.

B1.45–B1.64: Core science concepts: Physics

Introduction

Physics is the study of atoms, particles, energy, forces, mechanics and waves – in fact, the whole physical universe.

There is overlap with chemistry in places – atomic structure, for example. The overlap with biology is less obvious, but biophysics is an important part of modern biology. It uses physical methods to understand the interactions between biological molecules and within biological systems. Also, physics is based very firmly on a foundation of mathematics. In fact, mechanics is often an option in mathematics courses and the difference between theoretical physics and applied mathematics can be hard to spot! The field of medical physics is another important area of overlap, where physics contributes to treatment and diagnosis.

Whichever way you look at it, a good understanding of physics is important for work in many areas of science, healthcare and engineering.

Learning outcomes

The core knowledge outcomes that you must understand and learn:

Electricity
B1.45 the definitions of, and how to calculate, charge and current using $Q = It$
B1.46 the definitions of, and how to calculate, current, potential difference and resistance, using Ohm's law $V = IR$
B1.47 how to calculate total resistance of multiple fixed resistors in a series and parallel circuit
B1.48 the difference between alternating and direct current
B1.49 the properties of mains electricity in the United Kingdom

Magnetism and electromagnetism
B1.50 magnetism and magnetic poles
B1.51 magnetic fields
B1.52 the uses of electromagnetism and electromagnets

Waves
B1.53 the definition of a wave
B1.54 the relationship between frequency, wavelength and speed using the wave equation $v = f\lambda$
B1.55 the properties of longitudinal and transverse waves
B1.56 the uses of different types of waves

Particles and radiation
B1.57 the types and properties of ionising radiation
B1.58 the definitions of half-life and count-rate
B1.59 the main types of radioactive decay in relation to unstable nuclei
B1.60 how radiation interacts with matter
B1.61 the applications of radioactivity within the health and science sector

Units
B1.62 the use of the international system of units (SI)
B1.63 how to convert between units
B1.64 the importance of using significant figures and science notation.

Electricity

Electricity in the home, laboratory or industry is usually **alternating current (AC)**. However, low-voltage lighting circuits or anything that you plug into a 5 V USB power supply (like a phone charger) will use **direct current** or **DC**.

We now know that an electric **current** is caused by a flow of electrons, i.e. from negative to positive poles of a battery or power supply. However, electricity and electric currents were discovered long before electrons. Investigators realised that something was flowing – which they called **current** – but did not know what it was. They decided that it must flow from positive to negative.

Although we understand electricity better now, we still follow this convention. You will sometimes see this described as **conventional current**, to distinguish it from flow of electrons. There has been so much work done assuming that current flows from positive to negative that we would have to rewrite too many formulae and textbooks!

Reflect

Why are electrons negative and protons positive? What do we mean by positive and negative?

Those are philosophical questions that we could spend hours thinking about. But what is important is the fact that electrons and protons have *opposite* charges, and we just call one 'negative' and the other 'positive'.

B1.45 The definitions of, and how to calculate, charge and current using $Q = It$

The size of the **current** is the rate of flow of **charge**. That means that when current (I) flows past a given point in a circuit for a length of time (T), we can calculate the charge (Q) that has flowed past this point using the formula:

$$Q = I \times t$$

Where Q is in **coulombs**, I is in amps and t is in seconds. This can be rearranged to give:

$$I = \frac{Q}{t}$$

In other words, current equals charge divided by time. This is the amount of coulombs of charge per second, which is the rate of flow of charge, which is the definition of current!.

To give an example, if a battery charger passes a current of 3.0 A through a rechargeable cell (battery) for a period of two hours, the total charge transferred to the cell can be calculated (don't forget to convert hours to seconds!):

$$Q = I \times t = 3.0 \times (2 \times 60 \times 60) = 21\,600\,C$$

Key terms

Charge: a fundamental property of many subatomic particles. Electrons, by convention, have a negative charge. The unit of charge is the **coulomb (C)** and the symbol is Q.

Coulomb **(C):** the unit of charge. **Current** is the rate of flow of charge past a given point in a circuit, i.e. how fast it flows past. The unit of current is the ampere (A), often shortened to 'amp', and the symbol is I.

B1.46 The definitions of, and how to calculate, current, potential difference and resistance, using Ohm's law $V = IR$

The relationship between **current, potential difference** and **resistance** is one of the most useful concepts in electronics:

$$V = I \times R$$

Potential difference (**voltage**) is the driving force that causes charge to flow round a circuit. It is defined as the electrical work done per unit of charge flowing through components in the circuit. The unit of potential difference is the volt (V) and the symbol is also V. Potential difference is often abbreviated to 'p.d.'.

Resistance is the property of any component of a circuit that slows the flow of current. The unit of resistance is the ohm (Ω) and the symbol is R.

To calculate the current that is flowing in a circuit with resistance $3\,\Omega$ and a potential difference of 12 V, we simply rearrange the formula and substitute the values:

$$I = \frac{V}{R} = \frac{12}{3} = 4\,A$$

B1.47 How to calculate total resistance of multiple fixed resistors in a series and parallel circuit

For resistors connected in **series**, the total potential difference (p.d.) of the supply is shared between the components (see Figure 14.1) and the current through each component is the same (see Figure 14.2).

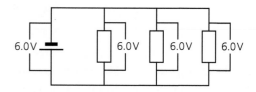

▲ Figure 14.3 Circuit diagram showing sharing of p.d.s in parallel circuits

Key terms

Series: circuits where the components are connected in line, end to end between the positive and negative terminals of the power supply. See Figure 14.1 for an example of a series circuit.

Parallel circuits: where the components are each connected separately to the positive and negative terminals of the power supply. See Figure 14.3 for an example of a parallel circuit.

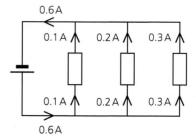

▲ Figure 14.4 Circuit diagram showing sharing of current in parallel circuits

When single resistors are connected in parallel, the potential difference across each will be the same, but the total resistance will be less than the sum of all the resistances. The total resistance is given by:

$$\frac{1}{R_{total}} = \frac{1}{R_1} + \frac{1}{R_2} + \frac{1}{R_n}$$

So, if three resistors of 5 Ω, 10 Ω and 15 Ω are connected in parallel to a power supply we can calculate the total resistance of the circuit by substituting the numbers in the equation:

$$\frac{1}{R_{total}} = \frac{1}{R_1} + \frac{1}{R_2} + \frac{1}{R_3} = \frac{1}{5} + \frac{1}{10} + \frac{1}{15} = 0.37$$

Therefore, rearrange this to find R_{total}:

$$R_{total} = \frac{1}{0.37} = 2.7\,\Omega$$

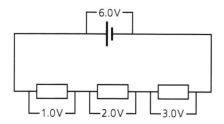

▲ Figure 14.1 Circuit diagram showing p.d. across resistors connected in series

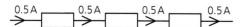

▲ Figure 14.2 Circuit diagram showing current in series circuits

When resistors are connected in series, the total resistance is equal to the sum of the individual resistors, so the total resistance of a circuit with n resistors is given by:

$$R_{total} = R_1 + R_2 + R_n$$

In **parallel circuits**, the p.d. across each route is the same (see Figure 14.3) and the total current through the whole circuit is the sum of the currents passing through each of these possible routes (see Figure 14.4).

B1.48 The difference between alternating and direct current

In **direct current**, DC, the **conventional current** constantly flows in one direction from the positive terminal to the negative terminal – although we now know that it is electrons flowing from negative to positive.

Alternating current, AC, as used in the mains electric supply in the UK and most other countries, has current that constantly changes direction alternating potential difference where the positive and negative ends alternating.

B1.49 The properties of mains electricity in the United Kingdom

By using alternating current, it is possible to transmit electricity over long distances at high voltages – between 275 kV and 400 kV (1 kV = 1000 V). This reduces the current and so less electrical energy is **dissipated** (scientific term for wasted) as heat.

The high voltage used for transmission can then be transformed to a lower voltage of 230 V for supplying to residences and businesses, and higher voltages can be supplied to businesses with a greater demand for energy.

The frequency of mains electricity in Europe is 50 Hz (see page 286), which means there are 50 cycles per second. This is the frequency at which electricity is generated.

Test yourself

1 What do the following terms mean?
   a current
   b potential difference (voltage)
   c resistance.
2 1.2 C of charge flows through a light bulb in a time of 30 s. Calculate the current flowing through the bulb.
3 A 9 V battery is connected to a 4 Ω resistor. Calculate the current flowing through the resistor.
4 Two more resistors of 5 Ω and 6 Ω are added in parallel with the 4 Ω resistor.
   a Calculate the total resistance.
   b What voltage battery would you need to use to maintain the same current as in question 3?

Magnetism and electromagnetism

We are all familiar with **magnets** and **magnetism**. The earth's **magnetic field** causes a compass needle to point towards the (magnetic) north pole. Magnetic fields are invisible, but we can see their effects all around us. A fridge magnet holds notes, family photos or children's artwork on a fridge door. Magnetic clasps are used on handbags and briefcases. Magnets have many other uses and **electromagnets** are particularly useful in science and engineering.

Key terms

Magnet: a material or object that produces a magnetic field.

Magnetism: the force experienced by some types of metals in the earth's magnetic field or in a magnetic field of a magnet. It is also defined as the attractive or repulsive force produced by a moving electric charge.

Magnetic field: a region where magnetic materials experience a force.

Electromagnet: produced when a current flows through a coil of wire.

B1.50 Magnetism and magnetic poles

All magnets have two **poles**, **north** (or north-seeking) and **south** (or south-seeking). These are determined by whether the pole points towards the earth's magnetic north pole (north-seeking) or south pole (south-seeking). For this reason, we call magnets **dipoles**. However, if you cut a magnet in half, you produce two smaller dipoles – you cannot produce a magnetic **monopole** (just a north or south pole).

The north and south poles of a magnet are where the magnetic forces are strongest because the **magnetic field** is strongest. When magnets are placed close together, they will **attract** or **repel** each other, even if they are not touching. For this reason, we say that magnetism is a **non-contact force**. Other types of non-contact force include:

▶ electrostatic force – opposite charges attract, even if they are not in contact

▶ weight – objects with mass attract each other and the greater the mass, the greater the attraction. A satellite falling out of orbit does not have to be in contact with the earth to feel the attractive force of the earth's gravity.

If we place two north poles or two south poles close together, they will repel each other. If we place north and south poles together, they will attract each other.

There are two types of magnet: **permanent** and **induced**. A permanent magnet produces its own magnetic field. If we bring a **magnetic material** close to a permanent magnet, the magnetic material becomes an induced magnet. It has its own induced poles and magnetic field (Figure 14.5).

N	permanent magnet	S

magnetic material

N	permanent magnet	S

N	induced magnet	S

▲ Figure 14.5 A permanent magnet causes magnetic material to become an induced magnet when they are placed close together. **N** and **S** are induced poles

If the induced magnet is removed from the magnetic field of the permanent magnet, it will quickly lose most or all of its magnetism.

Key terms

Permanent magnet: produces its own magnetic field.

Induced magnet: an object that can become a magnet when it is placed in a magnetic field.

Magnetic materials: such as iron, steel, nickel and cobalt will experience an attractive force when placed in a magnetic field.

Lines of magnetic flux: indicate the direction and strength of a **magnetic field**.

B1.51 Magnetic fields

We cannot see a magnetic field, but we can see its effect using iron filings (Figure 14.6). The small pieces of iron act as temporary magnets and line up along the magnetic field lines, also called **lines of magnetic flux**. This means that we can see the shape of the magnetic field.

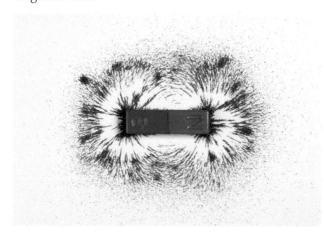

▲ Figure 14.6 Iron filings reveal the invisible lines of flux around a bar magnet

The iron filings allow us to see the shape of the field, but they do not show the direction of the lines of flux. We can plot the magnetic field lines around a bar magnet using a **compass needle**. The north pole of the magnet in the compass needle

will always point towards the south pole of the bar magnet and away from the north pole. We can use this to plot the flux lines of the field around a bar magnet (Figure 14.7). If we move the compass far enough away from the bar magnet, it will point to the earth's north pole.

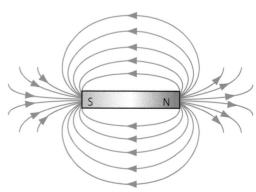

Field lines around a bar magnet

▲ Figure 14.7 Flux lines for a bar magnet. The lines are closest together near the poles, showing where the field is strongest

We follow the convention that the flux lines always go from north to south, indicated by the arrows on the lines in Figure 14.7. You can see how the flux lines are closest together near the two poles. This is where the magnetic field is strongest. Another way to describe the strength of the magnetic field is the **magnetic flux density**, which is defined as the number of magnetic flux lines that pass through an area of $1\,m^2$.

Reflect

The north pole of the magnet in a compass needle points towards the south pole of a bar magnet. But the north pole of the compass needle points towards the geographic north pole of the earth.

Does this mean that the earth generates its own magnetic field? If so, does it mean that the south pole of this 'magnet' is at the geographic north pole?

If you place a compass next to a wire carrying an electric current, you will see the compass needle move as you move the compass around the wire.

This must mean that the current flowing through the wire is generating a magnetic field; you are using the compass needle to trace the magnetic flux lines around the wire.

If you reverse the flow of current in the wire you will notice that the compass needle now points in the opposite direction. We can therefore tell that the direction of the magnetic field has reversed (Figure 14.8).

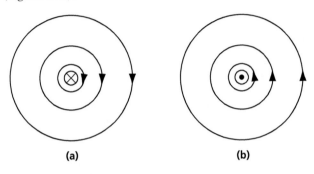

(a)   (b)

▲ Figure 14.8 The magnetic flux lines of a wire carrying a current. Symbols inside the wire indicate the direction of the current. In (a) the current is flowing into the page – away from you – and in (b) the current is flowing out of the page – towards you

From this we can conclude that moving charges (the electric current) generate a magnetic field. This phenomenon is of great importance in physics, engineering, electronics and many areas of our everyday lives.

Notice that the magnetic flux lines get further apart as the distance from the wire increases. This must mean that the strength of the field decreases as distance from the wire increases.

If we increase the size of the current flowing through the wire, we will see that the magnetic flux lines get closer together. Therefore, the greater the current, the stronger the magnetic field.

B1.52 The uses of electromagnetism and electromagnets

The magnetic field generated by a current flowing through a wire can be used to make magnets that can be switched on or off – these are **electromagnets**.

A **solenoid** is created by wrapping wire into a coil. This increases the strength (flux density) of the magnetic field when a current passes through the coil of wire (Figure 14.9). All the magnetic flux lines around each loop of wire line up with each other. This results in lots of flux lines all pointing in the same direction, very close to each other.

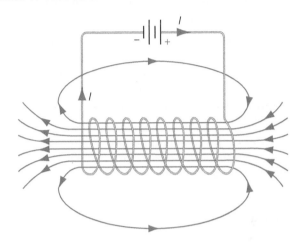

▲ Figure 14.9 The magnetic field generated by a solenoid

Note how close together the magnetic flux lines are in the centre of the solenoid. This means that this is where the magnetic field is strongest. Outside the coil, the magnetic field is just like the one around a bar magnet (Figure 14.7).

You can increase the strength of the magnetic field of the solenoid even more by placing an iron bar in the centre of the coil. This iron core becomes an induced magnet when the current flows – we have made an electromagnet. When the current is switched off, the magnetic field disappears.

A **portative** electromagnet is designed to hold material in place. An example is the type of electromagnet used for lifting materials made of iron or steel in a scrapyard.

A **tractive** electromagnet is one that applies a force and moves another object. An example is a simple solenoid where the coil surrounds a plunger. When the current is switched on, the solenoid applies a force to the plunger making it move. This can be used in many different ways, such as in valves or switches.

Electromagnetic induction

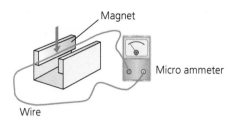

▲ Figure 14.11 Moving a wire into a magnetic field induces a potential difference

> ### Key terms
>
> **Ammeter:** measures the flow of current; always connected in series. **Voltmeters** measure the potential difference in a circuit and are always connected in parallel.
>
> **Electromotive force (emf):** like **potential difference**, except that it refers to power supplies such as cells (batteries), generators or mains power supplies. These transfer other forms of energy, such as light energy or kinetic energy, into electrical energy. The unit of emf is also the volt (V).
>
> **Generator effect:** when a **potential difference** (voltage) is induced in a wire that experiences a change in magnetic field.

Electromagnetic induction can be demonstrated using the apparatus shown in Figures 14.10 and 14.11.

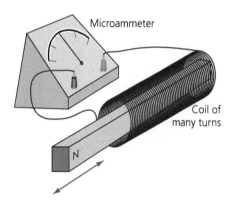

▲ Figure 14.10 Using a moving magnet to produce a potential difference

Figure 14.10 shows that if you move the bar magnet into the coil, you will see the needle on the micro **ammeter** flick in one direction and then in the opposite direction when the magnet is pulled out. The reading will be zero when the magnet is stationary. As the magnet moves, lines of magnetic flux are being crossed by the wires in the coil. Therefore, moving the magnet into the coil induces a potential difference. Providing the circuit is complete, this induces a current resulting in the reading on the microammeter. Moving the magnet back out causes the induced potential difference to change direction and therefore the current flow changes direction. The effect is the same if you move the coil and keep the magnet still.

Figure 14.11 shows that, as the length of wire moves between the two magnets, the micro ammeter will flick in one direction when the wire moves down and in the opposite direction when the wire moves up. In this case, a potential difference is induced in the wire because there is a moving electric charge (the electrons in the wire) **perpendicular** (at a 90-degree angle) to the magnetic field and they experience a force. This causes them to move towards one end of the wire, creating a potential difference across the wire.

The principle of electromagnetic induction is the basis of the **generator effect** and is used in dynamos and alternators to generate an electric current (Figure 14.12).

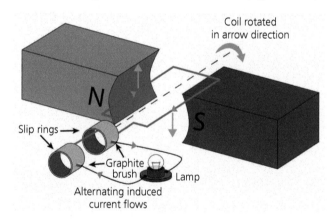

▲ Figure 14.12 A simple alternator

The motor effect

When a current passes through a wire placed in a magnetic field, it moves because a force acts on it. When a current passes through a wire, we know it induces a magnetic field. This results in the wire exerting a magnetic force onto the permanent magnet. When the current-carrying wire is placed in between the two poles of the magnet the magnetic fluxes combine to form what is known as a **catapult field**. This field exerts a force on the wire causing it to move. Figure 14.13 (a) shows the lines of magnetic flux between the poles of two magnets and Figure 14.13 (b) shows the lines of magnetic flux around the current-carrying wire.

(a)

(b)

= FORCE

(c)

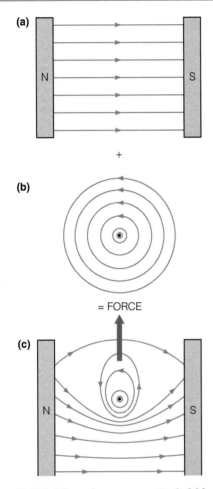

▲ Figure 14.13 (a) A uniform magnetic field between two poles of a magnet; (b) the field around a current-carrying wire; (c) the catapult field. The force is from the strong field (greater flux density) to the weak field (lower flux density)

You can use Fleming's left-hand rule (Figure 14.14) to work out the direction of the force on the wire.

Force, *F*

Magnetic fields, *B*

Current, *I*

Left hand

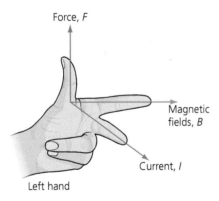

▲ Figure 14.14 Fleming's left-hand rule. Using your left hand, point your first finger in the direction of the field, your second finger in the direction of the current and your thumb will point in the direction of the force (motion)

As the name suggests, the **motor effect** is the basis of electric motors (Figure 14.15).

Force

Axis

+ve

−ve

Force

Split-ring commutator

Electrical contacts touching split ring

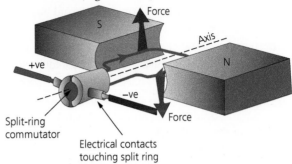

▲ Figure 14.15 A DC electric motor. The current flowing in the wires means they experience a force perpendicular to the magnetic field. The split-ring commutator reverses the current every half turn to ensure the motor keeps turning in the same direction

Key terms

Motor effect: when a current-carrying wire is placed between magnetic poles. The magnetic field around the wire interacts with the magnetic field it is placed in. This causes the wire and magnet to exert a force on each other and can cause the wire to move.

Reflect

Look at Figure 14.14 and use Fleming's left-hand rule to work out the direction of the magnetic field. Is that the direction you expect? It is always worth checking your answer!

Induction heating

Induction heating has many applications. Perhaps the most familiar is the 'induction hob' used to heat saucepans in domestic and commercial kitchens. An electronic oscillator passes a high-frequency alternating current through an electromagnet. This generates a rapidly alternating magnetic field. If a pan made of iron or steel is on the hob then currents, known as **eddy currents**, are generated inside the conductor (the pan). These currents generate heat which will then heat the contents of the pan.

Induction heating has the advantage that the heat is generated inside the object itself, so it is rapid. Also, it does not rely on conduction from an external heat source, such as a naked flame in a gas hob or a hot element in a traditional electric hob. This means that the hob becomes hot only because of being in contact with the hot pan and cools quickly once the pan is removed. It is therefore safer in many ways than using naked flame or a traditional electric hob, since heating does not occur without the conductor.

There are many other applications of induction heating, particularly in manufacturing, including:
▶ welding and brazing
▶ induction furnaces to produce molten metals
▶ cap sealing of containers in food and pharmaceutical industries
▶ heat treatment (e.g. hardening) of metals.

Research

There are many uses for permanent and temporary magnetic materials such as iron, steel, cobalt and nickel.

There are also many applications of electromagnets in electric and electromechanical devices:
▶ transformers
▶ motors, generators, alternators
▶ loudspeakers and microphones
▶ induction heating
▶ MRI machines
▶ cranes and sorting or separation equipment used in recycling
▶ relays.

Select a number of these applications and see if you can find others. For each, research the application and how our understanding of the topics covered in this section has allowed advances in technology. In particular, think about:
▶ the type of magnetic material used – permanent or temporary
▶ how the type of material relates to its function
▶ is this an example of the generator effect, motor effect or magnetic induction?
▶ for electromagnets:
  – does the material affect the properties of the electromagnet?
  – is the electromagnet tractive, portative or neither?

Test yourself

1 Explain the difference between a permanent magnet and an induced magnet.
2 What is the convention for drawing flux lines of a magnetic field?
3 How do flux lines indicate the strength of a magnetic field?
4 Describe how you would make an electromagnet.
5 Explain the difference between portative and tractive electromagnets.

Waves

We learn about waves from an early age – a toddler dropping a pebble into a still pond and watching the ripples is observing waves. Studying waves in water can help us understand a lot about how waves behave. However, watching waves crashing onto a shore, or even just watching the tide come in on the beach, can give us a misleading impression of what a wave is.

Key terms

Amplitude: the maximum displacement of any point from the equilibrium position (Figure 14.16).

Frequency: in Hz, the number of complete waves that pass a given point in one second (Figure 14.17). One complete wave is a **cycle**, so a frequency of 1 Hz corresponds to one cycle per second. This is a very low frequency, so you will often see frequency measured in kHz (kilohertz, 10^3 Hz), MHz (megahertz, 10^6 Hz) or GHz (gigahertz, 10^9 Hz).

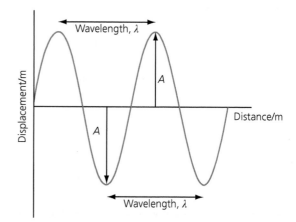

▲ Figure 14.16 Wave terminology. A represents the amplitude. This is an example of a transverse wave

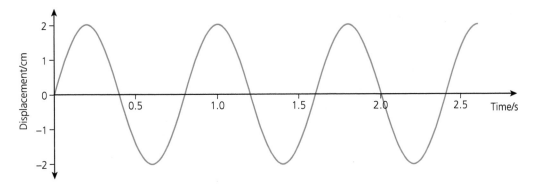

▲ Figure 14.17 If you measure from one peak to the next peak you can calculate that the **frequency** is 1.25 Hz. You will get the same answer if you measure from trough to trough

B1.53 The definition of a wave

Waves transfer **energy** from one energy store to another, they do not transfer **matter** (e.g. objects or water, for example). For example, electromagnetic waves transfer energy from the nuclear store of energy in the Sun to the thermal store of energy on Earth. This is why waves crashing onto the shore can be misleading. When waves travel through a medium (e.g. the ocean) the particles in the medium (i.e. water molecules) **oscillate** (move up and down). However, the particles stay in the same place, only the energy is transferred. When the wave hits the beach, things change, because now the particles of water are interacting with the particles of sand, and the wave is changed into a movement of the water – and anything floating in it, which is why things get washed up on the beach by the waves.

B1.54 The relationship between frequency, wavelength and speed using the wave equation $v = f\lambda$

The speed of a wave is a measure of how fast energy is transferred. More simply, it is the speed the wave is moving at. The relationship between wave speed, frequency and **wavelength** is the same for all types of wave and is given by the wave equation:

$$v = f\lambda$$

where:

v = wave speed in m/s

f = frequency in Hz

λ = wavelength in m.

For example, radio waves travel at the speed of light (approx. 3.0×10^8 m/s). A radio station transmits at a frequency of 92.3 MHz, calculate the wavelength of the radio waves.

92.3 MHz = 92.3×10^6 Hz = 9.23×10^7 Hz

Rearrange the equation above to give:

$$\lambda = \frac{v}{f}$$

So

$$\lambda = \frac{30 \times 10^8}{9.23^7} = 3.25 \, \text{m}$$

Key term

Wavelength: the distance between the same point in successive cycles. For example, the distance from the peak of one wave to the peak of the next wave (Figure 14.16). The standard unit of wavelength is the metre, m. However, **electromagnetic** waves can have wavelengths from 10^4 m to 10^{-15} m, so you will often see wavelengths expressed in units such as **nanometres**, nm. (1 nm = 1×10^{-9} m – see section B1.64, page 297 for more about units.)

B1.55 The properties of longitudinal and transverse waves

There are two types of wave, **transverse** and **longitudinal**.

Most waves are **transverse**, where the waves transfer energy in a direction at right angles to the direction in which the particles are vibrating. This means the oscillations are **perpendicular** (at right angles) to the direction of energy transfer (Figure 14.16). The particles move away from and towards the horizontal line – this is represented by the arrow 'A' (for amplitude) – so the energy transfer is in the forward direction even though the particles just move from side to side, or up and down, depending on how you look at the wave.

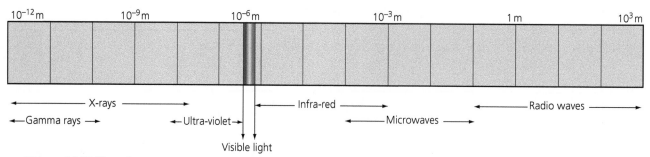

▲ Figure 14.18 The **electromagnetic spectrum**

> **Key terms**
>
> ***Electromagnetic waves:*** include gamma rays, X-rays, visible light, microwaves and radio waves. Their energy is carried by oscillating electric and magnetic fields.
>
> ***Electromagnetic spectrum:*** describes all the different types of electromagnetic waves. The properties of the different types of waves vary considerably, so we usually consider the spectrum as seven groups, with slight overlaps (Figure 14.18).

Examples of transverse waves include:
- all **electromagnetic waves**, e.g. light, radio waves, X-rays (Figure 14.18)
- ripples in a pond or waves in the ocean
- a wave on a string, e.g. a violin or guitar string that is made to vibrate when it is bowed or plucked.

Electromagnetic waves are a little more complicated because the wave represents changes in the electric and magnetic fields, but the principles are the same.

Longitudinal waves transfer energy in the same direction in which the particles are vibrating. This means that the oscillations are **parallel** to the direction of energy transfer. These oscillations create **compressions** (where the particles get closer together) and **rarefactions** (where the particles move further apart) (Figure 14.19).

Examples of longitudinal waves include:
- sound waves moving in air
- **ultrasound** (very high-frequency sound waves) that move through materials, for example:
  - metals, when used to detect cracks in components or structures
  - the body, when used in medical imaging such as scans in pregnancy
- **shock waves**, such as some types of **seismic** waves (produced by earthquakes).

> **Reflect**
>
> You can use a metal spring such as a Slinky to demonstrate both transverse and longitudinal waves (Figure 14.20).
> - If you lay the spring out on a surface, hold it at one end and wiggle it from side to side, you will see a transverse wave move along the length of the spring.
> - If you push the end of the spring quickly back and forward, you will see a longitudinal wave move along the length of the Slinky.
>
> Does a longitudinal wave in the Slinky explain why, when you speak, the sound waves travel through the air, but they do not create a vacuum in your mouth?

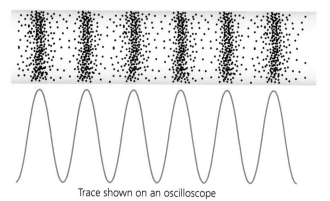

Trace shown on an oscilloscope

▲ Figure 14.19 Changes in air pressure at a microphone diaphragm, measured over a period of time

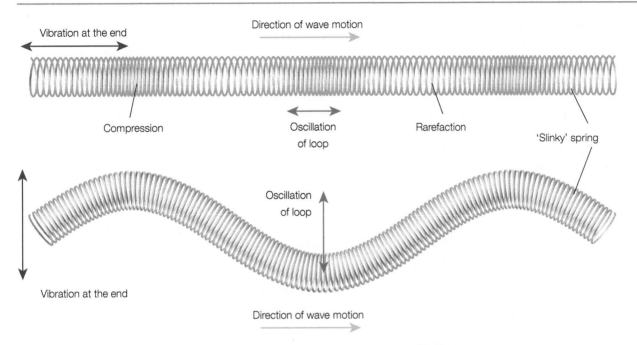

▲ Figure 14.20 Longitudinal (top) and transverse (bottom) waves in a Slinky spring

B1.56 The uses of different types of waves

Waves transfer energy, but they can also transfer information. The simplest example is signalling, using beacon fires to send warnings or flashlights to send signals using Morse code – light waves are being used to transfer information.

Communication

Radio waves are probably a better example of the use of waves in communication. Since the pioneering experiments of Marconi, we now use radio waves for many different types of communication. You can probably think of many more examples than these:

▶ TV and radio broadcasts (although not satellite TV – see below)

▶ wireless broadband (WiFi).

▶ Bluetooth® and other wireless technologies used in computing and control systems.

Microwaves have a slightly shorter wavelength/ higher frequency than radio waves but can also be used for short-range radio communication. A major use of microwaves now is in satellite communication, including satellite TV. This uses microwaves of a wavelength that is not absorbed by water molecules in the atmosphere.

Medical uses

There are numerous examples of the use of waves of different types in science and medicine:

▶ X-rays are used in different types of imaging from a simple X-ray taken to show a broken bone to the much more complex CT (computerised tomography or CAT) scan. A CT scan can build up a three-dimensional image of the whole body or part of the body.

▶ Gamma rays are used for cancer treatment, to kill cancer cells.

▶ Gamma rays can also be used to sterilise medical instruments and equipment.

▶ Ultrasound is used in scanning, particularly to create images of soft tissues that don't show up well on X-rays such as the heart, liver, kidneys, gallbladder and major blood vessels. This can be useful in diagnosis of some types of cancer.

▶ Ultrasound can also be used for cleaning. The high-frequency sound waves help to dislodge dirt from objects as diverse as jewellery, electronic components and medical equipment.

Food processing

We saw in section B1.52 how magnetic induction can be used for heating in both domestic and commercial food processing. Waves are also important in food processing:

▶ Infrared heating uses electromagnetic radiation with a longer wavelength than visible light:
  – Heat lamps to keep food hot before serving, for instance, in canteens.
  – Infrared ovens, particularly small ones, heat up more rapidly than conventional electric or gas ovens.
▶ Microwave heating can be used for cooking and reheating food. This uses microwaves of a different wavelength to satellite communication. In microwave heating, energy from the microwaves is absorbed by water molecules in the food. This transfers the energy to the water molecules, causing them to heat up. The energy is then transferred to the rest of the food by heating, which quickly cooks the food.
▶ Gamma radiation can be used in food preservation (see section B1.61).

Reflect

You are at a festival listening to a band and realise that the lead guitar produces high-frequency sounds, while the bass guitar produces low-frequency sounds. Also, you can tell that the drum kit is similar – the hi-hat cymbals produce high-frequency sounds and the bass drum produces low-frequency sounds. In spite of that, you hear all the different sounds at the right times – this band has rehearsed!

What does that tell you about the relationship between frequency and speed of sound?

Could you devise an experiment to test your hypothesis?

Test yourself

1 What is meant by the frequency of a wave?
2 What are the units of frequency used for waves?
3 A student was studying waves in a swimming pool of 25 m in length. They created a wave that had a frequency of 5 Hz and wavelength of 0.05 m. Calculate how long, in seconds, the wave would take to travel the length of the pool.
4 Give two examples of transverse waves and one example of longitudinal waves.
5 Give two examples of the use of microwaves.

Particles and radiation

This is an area where chemistry and physics overlap. You will have learnt about the structure of the atom in section B1.33 and about sub-atomic particles in section B1.35 in the chapter on chemistry. Knowledge of these sub-atomic particles helps us understand the basis of radiation and radioactive decay.

B1.57 The types and properties of ionising radiation

Key term

Ionising radiation: any form of radiation that interacts with matter, resulting in ionisation of that matter.

There are three types of **ionising radiation** that you need to know about: alpha (α), beta (β) and gamma (γ). The first two are types of particle, whereas gamma radiation is a form of electromagnetic radiation, mentioned in sections B1.55 and B1.56. It helps us understand the properties of these types of radiation if we understand their nature and origin.

Alpha radiation

Alpha particles are helium **nuclei** (plural of nucleus), meaning that they consist of two **protons** and two **neutrons** which give them a positive charge (+2). On the atomic scale, alpha particles are relatively large compared to beta particles (they have a relatively large mass). This means that they can easily remove electrons from atoms when they collide with them. This makes alpha radiation highly ionising.

However, because of their size, alpha particles do not penetrate materials very far – they are more likely to collide with atoms or nuclei of atoms. Alpha radiation can travel just 1–2 cm in air and can be absorbed by a sheet of paper.

Beta radiation

A beta particle is a fast-moving **electron**, therefore they have almost no mass (about 1800 times less than a proton) and a negative charge (−1). Beta particles are less ionising than alpha particles and can penetrate materials a moderate amount.

Beta radiation can travel approximately 15 cm in air and can be absorbed by a sheet of aluminium about 5 mm thick.

Gamma radiation

Unlike alpha and beta radiation, gamma radiation is a form of electromagnetic radiation – like X-rays or radio waves (see section B1.55). Gamma rays tend to pass through atoms rather than be absorbed by them. This makes them only weakly ionising, but with high penetrating power. Gamma rays have a range of many kilometres of air but can be absorbed by thick sheets of lead or several metres of concrete.

B1.58 The definitions of half-life and count-rate

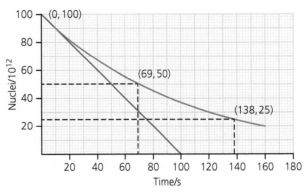

▲ Figure 14.21 A graph of radioactive decay showing how the number of nuclei decrease with time

> **Key terms**
>
> *Radioactive decay:* the random process that occurs when an unstable nucleus (see B1.34, page 266) loses energy by giving out **alpha** or **beta** particles or **gamma** radiation.
>
> *Ionisation:* the formation of charged particles from neutral molecules or atoms by adding or removing electrons.
>
> *Activity:* the rate at which a radioactive source decays. The unit of activity is the **becquerel** (Bq) where 1Bq = 1 decay per second. **Count-rate** is the number of radioactive decays recorded each second. You can see that activity and count-rate can be used interchangeably.
>
> *Half-life:* the time taken for half the unstable nuclei in a sample to decay.

Radioactive decay is detected and measured by using a **Geiger-Muller tube** and counter – usually referred to as a **GM tube** or **Geiger counter**. This measures the radiation such as alpha particles, beta particles or gamma rays that are emitted when a radioactive source decays.

The rate at which a radioactive source decays can be plotted in a graph of activity against time or number of nuclei against time (Figure 14.21).

There is a lot of useful information in Figure 14.21. First, we can see that the rate of radioactive decay (the **activity**) decreases with time. The tangent (blue line) is drawn at time = 0. If we measure the slope, we can calculate the rate of decay. Try drawing tangents at other times, such as 60 s and 120 s. You will see that the slope of the line is a maximum at time = 0 and then decreases. This shows that the rate of decay is decreasing. This is called an **exponential decay**.

Look at how the number of nuclei change with time. We start with 100×10^{12} nuclei but after 69 s there are 50×10^{12} nuclei remaining – the number has reduced by half. After another 69 s (at 138 s) the number has reduced by half again to 25×10^{12} nuclei. This is characteristic of exponential decay: the time it takes for the number of nuclei to halve is constant. We call this the **half-life**, sometimes written as $T_{1/2}$.

We can make the same calculation from a graph where the y-axis (vertical axis) is **activity** rather than number of nuclei.

B1.59 The main types of radioactive decay in relation to unstable nuclei

There are two important facts about radioactive decay that you need to know:
1. Radioactive decay is **spontaneous**. Radioactive nuclei are **unstable**, which is why they decay. However, there is nothing that triggers decay.
2. Radioactive decay is **random**. We cannot predict which nucleus in a radioactive source will decay nor can we predict when it will decay.

As we saw in section B1.58, we can measure the half-life of a radioactive source and then use this to make predictions about the behaviour of the radioactive source, even though the decay is a random process.

Alpha decay

We saw in section B1.57 that an alpha particle consists of two neutrons and two protons and is equivalent to a helium nucleus. It is represented by the symbol $_{2}^{4}$He in nuclear equations. The top number represents the mass number – the sum of the protons and the neutrons. The bottom number represents the atomic number (see section B1.34), i.e. the number of protons. You generally will not see atomic and mass numbers featured in chemical equations as they do not change in a chemical reaction. However, because nuclear equations can involve transformation of one element into another, it is useful to include these to show the changes that have taken place.

An alpha particle is formed when an unstable nucleus loses two neutrons and two protons and becomes more stable in the process. An example is the decay of uranium-238 into thorium-234, represented by the nuclear equation:

$$_{92}^{238}\text{U} \rightarrow {}_{90}^{234}\text{Th} + {}_{2}^{4}\text{He}$$

In this case, the uranium-238 has lost 2 neutrons and 2 protons, so the atomic number (number of protons) decreases by 2, forming thorium and the mass number decreases by 4, so the isotope of thorium is thorium-234. We can see that the mass and atomic numbers all balance, because the alpha particle (helium nucleus) has 2 protons and 2 neutrons, giving it an atomic number of 2 and a mass number of 4.

Beta decay

A beta particle is a high-speed electron. It is represented in nuclear equations by the symbol $_{-1}^{0}$e. This electron is formed and then ejected at high speed from the nucleus when a neutron turns into a proton. This means that the number of protons increases by 1, therefore the atomic number increases by 1 although the mass of the nucleus remains the same. An example is the decay of carbon-14 into nitrogen-14, represented by the nuclear equation:

$$_{6}^{14}\text{C} \rightarrow {}_{7}^{14}\text{N} + {}_{-1}^{0}\text{e}$$

Note that in both alpha and beta decay, a new element will be formed as the nucleus produced will always have a different number of protons. The atomic number determines which element it is, so this means the atomic number changes and therefore the element changes.

Gamma radiation

Gamma radiation is a form of electromagnetic radiation from the nucleus produced when excess energy is lost from the nucleus. When a nucleus decays by alpha, beta or other types of emission, the protons and neutrons in the nucleus are often left in an excited state. The protons and neutrons then return to a lower energy level and the difference in energy is emitted as gamma radiation. Unlike alpha and beta decay, there is no change to the atomic structure and so no new elements are formed.

Health and safety

Some radioactive sources have a short half-life and others have a long half-life. A source with a short half-life will usually decay rapidly – i.e. the nuclei will be very unstable and the source will have a high activity. This means it will emit a high level of radioactivity, which could be dangerous. However, it will become safe relatively quickly as the unstable nuclei decay quickly.

A long half-life means that the source will have a low activity and will emit a relatively low level of radioactivity. However, it could still be dangerous because it will go on emitting radiation for a long time – even for millions of years.

We also need to consider the type of radiation emitted. For example, an alpha source is the most dangerous via contamination; an alpha source absorbed into the body will do damage to any tissues it is in contact with. On the other hand, a beta source is more dangerous by irradiation as beta particles are more penetrating.

B1.60 How radiation interacts with matter

Radiation interacts with matter in two ways: **ionisation** and **excitation**.

Ionisation

Ionisation occurs when electrons are removed from atoms or molecules to produce positive ions. All forms of radioactive decay produce radiation that can cause ionisation – hence the term **ionising radiation**.

We saw in section B1.57 that alpha radiation is the mostly highly ionising while gamma radiation is the least ionising. Beta radiation is in between the two in its ability to cause ionisation.

Excitation

Excitation occurs when radiation transfers energy to atoms or molecules. Excitation involves moving an electron to a higher energy level (**shell** or **orbital**). If enough energy is transferred to the electron, it will be removed from the atom and ionisation will have occurred. Gamma radiation can cause excitation. In fact, other types of electromagnetic radiation such as X-rays and visible light can cause excitation of electrons. This is why some types of ultraviolet (UV) light can cause sunburn or, in the worst cases, skin cancer. The UV light causes excitation of electrons in the DNA molecules found in skin cells, leading to ionisation which can result in cancer-causing mutations.

B1.61 The applications of radioactivity within the health and science sector

Health and safety

Before we look at applications of radioactivity, it is worth considering the biological effects of radiation – how radiation interacts with biological materials, including the human body.

The human body is made up of many complex molecules. Removal or addition of an electron changes a molecule chemically – this means that it may behave differently in any interaction with other molecules. As you have learned from Biology, interaction between molecules is central to how the body works.

UV light has sufficient energy to ionise biological molecules. Alpha, beta and gamma radiation all have energy millions of times greater than that of UV light. This means that these types of ionising radiation can be highly dangerous because they can change the chemistry of the body. The function of enzymes can be changed, cells can be damaged and the DNA in cells can be damaged, which can lead to cancer.

Case study

Because radiation can be so damaging, we must exercise great care when handling radioactive sources.

Hasini is working as a technician in a college science laboratory. She is responsible for the safe storage and demonstration of radioactive sources.

Hasini decides that, for each source, she must consider the following:
▶ the activity of the source
▶ the type of radiation (see section B1.57).

Based on these two considerations, Hasini can decide what protection is required.
▶ Alpha radiation is highly damaging but has low penetration, so can be relatively easily screened. This makes it relatively harmless outside the body, but if a source emitting alpha radiation enters the body, it can be highly damaging.
▶ Beta and gamma radiation are less ionising, but they have much greater penetration and may require screening with thick sheets of lead.

The table shows the radioactive sources kept in the college laboratory. For each source, the type of radiation emitted is shown.

Source	Radiation emitted
cobalt-60	pure gamma
strontium-90	pure beta
americium-241	alpha and some gamma

There are strict regulations covering working with radioactive sources, including those described in Chapter A3 (page 48).
▶ What precautions should Hasini use for storing each source?
▶ What precautions should she take when using each source?

Radioactive tracers

A major use of radioactive tracers is in medical diagnosis (next section).

In industry, radioactive tracers can be used to detect the presence of materials such as dust, cellulose fibres, glass fragments or organic materials as these all adsorb radioactive tracers from solution.

Another use of radioactive tracers is in monitoring hydraulic fracturing ('fracking') used to extract oil and gas from rocks.

Medical diagnostic applications

Radioactive isotopes (radioisotopes) can be injected or swallowed and their course around the body followed using an external detector. One example is iodine-123. This is taken up by the thyroid gland, just like the non-radioactive isotope (iodine-127). The radiation given out can be detected and used to show whether the thyroid gland is absorbing iodine correctly.

Radioactive tracers are usually gamma emitters as these are weakly ionising but highly penetrating. This means that they are less likely to cause damage to the body but can be easily detected from outside the body. Radioisotopes used as tracers also need to have short half-lives so that their activity disappears soon after the procedure is completed.

Computerised tomography uses X-rays to build up a three-dimensional image of the body – known as a CT scan. More recently, gamma radiation detectors have been used to detect gamma emission of a radioactive tracer from many angles. A computer can then build up an image from the points of emission. This technique, known as **single photon emission computerised tomography (SPECT)** is now the main scanning technology used to diagnose a range of medical conditions.

Iodine-123 is an example of a **diagnostic radiopharmaceutical**. Various radioisotopes can be attached to biologically active substances, such as amino acids, hormones, therapeutic drugs, etc. These can be used together with SPECT to examine a wide range of processes:

▶ blood flow to the brain
▶ functioning of the liver, lungs, heart or kidneys
▶ assess bone growth.

Food preservation

Sufficiently high doses of radiation will kill micro-organisms in food. Some of these may be harmful (**pathogens**), so irradiation can kill the organisms that cause food poisoning, for example.

Other micro-organisms cause food to 'go off' – these are known as **spoilage** micro-organisms. Because irradiation will kill these spoilage micro-organisms as well, it can help to preserve food or extend the shelf-life of fresh or prepared foods.

Key term

Isotopes: atoms of the same element (they have the same number of protons) but with different number of neutrons.

Radioisotopes: unstable isotopes that undergo radioactive decay emitting radioactivity as they do so.

Radiopharmaceuticals: therapeutic drugs (medicines) that incorporate radioisotopes. Some radiopharmaceuticals are used to treat disease whereas **diagnostic radiopharmaceuticals** are used to help in diagnosis of disease.

Irradiation: the process of exposing an object to radiation. It does not make the object radioactive.

Research

The Food Standards Agency is responsible for ensuring the safety of the food that we buy and eat. Its website has a lot of information about the use of irradiation to preserve food.

Visit the website: www.food.gov.uk

Search for 'irradiated food', then research the following:
▶ Is irradiated food safe to consume?
▶ How does irradiation change food?
▶ What types of food can be irradiated and sold?
▶ How can you tell that a food has been irradiated?

Dating deceased organisms

Radiocarbon dating measures the age of any object that contains organic material. This includes dead organisms as well as anything made from dead organisms – such as a wooden table or pair of leather shoes.

Carbon-14 (^{14}C) is the radioactive isotope of carbon. The isotope is constantly made in the atmosphere from nitrogen using energy absorbed from **cosmic radiation**. This is the reverse of the reaction shown in section B1.59 illustrating beta-decay.

The carbon-14 then combines with atmospheric oxygen to produce carbon dioxide. This is taken up by plants and used in **photosynthesis** to produce sugars and other organic compounds. Plants are eaten by animals and so the carbon-14-containing organic compounds are incorporated into animal tissues as well. Both plants and animals respire and emit carbon dioxide. This means that the level of carbon-14 remains constant while the organism is alive.

Once the organism dies, it no longer exchanges carbon-14 with the environment and the carbon-14 undergoes radioactive decay. We can calculate how long ago the organism died by measuring the proportion of carbon-14 in a sample of bone, skin, fur, wood, etc.

The half-life of carbon-14 is about 5730 years. That means we can only date samples from organisms that died less than about 50 000 years ago. After that long, there will not be enough carbon-14 left to measure accurately.

Key terms

Radiocarbon dating: the process that uses a radioactive isotope of carbon, **carbon-14**, to determine the age of an object containing organic material.

Cosmic radiation: (also called cosmic rays) originates from the sun as well as from outside the solar system. It is a mixture of high energy protons (hydrogen nuclei), alpha particles (helium nuclei) and beta particles (electrons).

Photosynthesis: the process that plants use to make complex organic compounds such as sugars from carbon dioxide and water using light energy.

Test yourself

1   Explain how gamma radiation is different to alpha or beta radiation.
2   Nobelium-254, $^{254}_{102}$ No, undergoes radioactive alpha decay to form an isotope of the element fermium, Fm.
    a   What is meant by isotopes of an element?
    b   Write a balanced equation to show the radioactive (alpha) decay of nobelium-254.
3   A radioactive source had an activity of 500 000 Bq and a half-life of 2.5 years. Calculate the activity remaining after 10 years.
4   The only foods that can be legally irradiated for sale in the UK are dried herbs and spices. Explain what type of radiation would be most appropriate for irradiation of herbs and spices.

Units

You will have encountered units already in this chapter – for length (e.g. wavelength) as well as various electrical measurements (charge, current, voltage). There have been many different types of unit used over the years. The **imperial** system uses fluid ounces, pints and gallons for volume and feet, inches and miles for distance. The **metric** system uses millilitres and litres for volume and millimetres, metres and kilometres for distance. Getting measurements from these two systems mixed up can be confusing or worse. In 1999, NASA lost the $125 million Mars orbiter because of confusion between imperial and metric units.

B1.62 The use of the international system of units (SI)

The international system of units is known as SI, from the French *Système international*. It is a modern form of the metric system but extends to units used for all kinds of measurement, particularly in science and engineering.

The metric system originally used **standards** for several units, such as the standard **kilogram** and standard **metre**, both of which were made of platinum–iridium alloy and kept in Paris. These are no longer sufficiently accurate for modern measurements and have been replaced by definitions based on **defining constants**, such as the speed of light, the Planck constant and the Avogadro constant.

There are seven SI base units, as shown in the table.

Unit name	Unit symbol	Quantity name
ampere	A	electric current
candela	cd	luminous intensity
kelvin	K	temperature
kilogram	kg	mass
metre	m	length
mole	mol	amount of substance
second	s	time

There are many other SI units that are derived from these base units. Some that you may have come across include:

- hertz (Hz) for frequency
- volt (v) for electrical potential difference
- coulomb (C) for electric charge
- joule (J) for energy, work or heat
- watt (W) for power.

B1.63 How to convert between units

The metre and kilogram are both SI base units. That does not make them useful for measuring very short lengths or small masses. If you look at a ruler, the smallest division is usually the **millimetre** (mm). Paracetamol tablets are usually 500 **milligrams** (mg). The **prefix** 'milli' represents one thousandth, so we can work out the following conversions:

Length – metres (m) and millimetres (mm)

$1\,m = 1000\,mm$ or $10^3\,mm$

$1\,mm = 0.001\,m$ or $10^{-3}\,m$

Mass – grams (g) and milligrams (mg)

$1\,g = 1000\,mg$ or $10^3\,mg$

$1\,mg = 0.001\,g$ or $10^{-3}\,g$

Prefixes

You can see that millimetres use the prefix 'milli' to represent one thousandth. There are other prefixes used in SI units, as shown in the table.

Prefix name	Prefix symbol	Base 10
Tera	T	10^{12}
Giga	G	10^9
Mega	M	10^6
Kilo	K	10^3
Hecto	H	10^2
Deca	Da	10^1
Deci	d	10^{-1}
Centi	c	10^{-2}
Milli	m	10^{-3}
Micro	μ	10^{-6}
Nano	n	10^{-9}
Pico	p	10^{-12}

Many of these prefixes will be familiar, although not all of these examples are SI units:

- centimetre (cm) is common in everyday measurement
- micrometre (μm) is common in microscopy
- nanometre (nm) is commonly used to measure wavelength of visible light
- megabytes (MB), gigabytes (GB) and terabytes (TB) are used in computing for capacity of hard drives, memory modules and data transmission speeds. Unfortunately, these can be misleading because they can be calculated in **binary** as well as in **decimal**. This is the reason that a 400 GB hard drive (decimal) is shown by Microsoft Windows as only 372 GB (binary).

Notice that the base unit of mass is the kilogram, which is named as if the base unit is the gram.

Volume

The SI unit of volume is the cubic metre (m^3). This is too large to be useful in many situations – particularly in biology, chemistry and everyday life – it is much easier to ask for 1 litre of orange juice than asking for '$0.001\,m^3$ please'.

In chemistry, the most common units of volume are the litre (*l*) and millilitre (ml):

$1\,l = 1000\,ml$

$1\,ml = 10^{-3}\,l$

Using 'l' as the abbreviation for litre can be confusing – it can look like the number 1. That is why it has been printed in italics here. In the United States you will often see 'L' used as the abbreviation for litre or mL for millilitre.

B1.64 The importance of using significant figures and science notation

Powers of 10

You will have encountered several numbers in this chapter and elsewhere using powers of 10. This is very convenient in science (see **Standard form** below) because it allows us to write very large or very small numbers more easily. There is another advantage: when we multiply two numbers shown as powers of 10 we **add** the powers. This is illustrated in the following example:

$$100 \times 1000 = 100\,000$$

Using powers of 10, 100 becomes 10^2 and 1000 becomes 10^3. This means that we can rewrite the calculation as follows:

$$10^2 \times 10^3 = 10^5$$

Notice that when we multiply the numbers shown as powers of 10, we simply add the powers to get the answer. This makes life so much easier!

If you look at the table of prefixes in section B1.63 you will see a range of values from 10^{-12} (pico) all the way up to 10^{12} (tera). These are examples of scientific notation where we use powers of 10 rather than writing the number out in full. For example:

1 million can be written as $1\,000\,000$ or 10^6

$1\,nm$ is equal to $0.000\,000\,001\,m$ or $10^{-9}\,m$

It is not difficult to see that using powers of 10 makes it much easier to write (and understand) very large or very small numbers.

Standard form

When we use scientific notation, using powers of 10, we follow a convention known as **standard form**. A number in standard form has two parts. For example, $2\,650\,000$ would be written as:

$$2.65 \times 10^6$$

The first part is a number between 1 and 10. The second part is a power of 10. So we should not write that number as 26.5×10^5.

By using numbers in standard form, calculations become less cumbersome. Also, with a little practice, it is easier to write down and understand very large or very small numbers using standard form.

Significant figures

Because there is **uncertainty** in any measurement, we must take care not to imply a greater accuracy than is possible. In the case of the measurement of the line (75.405 mm), we would probably round it down to 75.4 mm, but is that the **true value**? We cannot estimate 0.4 of the smallest division.

Therefore, we use **significant figures**. These are the digits in a number that we believe are reliable. In the example, the first two digits (7 and 5) are reliable, but the third digit, after the decimal point, is not. We can be confident that the **true value** is closer to 75 mm than to 76 mm.

This value of 75 mm is quoted to two **significant figures**, the number of digits that we believe are reliable.

If the smallest division on the ruler was only 10 mm, we would have to give a value of 70 mm – this is **one** significant figure.

Here are some more examples of a different measurement (1257.59) to various numbers of significant figures.

Number	Significant figures
1257.59	6
1258	4
1300	2
1000	1

From this example, you can see that **trailing zeros** do not count as significant figures – we call them **placeholders** as they stand for the 1s and 10s.

Similarly, **leading zeros** (usually after the decimal point) do not count towards the number of significant figures – so 0.075 m has two significant figures. We could write it as 75 mm and it would be the same length with the same uncertainty.

Trailing zeros in a **decimal** do count as significant figures. So, a concentration of 0.0500 mol/dm^3 is to **three** significant figures.

One important feature of significant figures is that they help us to reduce the chances of data errors:

▶ making sure data is not recorded to more digits than the measurement allows (e.g. ruler, balance, burette)

▶ in calculations, ensuring that we report the same number of digits as the original measurements allow.

As a rule in **calculations**, we look at the number of significant figures in the items of data. A calculator may give an answer to 10 digits, but using all of them would give **spurious** digits – they would not all be reliable. We should not report the answer to more significant figures than are in the item of data with the **lowest** number of significant figures.

In a titration (see section B1.44) we might have a standard solution that is 0.0500 mol/dm^3 (three significant figures) and a titre of 24.5 cm^3 (three significant figures). This means that we can calculate the number of mol:

mol = concentration × volume

mol = 0.0500 × 0.0245 = 1.225 × 10^{-3} or 0.001225 mol

However, we should only report this answer to three significant figures, or 1.23 × 10^{-3} mol.

There are some exceptions to this rule. For example, if we have a set of data and calculate a mean, it can be acceptable to quote the mean to one more significant figure than the values in the data. This is justified because calculating a mean allows us to get closer to the **true value** than any individual data point would be.

Test yourself

1 Give the SI unit for the following measurements:
   a mass
   b length
   c temperature.

2 Which of the following is not an SI unit?
   a candlepower
   b coulomb
   c joule
   d watt.

3 Complete the following table of conversions.

Convert from	Convert to	Answer
1250 mm	m	
0.0005 kg	g	
1250 000 J	kJ	
0.005 W	mW	
2.5 MHz	Hz	

4 Convert the following to numbers in standard form to three significant figures:
   a 1256 000
   b 0.000 000 135 023

Project practice

You are working for a company that provides components for use in lateral flow diagnostic test kits, like those used for COVID-19 testing in schools. The kits include swabs used to collect a sample from the nose and throat. These are currently sterilised with ethylene oxide gas. People have been concerned that ethylene oxide is dangerous and that children should not be exposed to the risk.

Exposure to ethylene oxide in large quantities can have serious health consequences. However, you know that there is no ethylene oxide remaining on the swabs after sterilisation and ethylene oxide has been used safely for decades to sterilise medical equipment and devices, including swabs and dressings. There has never been any evidence of harm caused to patients or users.

You have been asked to investigate other sterilisation methods and prepare a report with recommendations for alternatives to ethylene oxide.

You will need to carry out the following:

1 Research the options:
   a Carry out a literature review of sterilisation methods.
   b Investigate sources of safety information.

2 Prepare a plan:
   a Make a shortlist of possible methods.
   b Justify your choice of methods.
   c Prepare risk assessments of the different methods.

3 Analyse the data in comparison with the current method (ethylene oxide) and reach conclusions:
   a comparison of effectiveness of different methods
   b relative costs, including any specialist equipment needed and consumable items, e.g. chemicals
   c possible damage to components caused by the different methods
   d risk factors associated with the different methods, either to people carrying out the tests or to end users/patients.

4 Present your analysis and conclusions in the form of a PowerPoint presentation.

5 Group discussion covering:
   a the relative effectiveness and safety of the different methods
   b would they be more or less effective than the existing method
   c the perception of risk by members of the general public.

6 Write a reflective evaluation of your work.

Assessment practice

1 Karen has an iPhone XR. She has found out that it has a battery with a capacity of approximately 2900 mAh. A charge of 1 mAh is transferred when a current of 1 mA flows for 1 hour.
   a Calculate the total electric charge, in coulombs, in the iPhone XR battery.
   b Karen sees that the charger supplied with the iPhone XR is marked '5 V, 1000 mA'. She also has a charger for an iPad mini that is marked '5 V, 2100 mA'. Karen believes that the iPad charger will charge the iPhone more quickly. Is Karen correct? Calculate the time taken to charge the iPhone using each type of charger. Give your answers in hours, minutes and seconds.

2 The figure shows a circuit with a 9.0 V battery and three resistors.

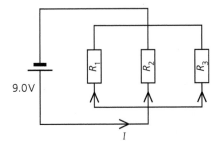

   a Is this an example of a series or parallel circuit?
   b The resistors are marked as follows: R1 = 10 Ω, R2 = 22 Ω, R3 = 47 Ω. Calculate the total resistance in the circuit. Give your answer to an appropriate number of significant figures.
   c Based on your answer to part b, calculate the current flowing from the battery. Give your answer to an appropriate number of significant figures.

3 Describe **two** ways you could use to make a piece of iron magnetic.

4 Electromagnets are used in the recycling industry.

  a What type of electromagnet would be found in a crane used for lifting scrap iron in a scrapyard?

  b Explain how electromagnets can be used to separate scrap iron from scrap copper.

  c A strong magnet will not attract aluminium. However, if a mixture of scrap aluminium and scrap plastic moves along a conveyor belt, eddy currents are created in the aluminium. These eddy currents cause the aluminium to be attracted to the magnet so it can be separated from the plastic. Explain how a current is formed in the aluminium.

5 Which of the following statements about waves is true?

  a Gamma radiation is a type of transverse wave.

  b Light waves transfer energy but sound waves transfer matter.

  c The displacement of particles in a longitudinal wave is perpendicular to the direction of travel.

  d The displacement of particles in a transverse wave is parallel to the direction of travel.

6 Make sketch graphs of transverse waves travelling along a Slinky. The y-axis should show the transverse displacement of the waves and the x-axis should show the distance along the Slinky.

  a Two waves with the same frequency but one wave has double the amplitude of the other.

  b Two waves with the same amplitude. One wave has double the frequency of the other wave.

7 Two radioactive sources were contained in glass bottles stored inside lead-lined containers. Both sources had approximately the same activity marked on the container. The bottles were removed from their containers and the following measurements taken using a Geiger counter:

  – Source A gave a very low reading.

  – Source B gave a very high reading.

  – When a sheet of aluminium was placed between source B and the Geiger counter, the reading fell by 75 per cent.

  – When a sheet of lead was placed between source B and the Geiger counter, the reading fell by 95 per cent.

Explain what type of radiation was emitted by each source. Justify your answer.

8 It is a Friday afternoon and there has been a spillage of a gamma-emitting radioactive material on the workbench in your lab. Examination of the data sheet for the material shows that it has a half-life of four hours. A radiation monitor shows that the level of radiation is ten times higher than the safe level. You have two options:

  – decontaminate the workbench immediately, or

  – seal the lab for the weekend and resume work on Monday.

Evaluate which option would be better. Your response should consider:

  – the concept of half-life

  – discussion of the two options

  – reasoned judgements and/or conclusions.

9 You are investigating sound waves moving in air or in water.

  a In air, the wavelength of the sound is 250 cm and its frequency is 131 Hz. Calculate the speed of the wave. Give your answer in the correct SI units to an appropriate number of significant figures.

  b Sound from the same source travels in water at 1480 m/s but the frequency remains the same. Calculate the new wavelength to the appropriate number of significant figures.

10 You have been asked to produce a wallchart showing the electromagnetic spectrum. You have been given the following table of values for the wavelength of the different types of electromagnetic radiation. Convert these values to metres (m) expressed in standard form so that they can be plotted more easily on the wallchart.

Type of radiation	Wavelength	Wavelength in standard form (m)
Gamma rays	1 pm to 10 pm	
X-rays	5 pm to 10 nm	
Ultra-violet	5 nm to 380 nm	
Visible light	380 nm to 750 nm	
Infra-red	750 nm to 1 mm	
Microwaves	0.1 mm to 10 cm	
Radio waves	10 cm to 2000 m	

B2: Further science concepts

Introduction

This chapter will build on the basic science concepts in biology that were discussed in B1: Core science concepts: Biology. We will explore human physiology – the study of the normal functioning of the body and its component systems – as well as how this relates to diseases and disorders that you are likely to encounter in your work.

Learning outcomes

The core knowledge outcomes that you must understand and learn:

B2.1 the components of the endocrine system; where they are located, their function and structure including how they are organised

B2.2 the components of the respiratory system; where they are located, their function and structure including how they are organised

B2.3 the components of the nervous system; where they are located, their function and structure including how they are organised

B2.4 the components of the musculoskeletal system; where they are located, their function and structure including how they are organised

B2.5 the components of the digestive system; where they are located, their function and structure including how they are organised

B2.6 the components of the cardiovascular system; where they are located, their function and structure including how they are organised

B2.7 the components of the reproductive system in males and females; where they are located, their function and structure including how they are organised

B2.8 the components of the renal system; where they are located, their function and structure including how they are organised

B2.9 the components of the integumentary system; where they are located, their function and structure including how they are organised

B2.10 the normal expected ranges for physiological measurements, how to identify when physiological measurements fall outside the normal expected ranges in adults, including factors that can contribute to measurement outside of usual parameters

B2.11 how physiological parameters are routinely measured including the equipment used

B2.12 the principles of homeostasis and how this links to maintaining the functions within the physiological systems which contribute to preserving a healthy body

B2.13 how failure of homeostasis mechanisms can impact the body and the subsequent development of disorders

B2.14 different classification systems and their purpose

B2.15 the most widely used classification systems of diseases and disorders

B2.16 examples of diseases and disorders and their relationship to the classification systems including the possible causes and symptoms

B2.17 injury and trauma and how the body reacts systematically as a response

B2.18 what is meant by epidemiology and some specific terminology that is used

B2.19 how epidemiology is used to provide information to plan and evaluate strategies to prevent disease

B2.20 how health promotion helps to prevent the spread and control of disease and disorder.

B2.1 The endocrine system

The **endocrine system** involves a series of **endocrine glands** (Figure 15.1) that secrete **hormones** into the blood. These act as chemical messengers because they are transported around the body in the blood and act on specific target cells or organs.

The endocrine system is involved in:
- regulation of growth and development
- regulation of the reproductive system
- **homeostasis** – the regulation of the internal environment of the body.

The reproductive system will be covered in more detail in section B2.7 and homeostasis in section B2.12.

There are two types of hormones, based on their chemical structure:
- **Steroid hormones** are based on cholesterol and include:
  - the sex hormones that regulate the reproductive system
  - the corticosteroid hormones that help regulate carbohydrate metabolism and mineral ions.
- Other hormones are amino acid derivatives, peptides or proteins.

Key terms

Endocrine system: a system of hormones that control many aspects of physiology (the normal functioning of the body).

Endocrine: glands **secrete** (release) their products directly into the blood. Examples are the alpha (α) and beta (β) cells in the pancreas that secrete the hormones glucagon and insulin respectively.

Gland: a group of cells that make chemicals such as hormones or enzymes.

Hormone: a chemical messenger released into the blood by an endocrine gland that acts on target tissues elsewhere in the body.

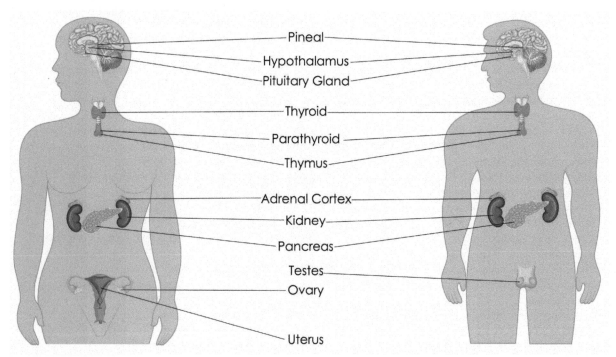

- Pineal
- Hypothalamus
- Pituitary Gland
- Thyroid
- Parathyroid
- Thymus
- Adrenal Cortex
- Kidney
- Pancreas
- Testes
- Ovary
- Uterus

▲ Figure 15.1 The human endocrine system showing the endocrine glands in females (left) and males (right)

Components and organisation of the endocrine system

Hypothalamus

The hypothalamus is located in the brain and is responsible for control of body temperature, water balance (**osmoregulation**) and secretion of hormones via the **pituitary gland**. The hypothalamus is responsible for control of most of the **homeostatic mechanisms** that regulate the internal environment of the body – with the exception of control of blood glucose concentration – either directly or by controlling other endocrine glands, such as the **thyroid** gland.

Pituitary

The pituitary is divided into **anterior** and **posterior** parts or lobes. Hormones produced in the hypothalamus are stored in the posterior lobe before secretion. The hypothalamus also produces releasing factors that stimulate the anterior lobe to secrete various hormones.

Thyroid and parathyroid

The thyroid is responsible for the regulation of **metabolic rate**. **Metabolism** is the term that describes all the chemical reactions that take place in the body. Metabolic rate is the rate at which the energy stored in our food is transferred by all the **metabolic reactions** that take place in the body. The thyroid is controlled by the releasing factor **TRH**, secreted by the hypothalamus.

The parathyroid works with the thyroid to control the levels of calcium in the body. **Parathyroid hormone (PTH)** is secreted by the parathyroid and increases the concentration of Ca^{2+} ions in the blood while **calcitonin**, secreted by the thyroid, reduces the concentration of Ca^{2+} ions in the blood.

Adrenals

The adrenals, located next to the kidney, have two parts:
▶ The adrenal **medulla** is the central part of the gland and produces the hormone **adrenalin** that prepares the body to respond to threat or danger – known as the 'fight or flight' response.

▶ The **adrenal cortex** produces several steroid hormones involved in regulation of different aspects of metabolism including carbohydrates and mineral ions. The general name for these hormones is **corticosteroids**. There are two classes of corticosteroids:
  – **glucocorticoids** (e.g. **cortisol**) help regulate carbohydrate metabolism
  – **mineralocorticoids** help regulate the balance of mineral ions such as Na^+ and K^+.

Ovaries

As well as their function in releasing egg cells (see section B2.7), the ovaries produce the female sex hormones, including **oestrogen** and progesterone, which are involved in the regulation of the **menstrual cycle**.

Testes

Like the ovaries, the testes have a dual function: production of **sperm cells** (see section B2.7) and secretion of the male **sex hormones** such as **testosterone**.

Pancreas

The pancreas has an important **exocrine** function producing digestive enzymes. The endocrine function of the pancreas is carried out by the **islets of Langerhans** which produce the hormones **insulin** and **glucagon**. These are the hormones responsible for the regulation of blood glucose concentration.

> **Key terms**
>
> **Exocrine:** glands release (secrete) their products into **ducts** or onto the body surface.
>
> **Ducts:** tubes that lead from an exocrine gland to the place where the products are used or needed. Examples include tear ducts in the eye, or salivary and pancreatic ducts in the digestive system (see section B2.5).

Functions of the endocrine system

To understand the way the endocrine system works we need to understand the relationship between the endocrine glands that produce hormones (chemical messengers) and the target cells or organs that respond to those hormones.

The production and activity of specific hormones

Hormone	Secreted by	Acts on
Thyroxine	Thyroid	Most body cells, to regulate metabolic rate.
Cortisol	Adrenal cortex	**Cortisol** is produced in the adrenal cortex in response to stress. Cortisol acts on liver and muscle cells and increases the blood glucose concentration.
Oestrogens	Ovaries	Pituitary and uterus. Oestrogen is involved in regulation of the menstrual cycle.
Testosterone	Testes	Muscle and bone cells. The **anabolic** action of testosterone increases muscle mass and bone density. Sex organs. The **androgenic** action of testosterone stimulates the development of the male sex organs and secondary sexual characteristics, such as facial hair. Testosterone is also required for production of sperm cells.
Gastrin	Stomach	Stomach. Gastrin has several actions in digestion involving the stomach and small intestine.
Growth hormone (GH)	Pituitary	Most body cells respond to GH, which is responsible for normal growth during infancy and childhood.
Follicle stimulating hormone (FSH)	Pituitary	Ovaries. FSH stimulates the growth and development of the egg follicle during the first half of the menstrual cycle. Egg follicles are located in the ovaries and contain the developing egg cell.

Practice point

The term **cortisone** is often misused to describe either any corticosteroid or specifically **hydrocortisone**, which is the name given to cortisol when it is used as a medication.

Try to always use the correct terminology.

The specificity of hormones in relation to target cells/organs

Hormones are transported throughout the body in the blood. However, only specific target cells will have **receptors** on their cell surface membranes. Each receptor is specific to a single hormone. Therefore, only cells with **insulin receptors** (e.g. muscle and liver cells) will respond to **insulin** and only cells with **ADH receptors** (kidney cells) will respond to **ADH** (**antidiuretic hormone**).

This represents an important difference between the organisation and function of two systems involved in controlling many body functions. The signal or message carried by a hormone is 'broadcast' throughout the body but only picked up by cells that carry the correct receptors. In contrast, the nervous system (see section B2.3) uses nerve cells to deliver impulses only to specific target cells or tissues.

The endocrine system is like satellite TV. The signals are broadcast over the whole of a geographical area and can be picked up anywhere within that area, but only if you have a satellite dish. Unlike satellite TV, cable TV is carried over copper wires or fibre optic cables to individual homes. However, if you do not live in an area supplied by cable, you cannot watch.

Reflect

Can you think of other examples that you could use to explain to someone how the endocrine system works? When you have covered the nervous system in section B2.3 think about the similarities between cable TV and the nervous system.

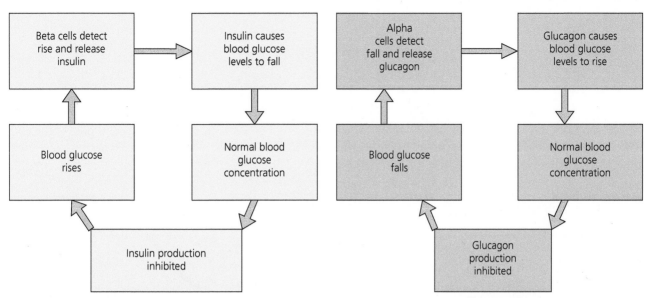

▲ Figure 15.2 Regulation of blood glucose concentration by insulin (left) and glucagon (right) These are both examples of negative feedback

The role of the pancreas in the regulation of blood glucose

The pancreas produces two hormones, insulin and glucagon, that are involved in the regulation of blood glucose concentration (Figure 15.2).

The actions of insulin and glucagon are **antagonistic** – they work in opposition to each other. They are also examples of **negative feedback** (we will cover this in more detail in section B2.12). Both are features of how other hormones help to regulate systems in the body.

The action of the antidiuretic hormone (ADH) in urine production

The renal system is covered in more detail in section B2.8. The **kidney** produces urine, but this has two main functions:

▶ **excretion** of nitrogenous waste in the form of **urea**
▶ **osmoregulation** – the regulation of the water balance in the body.

The process of **ultrafiltration** in the kidney produces a **filtrate** (filtered substance) that contains all the components of the blood, except for cells and large proteins. The process of converting the filtrate into urine involves reabsorption of useful substances such as glucose and amino acids, leaving a dilute solution of urea, which we call urine. Some water must also be reabsorbed, depending on the **water balance** of the

body. When we drink a lot of water, the blood has a high **water potential**. When we are dehydrated, the blood has a low water potential. The water potential of the blood is detected by osmoreceptors in the hypothalamus that control release of ADH by the posterior pituitary. This is illustrated in Figure 15.3 and is another example of a mechanism involving negative feedback.

Digestion

Gastrin is produced by cells in the stomach and its main target is also the stomach, where it stimulates release of hydrochloric acid (see section B2.5). Gastrin has other actions on the stomach, including:

▶ stimulates secretion of digestive enzymes
▶ stimulates contraction of stomach muscles which helps mix the food with acid and digestive enzymes
▶ stimulates emptying of the stomach into the **duodenum** (small intestine).

Gastrin also stimulates the release by the pancreas of secretions involved in digestion.

Growth

The pituitary gland controls growth through the secretion of growth hormone (GH). GH stimulates muscle and bone cells to divide and stimulates the intestines to absorb calcium, required for bone development. Lack of GH in childhood can lead to someone having reduced stature (i.e. being unusually short) while over-production leads to **pituitary giantism**.

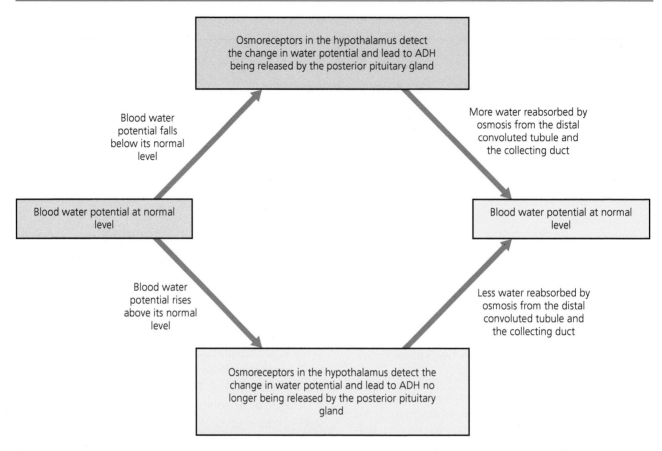

▲ Figure 15.3 Control of the water potential of the blood by ADH

Testosterone and oestrogen both stimulate the pituitary to secrete growth hormone. Increased production of these sex hormones during **puberty** explains the increase in growth rate around that time.

Effects of adrenalin

Adrenalin, together with the nervous system, is responsible for preparing the body to deal with danger or emergency situations by taking drastic action – the 'fight or flight' response. The actions of adrenalin include:

▶ increased heart rate
▶ stimulation of liver cells to convert glycogen to glucose, which increases blood glucose concentration
▶ increased blood flow to the muscles and brain
▶ decreased blood flow to the gut and skin
▶ increase in diameter of bronchioles (see section B2.2) to increase air flow into the lungs
▶ dilation of the pupils.

Reproductive cycle/function/puberty

Testosterone is required for production of sperm cells in males.

The menstrual cycle in females is more complex and involves hormones produced by the pituitary, the ovary and the uterus – see Figure 15.4.

The menstrual cycle takes about 28 days, although many people can have shorter or longer cycles or cycles that can be irregular.

Ovarian cycle

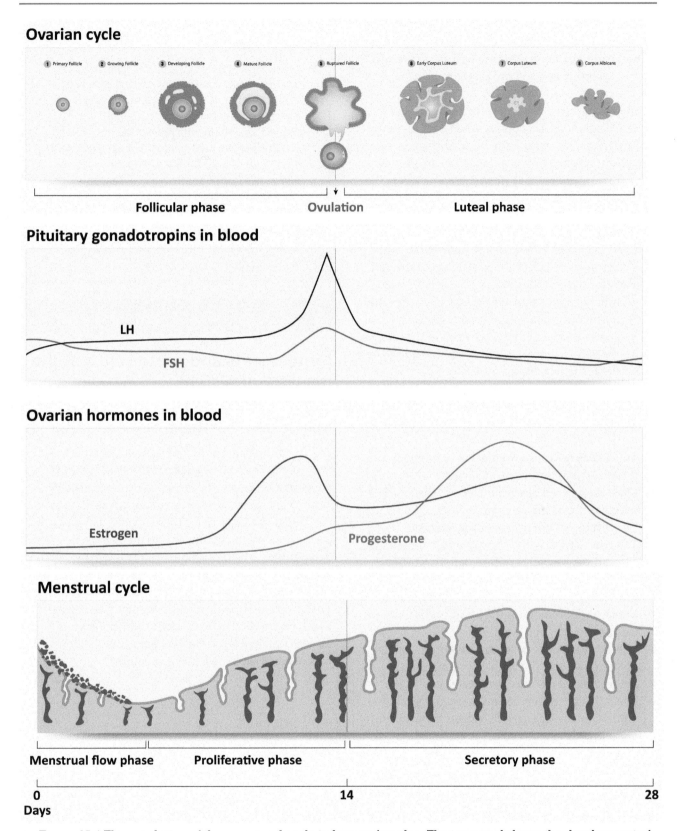

▲ Figure 15.4 The regulation of the menstrual cycle in human females. The top panel shows the development of the follicle and corpus luteum. The middle two panels show the levels of hormones in the blood. The bottom panel shows how the wall of the uterus thickens and then breaks down during the cycle

The cycle is regulated by two pituitary **gonadotropins** (hormones), **luteinising hormone** (**LH**) and **follicle stimulating hormone** (**FSH**) as well as the **steroid** hormones **oestrogen** and **progesterone**.

▶ The cycle starts (day 1) with the onset of **menstruation** (bleeding from the vagina, often called a period). This occurs when fertilisation of an egg cell has not occurred during the previous cycle and so the lining of the uterus breaks down. During the **menstrual flow** phase, the level of progesterone is low, which allows release of **FSH** from the pituitary. **LH** is also released by the pituitary.

▶ **FSH** stimulates growth of a **follicle** in the ovary.

▶ The growing follicle starts to produce **oestrogen**. The oestrogen produced:
  – inhibits production of FSH which ensures that normally only one egg matures each cycle
  – stimulates the growth and repair of the lining of the uterus, preparing it to accept a fertilised egg – the **follicular phase**.

▶ The concentration of oestrogen increases and just before day 14, the concentration reaches a high enough level to cause a surge in LH from the pituitary.

▶ This **LH surge** causes **ovulation** – the egg is released from the follicle on day 14.

▶ Once the egg cell has been released, the follicle becomes the corpus luteum.

▶ The corpus luteum releases **progesterone**.

▶ The concentration of progesterone in the blood rises and this inhibits release of LH and FSH by the pituitary – another example of negative feedback.

▶ Progesterone maintains the lining of the uterus ready to accept a fertilised egg.

▶ If fertilisation does not occur, the corpus luteum breaks down and the blood concentration of progesterone and oestrogen decreases.

▶ The fall in progesterone and oestrogen levels around, on average, day 28 triggers menstruation and the cycle begins again.

If fertilisation does occur, the placenta takes over the production of progesterone. This maintains the lining of the uterus during pregnancy, meaning that menstruation does not occur. A missed period can often be the first sign of pregnancy.

Test yourself

1 Most endocrine glands are the same in males and females. Name two endocrine glands that are present only in females and one that is present only in males.
2 Explain why hormones are carried throughout the body in the bloodstream but each hormone will act on only some types of cells.
3 Name two hormones involved in regulation of blood glucose concentration.
4 For the hormone ADH, state:
  a where it is produced
  b where it acts
  c its effect.

B2.2 The respiratory system

Components and organisation of the respiratory system

The respiratory system is contained largely within the **thorax** or chest cavity (Figure 15.5).

The two **lungs** almost fill the thorax. The mouth and nose lead to the **trachea** or windpipe, which is a wide tube kept open by C-shaped rings of cartilage. The trachea splits into two **bronchi**, one leading to each lung. The bronchi are also supported by rings of cartilage. The bronchi divide into many branches called **bronchioles**. The bronchioles lead to blind ends called **alveoli**. These are small air-filled sacs that have a wall consisting of a single layer of thin **epithelial cells**. The alveoli are the site of gas exchange (see section B1.10, page 238). The walls or the bronchioles and alveoli contain a lot of **elastic tissue**, which allows for expansion of the lungs during breathing.

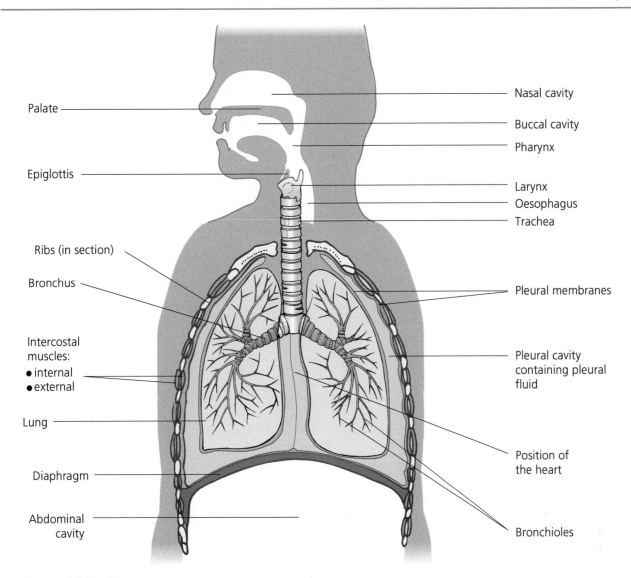

Palate

Epiglottis

Ribs (in section)

Bronchus

Intercostal
muscles:
● internal
● external

Lung

Diaphragm

Abdominal
cavity

Nasal cavity

Buccal cavity

Pharynx

Larynx

Oesophagus

Trachea

Pleural membranes

Pleural cavity
containing pleural
fluid

Position of
the heart

Bronchioles

▲ Figure 15.5 The human respiratory system

The lungs are surrounded by **pleural membranes**, a double layer that contains the lungs and also allows for expansion during breathing.

The chest cavity is enclosed by the **ribs**, which are connected to each other by two layers of **intercostal muscles**. The **diaphragm** is a sheet of muscle that forms the floor of the chest cavity. The diaphragm separates the chest cavity from the abdominal cavity and plays an important part in **ventilation** of the lungs (breathing).

Functions of the respiratory system

The properties of an efficient gas exchange surface were covered in section B1.10. In this section we will cover the ways in which the lungs are adapted for efficient gas exchange.

An important part of this is to maintain a high concentration gradient. The process of **ventilation** involves:
▶ **inspiration** or breathing in
▶ **expiration** or breathing out.

Ventilation of the lungs (Figure 15.6) ensures that fresh air high in oxygen is brought into the alveoli when we breathe in and carbon dioxide is removed when we breathe out.

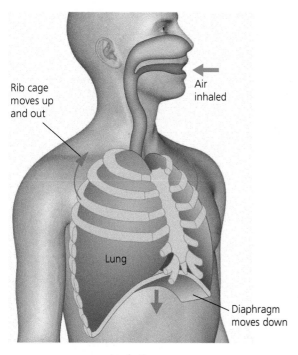

Inspiration

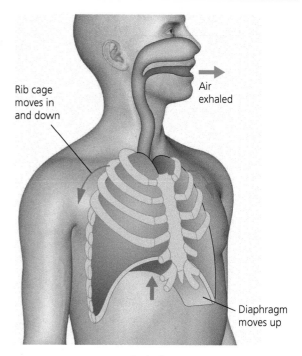

Expiration

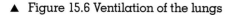

▲ Figure 15.6 Ventilation of the lungs

Inspiration (breathing in) involves contraction of two sets of muscles:

▶ the **diaphragm** contracts, which causes it to move down

▶ the **external intercostal** muscles contract, which causes the rib cage to move up and outwards.

As a result, the volume of the chest cavity increases and so the pressure in the lungs is reduced below the pressure of the air outside the body (atmospheric pressure). Air moves down a pressure gradient into the lungs, causing them to expand. This is assisted by the elastic tissue in the walls of the bronchioles and alveoli expanding.

Expiration (breathing out) when we are breathing at rest usually just involves relaxation of these two sets of muscles. As a result, the chest moves in and down and the diaphragm moves up. Therefore, the volume of the chest cavity decreases, the pressure increases and air is forced out down a concentration gradient. As well as this, the elastic tissue **recoils**, which also increases the pressure in the lungs, helping to force air out.

There is another set of muscles, the **internal intercostal** muscles. These are involved in **forced expiration**, which is what happens when you blow out candles, for instance. Contraction of the internal intercostal muscles causes the rib cage to be pulled in and down more forcefully, expelling air more rapidly from the lungs.

Key terms

Recoil: the process where elastic tissues or fibres return to their original length after having been stretched or expanded. This is what happens to an elastic band when you stretch it and then let go. Be careful not to use the term **contraction** to describe this process. Contraction is what muscles do, whereas elastic tissues recoil.

Epithelial: cells that line structures in the body and are usually thin, single layers.

Cilia: hair-like structures found on the plasma membranes of some types of epithelial cells. These are known as **ciliated epithelial cells**.

Ciliated epithelial tissue

The walls of the trachea and bronchi are covered with **ciliated epithelial cells** as well as **goblet cells** that produce mucus (Figure 15.7). The **cilia** contain proteins that can contract causing a wave-like movement. The mucus traps dirt and bacteria and the beating of the cilia moves the mucus back up the trachea to the throat where it is swallowed so that any bacteria are destroyed by the acid in the stomach.

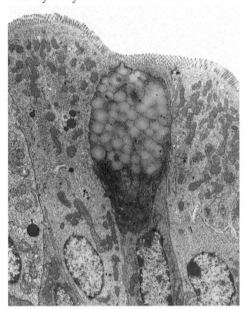

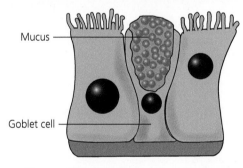

▲ Figure 15.7 A transmission electron micrograph (TEM) of a goblet cell with ciliated epithelial cells on either side (top); a diagram based on the TEM (bottom)

Pulmonary surfactant

This is produced by some cells in the wall of the alveoli and consists of a mixture of phospholipids and some protein. Surfactant acts like a detergent (for example, washing-up liquid). It coats the epithelial cells, reducing the **surface tension** of water. This makes it easier to inflate the lungs and stops the surfaces of the alveoli sticking together.

Proteins in the surfactant also help to protect against lung inflammation and infection.

How and where gaseous exchange takes place

So far, we have looked at the structure of the lungs and how the various parts are adapted to their function. We have also considered how ventilation of the lungs maintains a high concentration gradient of both oxygen and carbon dioxide in the alveolus. We now need to look at the detail of gas exchange in the alveolus (Figure 15.8).

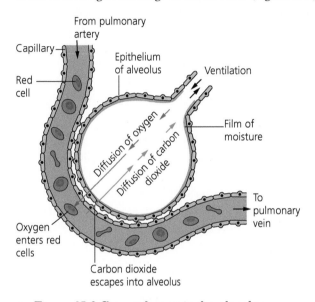

▲ Figure 15.8 Gas exchange in the alveolus

The pulmonary artery brings deoxygenated blood from the heart (see section B2.6) and the pulmonary vein returns oxygenated blood to the heart. In between, there is a network of capillaries surrounding the alveoli.

If you look back at 'Exchange and transport mechanisms' in Chapter B1: Core science concepts: Biology (page 238) you will see how the lungs have the three characteristics of an ideal exchange surface:

1   The wall of an alveolus is a single layer of epithelial cells. The wall of a capillary is a single layer of endothelial cells. This means that there is a short diffusion pathway for oxygen from the air in the alveoli to the red blood cells in the capillary – i.e. it makes it easy for oxygen to get into the red blood cells. The same is true for carbon dioxide dissolved in the blood moving in the opposite direction.
2   The many alveoli mean there is a large surface area for gas exchange – about $75\,m^2$ in an adult human.
3   Ventilation of the lungs (i.e. breathing) maintains a high concentration of oxygen and low concentration of carbon dioxide in the air in the alveoli. In addition, blood flow in the capillaries is continually bringing carbon dioxide to the lungs and removing oxygen, which also helps maintain the high concentration gradient.

How breathing rate can be increased or decreased

Regulation of breathing rate is performed by the **medulla oblongata** (sometime called just **medulla**), which is located at the base of the brain where it joins the spinal cord (see section B2.3). Carbon dioxide increases the acidity of the blood. This can be detected by **chemoreceptors** in arteries in the neck and in the medulla. As the acidity of the blood increases, the **respiratory centre** in the medulla sends nerve impulses to the muscles that control breathing to increase the breathing rate. As the acidity of the blood decreases, this is also detected and other nerves send impulses to slow down the rate of breathing.

A similar mechanism controls the heart rate (see section B2.6) so that the two systems work together. For example, when we exercise, the tissues produce more carbon dioxide and require more oxygen, so the heart rate increases. This increases blood flow to the tissues which delivers more oxygen to the tissues and removes more carbon dioxide. At the same time, an increase in breathing rate means that more oxygen can diffuse (see 'Exchange and transport mechanisms', page 238) into the blood in the lungs and more carbon dioxide can be removed.

The nose

The nose and nasal passages represent much more than just an alternative to the mouth for air entering the lungs, as you can see from Figure 15.9.

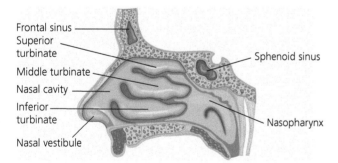

▲ Figure 15.9 The nose and nasal passages

Nasal passage

The nasal passage allows air to flow into the throat and then to the lungs. As it flows through, the air is warmed, filtered and humidified.

The following structures are located in the nasal passage:

- **Nasal turbinates** are located on the outer walls of the nasal passage and consist of a network of bones, vessels and tissues. They are primarily responsible for warming, filtering and humidifying the incoming air. The turbinates swell and shrink to regulate airflow through the nose. Infections such as the common cold or allergies such as hay fever can lead to inflammation and congestion of the turbinates.
- **Nasal sinuses** are air pockets in the bones surrounding the nose. They drain into the nasal passage and deliver clear mucus that also helps to humidify the air and trap dust and dirt. Inflammation of the sinuses (**sinusitis**) can occur when the drainage pathway becomes blocked. This can lead to infection of the sinuses.

Swallowing

If you look again at Figure 15.5 you will see the two remaining structures in the respiratory system that we need to consider. In fact, these are relevant more to the process of swallowing food than to breathing.

The **oropharyngeal passage** connects the back of the mouth or **buccal cavity** with the lower part of the **pharynx** leading to the throat. The pharynx connects the nasal cavity and buccal cavity with the **trachea** (towards the lungs) and **oesophagus** (towards the stomach).

The **epiglottis** is a flap of cartilage covered with a membrane. The epiglottis remains open during breathing to allow air into the larynx so that it can pass into the trachea towards the lungs. When we swallow, the epiglottis closes, shutting off the larynx and forcing food to pass into the oesophagus and on towards the stomach.

Test yourself

1   State the two groups of muscles involved in breathing (ventilation).
2   Describe three ways in which the human lungs show the properties of an ideal exchange surface.
3   Describe the function of:
    a   ciliated epithelia
    b   pulmonary surfactant
    c   nasal turbinates
    d   nasal sinuses.
4   Explain why breathing out at rest is sometimes described as a passive process compared with forced expiration.

B2.3 The nervous system

The nervous system controls and coordinates our movement. It allows us to interact with our surroundings by use of **receptors** and **effectors** (such as muscles). It also controls many of the **autonomic** functions of the body – those over which we have no conscious control. These include the movement of food along the gut in digestion (section B2.5), regulation of breathing rate (section B2.2) and regulation of heart rate (section B2.6).

Components and organisation of the nervous system

The main distinction in the nervous system is between the **central** and **peripheral nervous systems** – the **CNS** and the **PNS** (Figure 15.10).

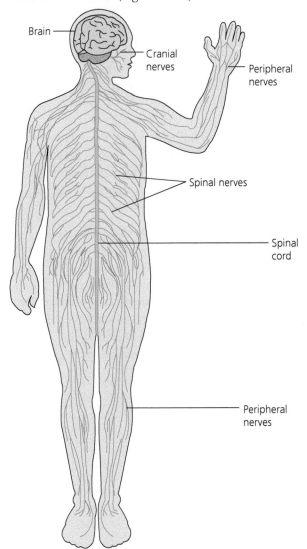

▲ Figure 15.10 The structure of the human nervous system

Central nervous system (CNS)

The CNS consists of the **brain** and the **spinal cord**. The brain is where sensory inputs (hearing, touch, vision, etc.) are processed and responses (such as movement) are initiated. The spinal cord is important in reflex actions, for example moving your hand away from a hot plate.

Peripheral nervous system (PNS)

The PNS consists of all the **sensory** **neurones** that connect receptors with the CNS as well as the **motor neurones** that connect to muscles or glands and bring about responses such as movement.

Figure 15.11 illustrates the structure of a motor neurone seen in mammals.

> ### Key terms
>
> **Neurone:** a nerve cell.
>
> **Nerves:** usually bundles of many neurones.

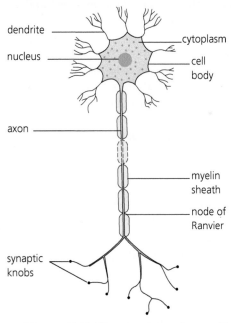

▲ Figure 15.11 The structure of a myelinated motor neurone

Motor neurones transmit **nerve impulses** in only one direction (away from the cell body) and have the following features:
▶ **dendrites** that make connections with other neurones, mostly within the CNS
▶ the **cell body** containing the **nucleus** and other **organelles**
▶ the **axon** which carries the nerve impulse from the cell body.

The **myelin sheath** consists of Schwann cells, a specialised type of cell wrapped around the axon (see Figure 15.12) which acts in a similar way to the insulation on an electric cable.

There are small gaps between the Schwann cells called **nodes of Ranvier**. The combination of the myelin sheath and nodes of Ranvier helps to significantly increase the rate at which the nerve impulse is carried along the axon.

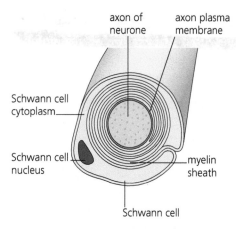

▲ Figure 15.12 A section across an axon showing the structure of the myelin sheath

At the end furthest from the cell body, the axon branches to form **axon endings** or **terminals** that make connections, usually with muscle cells. These are called **synaptic ends** or **synaptic knobs**.

Functions of the nervous system

The role of the PNS

The PNS carries nerve impulses from **receptors** that act as the body's **sensors** towards the CNS along sensory neurones. This is similar to the way in which a cable carries a message from a microphone to a loudspeaker. However, we should really refer to nerves carrying **impulses** and not messages.

The role of the CNS

The CNS takes all the information contained in inputs from sensory neurons and processes it. It then sends impulses via **motor neurones** to **effector organs**. Effector organs are usually muscles, but they can also be **glands** (see section B2.1).

As well as this coordinating function, the brain is where we store memories, feel emotion and generally experience what we call **consciousness**.

Motor neurones and synaptic transmission

Key terms

Depolarisation: the reversal of the charge difference.

Polarisation: of a nerve or muscle cell refers to the different electrical charges on either side of the plasma membrane caused by active transport of ions.

Repolarisation: the restoration of the original charge difference.

Nerve impulses are electrical signals transmitted from the cell body towards the axon terminals. When a neurone is 'at rest' there is a small potential difference across the plasma membrane of about $-60\,mV$. In other words, the inside of the neurone is slightly more negative than the outside due to positive Na^+ ions which have been pumped out of the neurone. This **polarisation** of the plasma membrane neurone is described as the **resting potential**.

A nerve impulse involves a rapid change in the membrane potential so that the membrane is **depolarised** – the inside is now slightly positive compared with the outside. This process is rapidly reversed within a few milliseconds and the membrane becomes **repolarised**. This is known as an **action potential**. An action potential is **propagated** or transmitted along the axon – this represents a nerve impulse.

Motor neurones are known as **myelinated** because they have a myelin sheath. In myelinated neurones, the action potential **jumps** from one node of Ranvier to the next. This makes propagation of the nerve impulse much faster. Speed is important when you consider that a motor neurone could start at the base of the spinal cord and travel all the way down to your big toe – that is quite a large distance for a single cell!

Connections between neurones are known as **synapses**. Electrical transmission of the nerve impulse across the synapse is not possible because there is a physical gap between the cells. The nerve impulse is carried across the synapse by chemicals known as **neurotransmitters**.

Figure 15.13 illustrates the structure of a synapse.

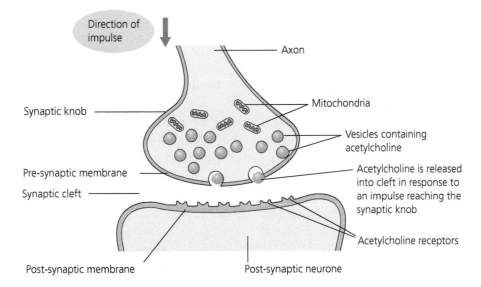

▲ Figure 15.13 The structure of a synapse

The synaptic knob makes a connection with a muscle or another neurone. When the nerve impulse arrives at the synaptic knob it causes release of neurotransmitters from membrane-bound **vesicles**. The most common neurotransmitter is **acetylcholine**. This diffuses across the synaptic cleft (see Figure 15.13) and then binds to **receptors** on the membrane of the muscle cell or the next neurone. If enough neurotransmitter binds, then the **post-synaptic** membrane will become depolarised and a new nerve impulse will be generated in the next neurone. The process is similar in muscle cells, except that the result is muscle contraction and not a new nerve impulse.

Different sensors in the body

We rely on our senses to tell us what is happening in the world around us. These work in different ways, depending on type, but they all have receptors connected to **nerve endings** of sensory neurones.

Pressure receptors detect, among other things, changes in blood pressure.

Temperature receptors are located in the skin, where they detect the external temperature, and in the CNS, where they detect the core body temperature.

Sound receptors in the inner ear detect sound waves and so allow us to hear.

Light receptors are located in the retina of the eye and are involved in vision.

Touch receptors are a type of pressure receptor located in the skin and allow us to experience a range of sensations, from a gentle caress to a sharp slap, or to explore our surroundings using touch.

Pain receptors are located throughout the body. Their function is to signal to the CNS when injury has occurred. The ability to feel pain gives us an important survival advantage, particularly if it means that we can avoid more serious injury. Interestingly, there are no pain receptors in the brain – which is why some types of brain surgery can be performed using just a local anaesthetic.

Taste receptors are of two types:
▶ Receptors on the tongue (taste buds) can detect the five main types of taste:
  – sweet
  – sour
  – bitter
  – salt
  – umami (this is the savoury taste we get from fried foods, fish sauce or mushrooms).
▶ **Olfactory** receptors, located in the nasal passage, detect smells or scents. Most of what we experience when we 'taste' food depends on our sense of smell rather than just taste.

Test yourself

1 Describe the components of:
  a the central nervous system
  b the peripheral nervous system.
2 Describe the structure of the myelin sheath and explain why nerve impulses are transmitted faster in myelinated neurones.
3 Explain the difference in the way that a nerve impulse is transmitted along a nerve cell and the way it is transmitted between nerve cells.
4 Describe the location of temperature receptors.

B2.4 The musculoskeletal system

The term **musculoskeletal** refers to the skeleton and the muscles attached to the skeleton. The musculoskeletal system is involved in support of the body and in movement. The human skeleton is made up of 206 bones connected by various types of **joints**.

Skeletal or **striated** muscle is the type of muscle attached to the skeleton and involved in movement. The name striated refers to its striped appearance when viewed with a microscope (see Figure 15.19). Another name you might see is **voluntary** muscle because when we move, we have conscious or voluntary control over the muscle.

There are two other types of muscle:
- **Smooth** or **involuntary** muscle is found in the gut (section B2.5) and blood vessels (section B2.6)

and, as the name suggests, is involved in all the processes over which we have no conscious control, such as movement of food along the gut or constriction of dilation of blood vessels.
- **Cardiac** muscle is found in the heart (section B2.6).

Key terms

Joint: the area where two or more bones connect.

Skeletal: the main type of muscle involved in movement because it is attached to the **skeleton**.

Cartilage: another type of connective tissue that contains, among other components, collagen and the elastic protein **elastin**. Cartilage is more flexible than ligaments and muscles, but not as hard and rigid as bone.

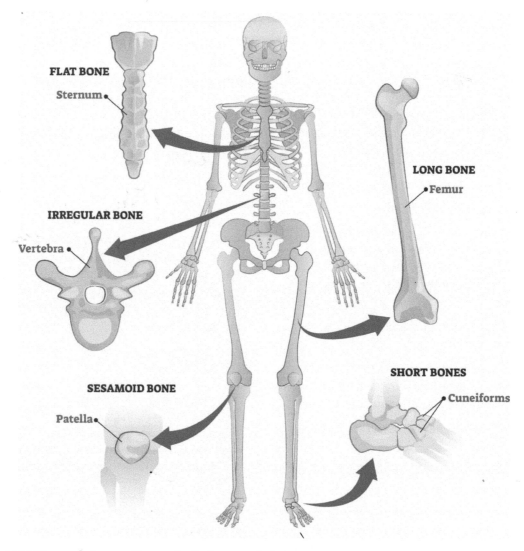

FLAT BONE
Sternum

IRREGULAR BONE
Vertebra

SESAMOID BONE
Patella

LONG BONE
Femur

SHORT BONES
Cuneiforms

▲ Figure 15.14 The main types of bones in the human skeleton

Components and organisation of the musculoskeletal system

Figure 15.14 shows the main types of bones in the human skeleton.

Joints can be classified according to their **structure**:
▶ **Fibrous** joints (also called immovable joints) are where bones are fused together, usually to create a structure. A good example is the **skull**, which consists of a number of bones fused together.
▶ **Cartilaginous** joints have bones connected by relatively flexible **cartilage** that allows some degree of movement. An example is the rib cage (see section B2.2) where the ribs are joined together by cartilaginous joints that allow the ribs to move during breathing.
▶ **Synovial** joints are the most common type. They are flexible and movable in a range of ways. The hip joint (Figure 15.15) is a good example of a synovial joint.

Synovial joints all have cartilage providing cushioning between the bones that are joined. They also have a **synovial capsule** consisting of connective tissue containing **synovial fluid**. This helps to lubricate the joint, allowing smoother movement and reducing wear

on the bones. **Ligaments** hold the bones together while allowing a degree of movement and flexibility.

Synovial joints can be classified according to their function. This functional classification of joints is based on the type of movement and degree of movement they permit. Figure 15.16 shows the main types of joint in the human skeleton. The full skeletal structure is shown in Figure 15.17.

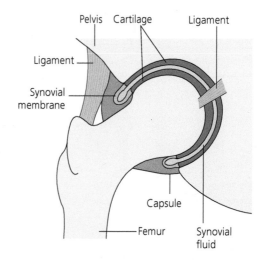

▲ Figure 15.15 The hip, a synovial joint

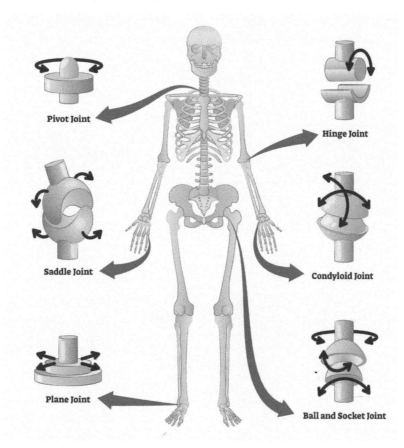

▲ Figure 15.16 The main types of synovial joint

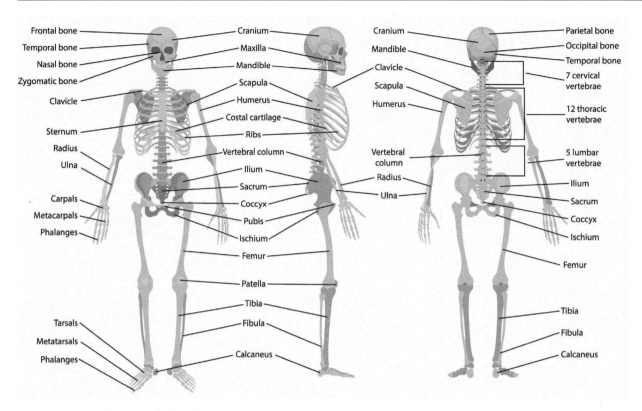

▲ Figure 15.17 The full skeletal structure

Besides bone and **ligaments**, the other main component of the musculoskeletal system are the muscles and associated **tendons**. These muscles are known as skeletal or striated muscles (Figure 15.18).

> ### Key terms
>
> **Ligaments:** made of **connective tissue** containing the protein **collagen**. Their function is to join bones together and to strengthen joints.
>
> **Tendons:** similar in structure and composition to ligaments. Their function is to attach the muscles to the bones that make up the skeleton.

Muscle fibres are the individual muscle cells. They contain many **myofibrils**, which are responsible for muscle contraction. The muscle fibres are held together in bundles by a sheath of connective tissue and several of these bundles will make a single muscle. **Tendons** at each end of the muscle attach it to the bones.

Skeletal muscle viewed in the light microscope has a characteristic striped appearance (Figure 15.19). These striations give an insight into the way in which skeletal muscle contracts and forms the basis of the **sliding filament hypothesis** (see page 316).

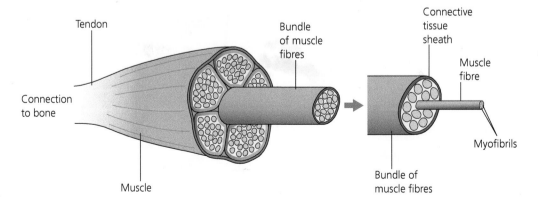

▲ Figure 15.18 The arrangement of muscle fibres in skeletal muscle

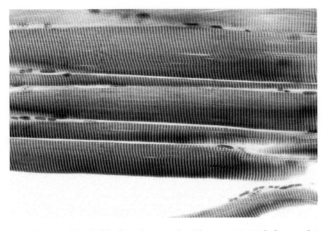

▲ Figure 15.19 Skeletal muscle fibres viewed through an optical microscope showing the striations

Functions of the musculoskeletal system

The skeletal system provides support for the body, protection of organs such as the brain and also allows for attachment of the ligaments holding joints together and the muscles involved in movement.

> ### Reflect
>
> Think about how the following parts of the skeleton provide protection. Which organs do they protect?
> ▶ skull
> ▶ backbone (vertebrae)
> ▶ pelvis
> ▶ ribs.

There are also some less obvious functions of the skeletal system.

Blood production

The long bones (see Figure 15.14) contain a spongy tissue in the centre called the **bone marrow**. This contains many **stem cells** that can develop into all the different types of blood cells, including **erythrocytes** (red blood cells) and the various types of **lymphocytes** (white blood cells) that are involved in the immune response, covered in section B1.30.

Minerals

Bone is a complex structure of cells embedded in a hard material consisting of the protein **collagen** and the inorganic compound **calcium phosphate**. This makes bone a bit like the kinds of **composite materials** that we covered in section B1.33.

This presence of large amounts of calcium phosphate allows bone to act as a reservoir of both of the minerals (calcium ions and phosphate ions) that are important for many processes in the body. Calcium is particularly important as it is involved in nerve conduction, muscle contraction and blood clotting. Phosphate is important as it is a major component of **DNA** and is also involved in energy metabolism. The main source of both calcium and phosphate is the diet. **Vitamin D** stimulates uptake of calcium from the gut and its incorporation into bone. However, the bones act as a **store** or **buffer** of both calcium and phosphate. The hormones **PTH** and **calcitonin** (section B2.1) regulate the levels of calcium and phosphate in the blood.

Movement (locomotion) and support

Figure 15.20 shows the two main muscles, **biceps** and **triceps**, involved in movement of the lower arm.

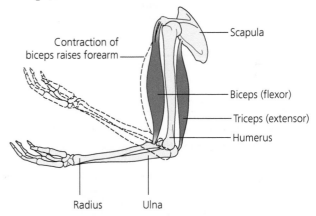

▲ Figure 15.20 Movement at the elbow showing the main bones and muscles involved

This shows an important principle of movement: muscles are generally arranged in **antagonistic** or **opposing pairs**. When the biceps contracts and the triceps relaxes, the forearm is raised. When the triceps contracts and the biceps relaxes, the forearm is lowered.

The sliding filament theory

Muscles contain two main proteins involved in muscle contraction, **actin** and **myosin**. These proteins make up the two types of **muscle filament** found in **myofibrils**.

▶ **Thick** filaments contain myosin.
▶ **Thin** filaments contain actin, as well as two other proteins.

These filaments are arranged in the myofibrils in a repeating pattern known as **sarcomeres**. It is this repeating pattern that gives striated muscle its striped appearance.

When muscles contract, we can see that the sarcomeres **shorten**. You might expect, therefore, that the filaments shorten. However, this is not the case. We now know that the sarcomere shortens because the filaments slide over each other (Figure 15.21).

Relaxed

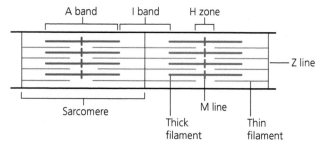

Contracted

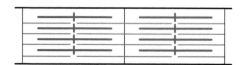

▲ Figure 15.21 The arrangement of thick and thin filaments in a relaxed and contracted myofibril

Figure 15.22 shows the structure of the thick and thin filaments. Thin filaments consist of long chains of actin molecules while thick filaments are bundles of myosin molecules arranged so that the 'head' groups protrude

all around the bundle. These head groups bind to actin molecules. When this happens, a change in the shape of the myosin head pulls the thin filament towards the centre of the sarcomere. The myosin head then detaches and energy transferred from the hydrolysis of adenosine triphosphate (ATP, see section B1.3) is used to change the myosin head back to its original shape ready to bind to another actin molecule. This process is repeated many times, leading to shortening of the sarcomere. As a result of shortening of all the sarcomeres, the muscle contracts.

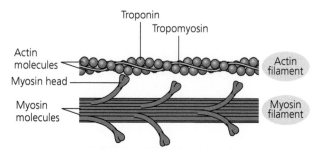

▲ Figure 15.22 The structure of thick and thin filaments

Test yourself

1 Name and describe the three types of joint structure.
2 Give one example of each of the following types of joint:
   a ball and socket joint
   b hinge joint
   c condyloid joint
   d pivot joint.
3 Describe one similarity and one difference between ligaments and tendons.
4 Name the three types of muscle.
5 Name the main protein found in each of:
   a thick filaments
   b thin filaments.

B2.5 The digestive system

Components and organisation of the digestive system

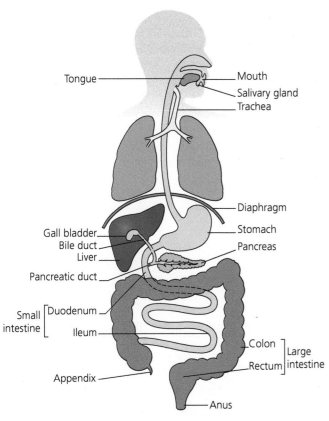

▲ Figure 15.23 The human digestive system

Figure 15.23 shows the human digestive system. You need to be familiar with the following parts:
▶ mouth
▶ oesophagus
▶ stomach
▶ pancreas
▶ liver
▶ small intestine, consisting of:
   – duodenum
   – ileum
▶ large intestine (colon).

The **gastrointestinal tract** (**GI tract**) consists of the oesophagus, stomach, and small and large intestines. The wall of the GI tract has four layers (Figure 15.24). The figure shows the stomach wall, but other parts of the GI tract have a similar arrangement of layers.

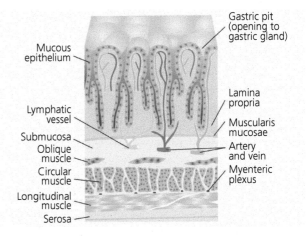

▲ Figure 15.24 The four layers of the wall of the GI tract: the mucosa, submucosa, muscularis and serosa

▶ The **mucosa** is the innermost layer, surrounding the **lumen** – the open space within the tube of the GI tract. The structure of the mucosa varies in the different parts of the GI tract according to the function of each part.
▶ The **submucosa** consists of a dense layer of connective tissue with blood vessels, **lymphatic vessels** and nerves.
▶ The **muscularis** or muscle layer has an inner oblique layer, a middle **circular** layer and an outer **longitudinal** layer.
▶ The **serosa** forms the outer layer and consists of several layers of connective tissue.

There are also glands linked to the components of the GI tract that play an important part in digestion, including **salivary glands** in the mouth, **gall bladder** and **bile duct**.

Functions of the digestive system

The digestive system breaks down food by **mechanical** and **chemical** digestion.

Mechanical digestion

This refers to the way in which food is broken up into smaller pieces, which increases the efficiency of chemical digestion.

The process starts with chewing the food (**mastication**). This begins the mechanical breakdown and mixes the food with **saliva**. The saliva helps lubricate the chewed food and contains the enzyme **salivary amylase**.

Mechanical digestion continues in the stomach where contraction of **smooth muscle** in the stomach wall causes a churning action, continually mixing the food with digestive enzymes and acid. This process can last for several hours.

Peristalsis describes the rhythmic movement of the wall of the gut that moves the food along the whole length of the GI tract. This is circular muscle behind a mass of food which contracts, pushing it forward. At the same time, longitudinal muscle around and ahead of the mass of food also contracts. This shortens the passage in front of the food. This process is controlled by the **autonomic nervous system**.

Key terms

Smooth (or **involuntary**) **muscle:** (see section B2.4) is not under conscious control. It is controlled by the **autonomic nervous system** and **hormones**.

Autonomic nervous system: part of the peripheral nervous system that controls many of the processes in the body over which we have no conscious control.

Chemical digestion

This involves digestive **enzymes** that catalyse (speed up) the **hydrolysis** reactions that break down the large molecules in food (proteins, lipids and polysaccharides such as starch) into smaller, simpler molecules. In sections B1.7 and B1.8 we saw how proteins and polysaccharides are formed by joining smaller molecules (amino acids and sugars) in **condensation** reactions. Hydrolysis is the reverse process.

Each type of food molecule is broken down by a specific type of enzyme, as shown in the table. A major source of digestive enzymes is the pancreas. Pancreatic fluid is made by the pancreas and released into the duodenum via the pancreatic duct.

Enzyme	Location/source	Action
Salivary amylase	Saliva (in the mouth)	Begins the digestion of starch (a polysaccharide) into maltose (a disaccharide)
Pancreatic amylase	Pancreatic fluid	Completes digestion of starch into maltose
Disaccharidases: • maltase • sucrase • lactase	Duodenum	Convert disaccharides into their constituent monosaccharides: • Maltase completes the digestion of starch by converting maltose into two molecules of glucose. • Sucrase converts sucrose into glucose and fructose. • Lactase converts lactose into glucose and galactose.
Proteases	Pepsin is located in the stomach. Trypsin, chymotrypsin and carboxypeptidase are contained in pancreatic fluid	Convert proteins into smaller fragments: peptides and eventually amino acids
Lipases	Pancreatic fluid	Break down lipids into fatty acids and glycerol

Reflect

Enzymes – what's in a name?

If you look at the enzymes listed in the table, you may notice a pattern. Most of them end in 'ase' and the first part of the name is linked to the function of the enzyme, so we have maltase, sucrase and lactase. Amylase is so called because it digests a type of starch called amylose. Protease and lipase are general names that follow the same pattern. Pepsin, trypsin and chymotrypsin are exceptions to this rule – but you can usually tell what an enzyme does from its name.

Find other enzyme names and see if you can match the name and the function.

There are two other important components of chemical digestion:

▶ **hydrochloric acid**, secreted by glands in the stomach wall – this helps to sterilise the food and provides the acidic conditions required by stomach proteases such as pepsin

▶ **bile**, which is produced in the **liver**, stored in the **gall bladder** and released into the duodenum via the **bile duct** and the **pancreatic duct**. Bile acts as a surfactant (like a detergent) and helps to break up large fat globules into smaller droplets so that lipases can work more effectively.

Absorption processes

Digestion of the main food types can be summarised as:

proteins → amino acids

polysaccharides → monosaccharides

lipids → fatty acids and glycerol.

Absorption of these products of digestion occurs mainly in the ileum and occurs in the **epithelial cells** lining the wall of the gut.

Section B1.10 (see page 238) covers the principles of efficient exchange surfaces, in particular the need for a large surface area. This is achieved in the ileum by folding of the wall of the gut into finger-like projections called **villi** (singular = **villus**). The epithelial cells on villi have microvilli on their surface, which increases still further the surface area for absorption (Figure 15.25).

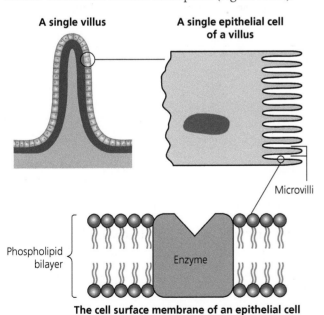

A single villus   **A single epithelial cell of a villus**

Microvilli

Phospholipid bilayer

Enzyme

The cell surface membrane of an epithelial cell

▲ Figure 15.25 The lining of the small intestine showing a villus, microvilli on the surface of an epithelial cell and its cell surface membrane incorporating an enzyme such as maltase.

Section B1.11 (see page 239) covers the principles of transport across membranes.

Remember that **polar** molecules cannot cross the phospholipid bilayer, such as the one in the plasma membrane of the epithelial cells lining the ileum. Fatty acids are non-polar and can, therefore, pass into the epithelial cells by simple diffusion.

All the other products of digestion are polar molecules (monosaccharides, amino acids, etc.) and are absorbed into the epithelial cells by **active transport** and **facilitated diffusion**. The process of glucose absorption is covered in section B1.11 (see page 239) and amino acids are absorbed by a similar mechanism.

Key term

Polar: a polar (hydrophilic) substance will dissolve in or mix with water. Polar molecules have a slight separation in electrical charge. Therefore, one part of the molecule will have a slightly positive charge and another, a slightly negative. This makes the molecule hydrophilic, meaning it will interact with and dissolve in water.

The role of micro-organisms

A recent study estimated the total number of cells in the human body to be 3.0×10^{13} while there are about 3.8×10^{13} bacterial cells. In terms of number of cells, we are all more bacteria than human!

Most of these bacteria reside in the **colon** and make up what is known as the **microbiome**. In **herbivores** such as cattle, horses and sheep, these gut bacteria play an important role in digestion of **cellulose** (the structural polysaccharide of plant cell walls) that cannot be digested by the animal's own enzymes. However, it is now understood that gut bacteria in humans also aid digestion, particularly for complex carbohydrates that are not broken down by enzymes such as amylase.

Test yourself

1 Name the four parts of the gastrointestinal tract.
2 Name the four layers of the wall of the gut.
3 Name two sites of mechanical digestion.
4 State the location and function of each of the following digestive enzymes:
   a salivary amylase
   b lactase
   c pepsin.
5 State the precise location of the absorption of the products of digestion.

B2.6 The cardiovascular system

Components and organisation of the cardiovascular system

The cardiovascular system consists of the heart and blood vessels.

Blood vessels

Figure 15.26 illustrates the structure of each of the three main types of blood vessel.

Arteries

The **arteries** carry blood away from the heart. The largest artery is the **aorta** that leads directly from the left ventricle (see below) of the heart. The aorta divides into smaller arteries supplying all the organs of the body. The smallest arteries are called **arterioles**. Arteries have an outer layer of connective tissue that provides strength and support. However, they also have a thick layer of **muscle** and **elastic tissue**. The muscle allows **constriction** (narrowing) or **dilation** (widening) of the arteries to regulate blood flow to different parts of the body. The elastic tissue allows the artery to expand, helping to withstand the pressure caused by the pumping of the heart.

Capillaries

The arterioles lead to the **capillaries**. These are the smallest vessels in the cardiovascular system and have a wall that is just a single cell thick.

Veins

The capillaries come together to form **venules** that merge to form larger **veins**. The blood is at a much lower pressure in the veins because it has had to force its way through the narrow capillaries, so the **lumen** (the space in the middle) of a vein is much larger than that of an artery. Veins also have thinner walls as they do not need to absorb the pressure of the pumping of the heart.

The heart

The heart is a pump. The blood enters via the **atria** and passes into the **ventricles**. The ventricles have thick muscular walls that contract to pump the blood to the lungs (right ventricle) or around the body (left ventricle). To ensure that blood only flows in the right direction, the heart also contains **valves** that prevent back-flow. Figure 15.27 illustrates the structures of the heart that you need to be familiar with.

You should take note of some of the features of the heart.

▶ The right ventricle is on the left as you look at Figure 15.27 and the left ventricle is on the right. That is because we label them from the viewpoint of the animal (in this case, the human). This is just like when you look at someone and their left arm is on the right as you look at them.

▶ The left ventricle has a thicker, stronger muscle wall. This is because it has to pump blood around the whole body. The right ventricle only has to pump blood a short distance to the lungs.

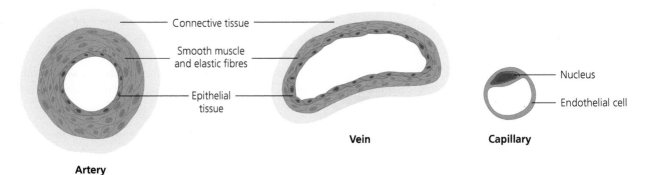

▲ Figure 15.26 Cross sections of an artery, a vein and a capillary. Capillaries are often single cells wrapped into a tubular shape

The **atria** have relatively thin walls as they only need to pump blood into the adjacent ventricle.

The **bicuspid** and **tricuspid** valves (also known as **atrioventricular** or **AV** valves) prevent blood flowing backwards from the ventricle into the atrium. When the pressure is higher in the atrium than in the ventricle, the valves are pushed open. When the pressure is higher in the ventricle than in the atrium, the valves are pushed closed. The tendons prevent the valves from being pushed too far so that they make a good seal.

The **semi-lunar valves** have a different structure, but they perform a similar function to the bicuspid and tricuspid valves. Because the semi-lunar valves are located at the entrance to the pulmonary artery and the aorta they prevent back-flow from these blood vessels into the ventricles.

Composition of the blood

The blood is made up of:

- plasma
- platelets
- red blood cells
- white blood cells.

Plasma is the straw-coloured fluid that is left if all the cells are removed. It contains proteins, known as **plasma proteins**, hormones, and all the small molecules (carbon dioxide, glucose, amino acids) and ions transported in the blood.

Platelets are small disc-shaped cell fragments without nuclei that are also called **thrombocytes**. They are present in large numbers in the blood and play an important role in blood **clotting**.

Red blood cells or **erythrocytes** are differentiated cells without a nucleus or the majority of their organelles. They are filled with **haemoglobin**, the protein that transports oxygen from the lungs to the tissues.

White blood cells or **leucocytes** are cells that are mostly involved in protection against infection, including the immune response (see section B1.30).

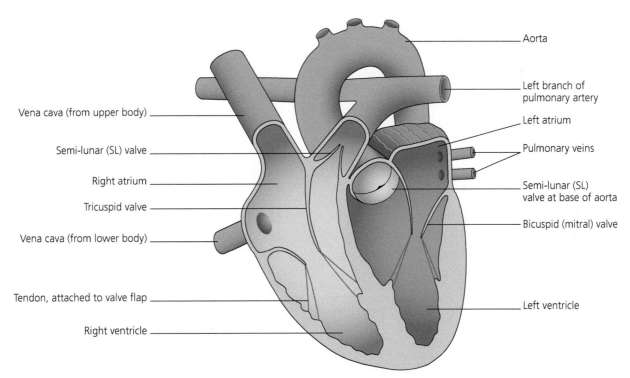

▲ Figure 15.27 Cross section through the human heart

Functions of the cardiovascular system

The cardiovascular system facilitates the circulation of blood to transport:

- nutrients (glucose, amino acids, lipids, vitamins, etc.), required for cell growth and repair
- oxygen, required for cellular respiration
- carbon dioxide, transported to the lungs to be eliminated from the body
- hormones (see section B2.1), transported to target cells
- blood cells:
  - erythrocytes for transport of oxygen
  - leucocytes as part of the immune system.

The human circulatory system is known as a **double** circulatory system. This is because the blood passes through the heart twice for every circuit of the whole body.

The first loop is from the heart to the lungs, then back to the heart. The second loop is from the heart, through all the other organs and back to the heart (Figure 15.28). This means that, with very few exceptions, the heart will only have to pump through one set of capillaries at a time.

The main exception to this is the digestive system, where blood flows via the **mesenteric artery** to the capillaries surrounding the **gut**. It then flows via the **hepatic portal vein** to the **liver**, which is where most of the products of digestion are processed and **metabolised**. The **hepatic vein** then takes blood from the liver back to the heart.

The cardiac cycle

The heart pumps blood through a series of muscle contractions and relaxations called the **cardiac cycle**. One way to understand this is to trace the path taken by the blood through the heart:

- The blood enters the right atrium from the vena cava.
- It then flows via the bicuspid valve into the right ventricle.
- From the right ventricle it is pumped into the pulmonary artery to the lungs.
- Returning from the lungs via the pulmonary veins, the blood enters the left atrium.
- It then flows into the left ventricle.
- From the left ventricle, blood is pumped into the aorta and around the body.

You can trace this 'journey' taken by the blood using a very simple diagram (Figure 15.29).

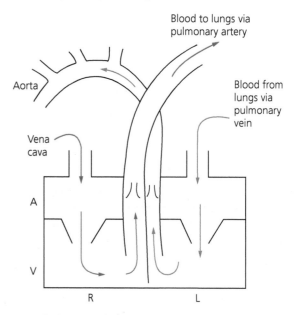

▲ Figure 15.29 Simplified diagram of the heart showing the main chambers, valves and blood vessels illustrating the route taken by blood through the heart. A = atria, V = ventricles, R = right, L = left

We can also understand the working of the heart by thinking about the pressure changes that occur during the cardiac cycle. This is illustrated in Figure 15.30.

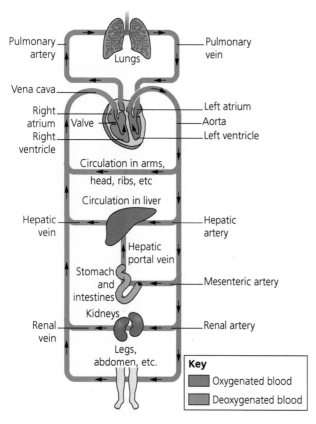

Key

Oxygenated blood

Deoxygenated blood

▲ Figure 15.28 The organisation of the human cardiovascular system

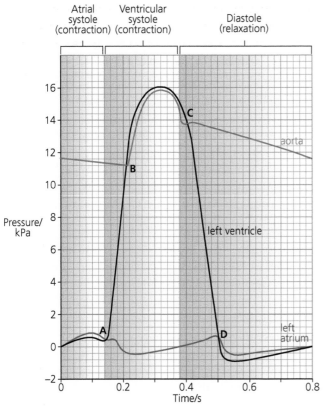

▲ Figure 15.30 A graph showing how pressure changes in the left atrium, left ventricle and aorta during one cardiac cycle

This might appear complicated at first. However, once you learn to read the graph it really does help understand what is happening. The graph shows how the pressure changes in the left atrium and left ventricle during one complete cardiac cycle.

Key terms

Systole: refers to the contraction of either atrium or ventricle. Hence the terms **atrial systole** and **ventricular systole** respectively.

Diastole: refers to the relaxation of either atrium or ventricle.

It is probably easiest to follow what is happening if we start towards the end of cycle, about 0.6 s on the graph.

▶ Blood is flowing back from the lungs into the left atrium. The pressure in the **atrium** is higher than in the **ventricle**, so the **bicuspid** valve is open and blood flows into the ventricle. We can think of this as the heart filling with blood.

▶ During **atrial systole**, the atrium contracts. This completes the emptying of blood from the atrium into the ventricle in preparation for the next stage.

▶ **Ventricular systole** is when the ventricle contracts. Its thick muscle wall means that the pressure in the ventricle rises rapidly. At point A on Figure 15.30 the pressure in the ventricle is higher than in the atrium and this pushes the **bicuspid valve** closed, preventing back-flow.

▶ As the pressure in the ventricle rises, it quickly exceeds the pressure in the **aorta**. This has happened at point B on Figure 15.30 and this pushes the semi-lunar valve open so that blood flows into the aorta.

▶ This causes the ventricle to empty.

▶ The cycle then moves to **diastole** (relaxation) and, at point C on Figure 15.30, the pressure in the ventricle falls below that in the aorta.

▶ This causes the semi-lunar valve to close, again preventing back-flow.

▶ Closure of the semi-lunar valve causes a drop in pressure in the aorta (the **dicrotic notch**) followed immediately by a slight increase in pressure (the **dicrotic wave**) that is caused by recoil of the elastic tissue in the wall of the aorta.

▶ The pressure in the ventricle continues to fall until, at point D on Figure 15.30, the pressure falls below that in the atrium. This causes the bicuspid valve to open, allowing blood to flow into the ventricle, and the whole cycle can begin again.

Something else you will notice in Figure 15.30 is the spike in pressure in the aorta as the left ventricle contracts and forces blood into the aorta and around the body. This spike can be felt as the **pulse** in many arteries, for example, in the wrist or neck. As there is one spike in pressure for each heart contraction, the pulse can be used to measure heart rate.

You will also see how the pressure in the aorta reaches a maximum during ventricular systole and falls during diastole. This pressure can be measured and forms the basis of widely used blood pressure measurements (see section B2.10).

The regulation of heart rate

The heart contains a specialised type of muscle known as **cardiac muscle**. Other types of muscle (skeletal and smooth muscle) require nerve impulses to cause them to contract. In contrast, cardiac muscle is **myogenic** – it will contract in a regular pattern without any nerve input.

Contraction of heart muscle is initiated by a small patch of specialised cardiac muscle on the wall of the right atrium known as the **sinoatrial node** or **SAN** (Figure 15.31). This is also known as the pacemaker because it maintains the regular contraction of the heart.

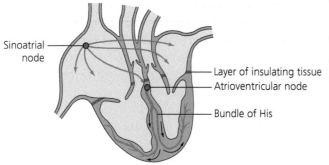

▲ Figure 15.31 Electrical activity in the heart that coordinates the heartbeat

The SAN generates electrical signals that spread out over the surface of the right and left atria, causing them to depolarise, leading to contraction (atrial systole). This electric activity is unable to pass directly to the muscle of the ventricles as there is a layer of collagen that acts as an electrical insulator between the atria and the ventricles.

However, these electrical signals reach another patch of specialised cardiac muscle known as the **atrioventricular node** or **AVN**. After a brief pause, the AVN generates more electrical signals that pass along another type of specialised muscle cells that act like nerve fibres. These are known as the **bundle of His** because they were discovered by the anatomist

Wilhelm His. The electrical activity (depolarisation) generated passes down the muscle separating the two ventricles and then passes up the walls of the two ventricles. As it does, it initiates contraction of the ventricles.

There are two important consequences of this complex arrangement:
1   The pause caused by the AVN means that the atria can complete their emptying into the ventricles before the ventricles start to contract.
2   Contraction of the ventricles from the base of the heart upwards, towards the pulmonary artery and aorta, means that the ventricles are not trying to pump blood against a blind end.

Left to itself, the heart would maintain a regular heartbeat. However, we know that heart rate increases in times of stress or when we exercise. This is under nervous control, coordinated by the **cardioregulatory centre** in the medulla, as shown in Figure 15.32. Two types of receptors, **chemoreceptors** and **pressure receptors**, detect changes in the acidity of the blood and blood pressure. These are located in the aorta and in the **carotid arteries** that pass through the neck to the brain. The cardioregulatory centre responds to inputs from these receptors and sends nerve impulses to the SAN that either speed up or slow down the heart rate.

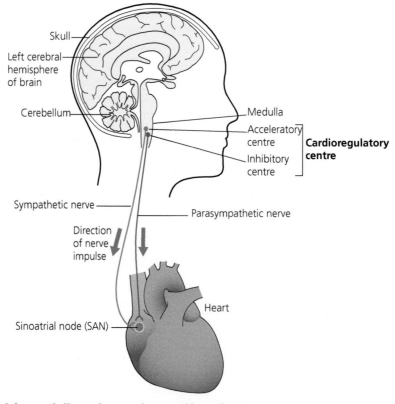

▲ Figure 15.32 Role of the medulla in the regulation of heartbeat

Use of electrocardiography (ECG) to monitor heart activity

The electrical activity of heart muscle that causes the heartbeat can be detected using electrocardiography (ECG). Electrodes are placed on the skin to detect electrical signals and produce an electrocardiogram (also abbreviated to ECG). Figure 15.33 shows an ECG of a healthy heart.

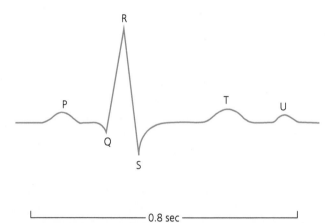

▲ Figure 15.33 ECG showing one beat of a healthy heart

This shows several distinctive waves caused by the heart activity:

▶ The **P wave** is caused by depolarisation of the atria initiated by the electrical signals generated by the SAN (atrial systole).
▶ The **QRS complex** is caused by depolarisation of the ventricles initiated by the electrical signals generated by the AVN and transmitted along the bundle of His (ventricular systole).
▶ The **T wave** is caused by repolarisation of the ventricles (diastole).
▶ The cause of the **U wave** is not certain and it is not always present in normal patients, although it can be exaggerated in some forms of cardiac disease.

Figure 15.34 shows a normal ECG trace together with examples of types of heart disease.

Atrial fibrillation is a faster and more irregular heartbeat caused by disorganised electrical signals in the atria. It is the most common serious abnormal heart rhythm that affects more than 33 million people worldwide.

Ventricular fibrillation is caused by disorganised electrical signals in the ventricles causing them to twitch randomly rather than contracting in an organised way. If it is not treated it can rapidly lead to cardiac arrest (the heart stops beating) and death.

Normal Sinus Rhythm

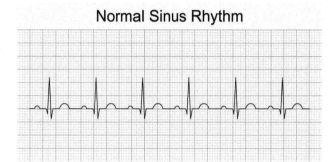

Atrial Fibrillation (AF)

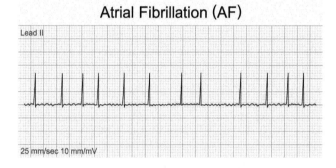

Ventricular Fibrillation (VF)

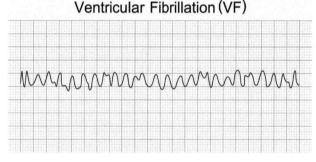

▲ Figure 15.34 ECGs of normal heart rhythm (top), atrial fibrillation (middle) and ventricular fibrillation (bottom)

Other abnormalities can also be diagnosed by ECG, including:

▶ **tachycardia**, where the heart beats too rapidly – a resting heart rate greater than 100 beats per minute (bpm). The peaks on the ECG are too close together
▶ **bradycardia**, where the heart beats too slowly – a resting heart rate less than 60 bpm. The peaks are too far apart
▶ **ectopic heartbeat**, where the heart beats too early, followed by a pause. This is quite common and usually does not require any treatment.

Note that a resting heart rate of less than 60 bpm is not necessarily a sign of heart disease. Highly trained athletes can have resting heart rates of 50 bpm or less.

Blood groups

We saw in section B1.29 how all body cells have **antigens** on their plasma membranes that allow the immune system to distinguish between self and non-self.

Two types of these antigens are found in the plasma membranes of erythrocytes and form the basis of the two most important types of blood group: **ABO** and **Rhesus (Rh)**.

The **ABO system** is used to indicate the presence of one, both or neither of the A and B antigens on erythrocytes.

▶ Group A blood only has the A antigen.
▶ Group B blood only has the B antigen.
▶ Group AB blood has both antigens.
▶ Group O blood has neither antigen.

This system is of great importance in **blood transfusion**. You would normally be given blood of the same **blood type** as your own, otherwise your immune system will recognise it as foreign. However, a person with type AB blood will have both antigens, so their immune system will not recognise A, B or O types of blood as foreign. Similarly, because type O blood does not contain either antigen, it can be given to recipients of any ABO blood type. Fortunately, type O blood is the most common type in Western Europe.

The **Rh system** is based around another set of antigens on erythrocytes. There are 49 defined Rh antigens, of which the **RhD** is by far the most common. According to the NHS (**www.nhs.uk/conditions/blood-groups**), about 85 per cent of the UK population have the RhD antigen and are described as **Rh positive** while about 15 per cent lack the antigen and are described as **Rh negative**.

As group O and Rh positive are the most common, it is not surprising that O positive is the most common blood type. However, O negative is probably the most useful. Because these individuals do not carry ABO or Rh antigens, they are known as 'universal donors' as their blood can be given to almost all recipients. Although they form only about 8 per cent of the UK population, about 13 per cent of blood donors in the UK have O negative blood, so the donation rates are higher than average in response to this demand for their blood type.

Test yourself

1 Blood vessels have similarities and differences.
   a Name one feature that is common to arteries, veins and capillaries.
   b Give one difference between the structure of arteries and the structure of veins.
2 Describe the path through the heart taken by blood from the vena cava via the lungs to the aorta. Include all the valves and the main blood vessels in your answer.
3 Explain why the human cardiovascular system is described as a double circulation system.
4 Describe:
   a the role of the sinoatrial node (SAN) in how the heart maintains a steady rate of contraction without nerve impulses
   b the role of the AVN and bundle of His.

B2.7 The reproductive system in males and females

At its simplest, **sexual reproduction** involves formation of male and female **gametes**. Male gametes are **sperm cells** (also known as **spermatozoa**). Female gametes are **egg cells** (also known as **ova**). In the process of **fertilisation**, the gametes fuse to form a **zygote** (fertilised egg cell). The zygote develops into an **embryo** and then a **foetus**. This is covered in more detail below.

First we have to consider the components of the female and male reproductive systems (Figure 15.35).

Key terms

Gametes: haploid cells (half the number of chromosomes) that are produced by **meiosis**, a type of cell division that halves the number of chromosomes.

Fertilisation: involves fusion of haploid gametes (sperm and egg) to form the **diploid** zygote with the full number of chromosomes.

Components and organisation of the female reproductive system

Ovaries

The ovaries produce the female gametes (egg cells). Usually, one egg is released in every menstrual cycle. For more detail on the menstrual cycle, see section B2.1.

Fallopian tubes

The fallopian tubes connect the ovaries with the **uterus**. An egg cell that is released from the ovary is drawn into the fallopian tube where it may meet a sperm cell and fertilisation may occur. The fertilised or unfertilised egg cell passes down the fallopian tube to the uterus. A fertilised egg will have become an embryo by this stage and will become implanted in the wall of the **uterus**. An unfertilised egg will pass out of the uterus with the **menstrual flow**.

Uterus and cervix

The **cervix** is a ring of muscle that acts as a barrier to the **uterus**. Cervical mucus helps to either block or promote passage of sperm from the vagina to the uterus at different stages in the menstrual cycle. If an egg is fertilised and becomes an embryo, it will implant in the wall of the uterus and will develop into the foetus. The cervix remains closed during pregnancy and a plug of cervical mucus helps keep pathogens from infecting the fetus. At the end of pregnancy, the hypothalamus (see B2.1, page 302) releases the hormone **oxytocin**. This stimulates contraction of the muscular wall of the uterus, which causes pressure of the baby's head on the cervix, causing the cervix to start to **dilate** (get wider). This leads to the release of more oxytocin, stimulating even more contraction of the uterus. This is an example of **positive feedback** where movement away from a normal level (in this case, contraction of the uterus) leads to movement even further away from the normal level. This usually leads to rapid delivery of the baby.

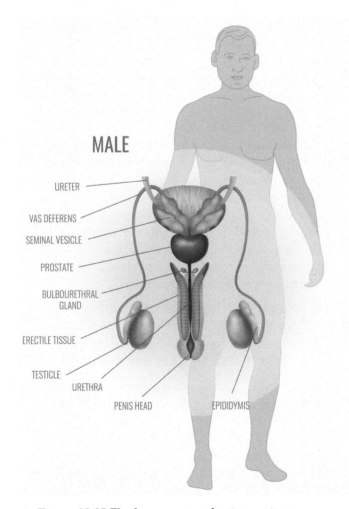

MALE

URETER
VAS DEFERENS
SEMINAL VESICLE
PROSTATE
BULBOURETHRAL GLAND
ERECTILE TISSUE
TESTICLE
URETHRA
PENIS HEAD
EPIDIDYMIS

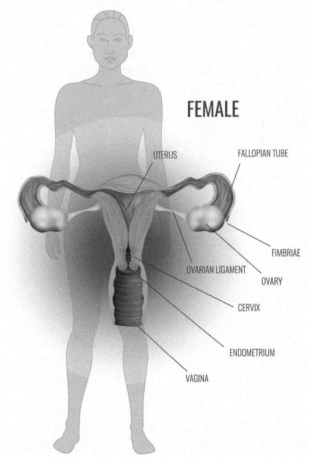

FEMALE

UTERUS
FALLOPIAN TUBE
FIMBRIAE
OVARIAN LIGAMENT
OVARY
CERVIX
ENDOMETRIUM
VAGINA

▲ Figure 15.35 The human reproductive system

Vagina

The **vagina** is the elastic, muscular part of the female reproductive system. It stretches from the **external genitalia** or **vulva** to the cervix. The vagina fulfils three functions:

▶ It receives sperm during sexual intercourse.
▶ It forms the **birth canal** along which the baby moves during childbirth.
▶ It allows loss of menstrual blood when the lining of the uterus breaks down during each cycle.

> **Key term**
>
> **Genitalia**: the male and female sex organs.

Components and organisation of the male reproductive system

While the female reproductive system is mostly internal (inside the body), the male reproductive system is largely external (on the outside of the body).

External organs

Penis and urethra

The **penis** has a dual function. The **urethra** connects to the **bladder** and provides an exit from the body for **urine** (see section B2.8). The urethra is also connected, via the **vas deferens**, to the testes (see section B2.1), which is where sperm is produced. During sexual arousal, the erectile tissue of the penis fills with blood which causes the penis to become erect. This allows it to be inserted into the vagina of the female during sexual intercourse. **Semen**, which contains sperm, is expelled through the end of the penis (a process called **ejaculation**) when the man reaches a **sexual climax** or **orgasm**. (When the penis is erect, the flow of urine into the urethra is blocked so that only semen is ejaculated.)

Scrotum and testes

The **testes** produce sperm and are contained within the **scrotum**. This is a relatively loose sac of skin that hangs below and behind the penis. By holding the testes outside of the core body, they are maintained at a slightly lower temperature than normal body temperature; this is essential for normal sperm development.

Internal organs

Vas deferens and seminal vesicles

The **vas deferens** is a long, muscular tube which carries sperm from the testis to the urethra. There is one on each side. Each vas deferens meets the **seminal vesicles** just before it enters the urethra at the base of the bladder. The seminal vesicles produce a fluid rich in the sugar fructose that provides sperm with a source of energy to help them move once they reach the vagina.

Prostate

The **prostate gland**, which surrounds the urethra just below the bladder, also contributes fluid that helps to nourish the sperm. The combination of sperm with the seminal fluid and fluid from the prostate forms **semen** (also known as **ejaculate**).

> **Practice point**
>
> The prostate gland is often misspelled as the 'prostrate gland'. 'Prostrate' means 'lying with the face down' and is nothing to do with the male reproductive system.

Functions of the reproductive system

Sexual reproduction involves male and female gametes fusing in the process of fertilisation. In one sense, it provides a mechanism for the survival of the species by producing offspring through the combination of gametes (eggs and sperm). However, you will have learned from studying genetics in section B1.13 (page 244) that sexual reproduction means that offspring inherit characteristics from both parents. This leads to greater variation, meaning that some organisms can become better adapted to their environments. This gives some a survival advantage and is the basis of **evolution**.

The female reproductive system has two functions:

▶ to produce egg cells – this occurs during the menstrual cycle and has been covered in section B2.1
▶ to protect and nourish an offspring until birth.

The second function is carried out by the **uterus** and the **placenta**. As the embryo develops, part of the embryo grows into the wall of the uterus. This is the placenta, and it has a rich blood supply that is in very close contact with the mother's blood supply. This allows for exchange of gases (oxygen and carbon dioxide), supply of nutrients (glucose, amino acids, etc.) and removal of waste products via the mother. The foetus is also contained within protective membranes in the fluid-filled amniotic sac that provides additional protection.

The male reproductive system has one function: to produce and deposit sperm, as described above.

B2.8 The renal system

The renal system has two main functions:
▶ **excretion** or removal from the body of **nitrogenous waste** in the form of **urea**
▶ **osmoregulation** or regulation of the water balance of the body. This aspect was covered in section B2.1.

Proteins and nucleic acids both contain nitrogen. We normally take in more nitrogen-containing compounds in our food than we need daily. Any excess is converted by the **liver** to **urea**. The urea is transported in the blood to the kidneys where it is removed from the blood during the process of formation of **urine**.

The renal system is sometimes called the **urinary system** and is closely connected with the reproductive system. For this reason, the two systems are sometimes referred to as the **genitourinary system**.

Components and organisation of the renal system

Kidney

The **kidneys** form the main part of the renal system. If you look at Figure 15.36 you will see that the kidneys are supplied by the left and right **renal arteries**. Blood leaves the kidney via the **renal veins**. Urine, formed in the kidney, is transported via the **ureter** to the **bladder** where it is stored prior to **urination**.

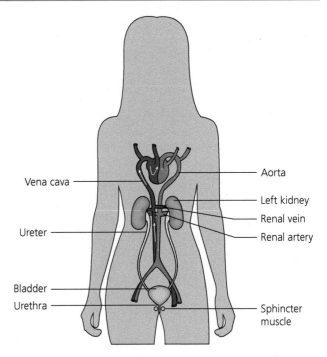

▲ Figure 15.36 The urinary system

Nephron

Each kidney contains about 1 million nephrons. The **nephron** is the main functional unit of the kidney. It is like a long, U-shaped tube surrounded by capillaries. Many nephrons connect with collecting ducts that take what has become urine towards the ureter and then the bladder. The nephron is where the blood is filtered and where water and other useful substances are reabsorbed, leading to the production of urine.

The length of the nephron means that there is a large surface area for exchange. The wall of the nephron is a single layer of **epithelial** cells that is in close contact with capillaries whose walls are a single layer of **endothelial** cells. This means that there is a short diffusion pathway. Finally, the unusual layout of the nephron, with **the loop of Henle** (Figure 15.37), helps to maintain a concentration gradient. We can see, therefore, that the nephron has all the characteristics of a good exchange surface as described in section B1.10. This will be covered in more detail below.

Ureter, bladder and urethra

The left and right ureters take urine from each kidney to the bladder where it is stored until the bladder is emptied via the urethra in the process of **urination**.

In males, the urethra is intimately connected with the reproductive system described in section B2.7. In females, the urethra is shorter and leads to an opening within the vulva next to the vaginal opening.

The functions of the renal system

Filtration of the blood to remove urea and reabsorption of water, glucose, amino acids and other useful substances all occur in the nephron (Figure 15.37).

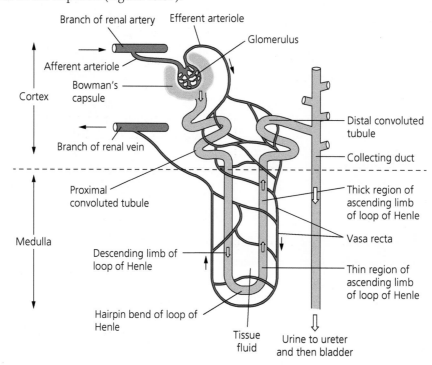

▲ Figure 15.37 One nephron and associated blood vessels. The flow of blood is shown with black arrows and the flow of filtrate and urine with white arrows

Removal of waste products from the body

Urea is removed from the blood by the process of **ultrafiltration**. This occurs at the start of the nephron in **Bowman's capsule**. If you look at the blood vessels in Figure 15.37 you will notice how a branch of the renal artery leads to an **afferent arteriole**. This then divides into many capillaries in the space surrounded by Bowman's capsule. This knot or tangle of capillaries is known as the **glomerulus**. The capillaries of the glomerulus come together to form the **efferent**

arteriole. The efferent arteriole leads to another network of capillaries that surround the rest of the nephron before joining a branch of the renal vein. The term afferent means 'leading in' and efferent means 'leading out'.

Because the diameter of the efferent arteriole is smaller than that of the afferent arteriole, high pressure develops in the glomerulus. This pressure forces out fluids from the capillaries and into the lumen (space inside) of the nephron, forming the **filtrate** (i.e. the product of filtering). The filtrate contains water, small molecules such as glucose and amino acids, mineral ions such as sodium, potassium and chloride, and also urea. Only red blood cells and large proteins are unable to pass into the filtrate.

Process of urine production

The filtrate then moves along the length of the nephron. The changes to the composition of the filtrate in the nephron lead to it eventually becoming urine. The urine enters the collecting duct and from there is taken via the ureter to the bladder.

Reabsorption

Many of the substances dissolved in the blood are required by the body and so must be reabsorbed. These include glucose and amino acids. These are reabsorbed by a mechanism of co-transport that is very similar to the mechanism illustrated in Figure 12.17, page 242 in section B1.11. This occurs in the first part of the nephron called the **proximal convoluted tubule** (**PCT**).

Mineral ions, such as sodium, potassium, calcium and chloride, may also need to be reabsorbed. This depends on whether there is an excess of them present in the blood or not. This reabsorption takes place mostly towards the end of the nephron in the **distal convoluted tubule** (**DCT**) and is controlled by the mineralocorticoid hormones (mentioned in section B2.1) that regulate the concentrations of mineral ions in the body.

Water is also reabsorbed. However, how much water is reabsorbed depends upon the water balance of the body and this part of the system known as **osmoregulation**.

Role in osmoregulation

Reabsorption of glucose and amino acids occurs in the PCT. As a result of the molecules entering the epithelial cells, the water potential of those cells falls. Therefore, water moves out of the filtrate down a water potential gradient by **osmosis** (see sections B1.11 and B2.1).

Most of the reabsorption of water occurs in the **collecting duct** that passes through the **medulla**. If you look at Figure 15.37 you will see that the loop of Henle is shaped like a hairpin, i.e. folded back on itself. As the filtrate passes **up** the **ascending limb**, Na^+ and Cl^- ions are pumped out into the surrounding medulla, from where they diffuse into the **descending limb**. The effect of this is to cause the highest concentration of ions in the filtrate at the bottom of the loop of Henle. This means that, moving down the medulla, the concentration of ions in the medulla surrounding the collecting duct **increases**. The water potential **decreases** in the same direction.

As a result, there is a constant water potential gradient from the collecting duct to the surrounding medulla. As water moves out of the collecting duct by osmosis, the water potential of the filtrate in the collecting duct falls. However, as it moves further down the collecting duct it meets medulla where the water potential is even lower. Therefore, there is a constant water potential gradient that moves water out of the filtrate by osmosis.

This is how water is reabsorbed in the collecting duct. At the end of this process the filtrate has become **urine**.

The urine will be more or less concentrated, depending on how much water is reabsorbed. This is controlled by the hormone **ADH**; the mechanism of this is described in section B2.1. ADH acts by stimulating an increase in aquaporins in the epithelial cells of the collecting duct, thereby increasing the permeability of the collecting duct leading to greater water reabsorption. This also explains how drinking alcohol can lead to dehydration as alcohol inhibits ADH and so inhibits reabsorption of water.

Role in homeostasis

Homeostasis is the regulation of the internal environment of the body. **Osmoregulation** is an important part of this. Regulating the water balance of the body also plays a part in maintaining blood pressure. A rise in blood pressure can be caused by a rise in blood volume. More water is removed by the kidney when release of ADH by the pituitary is inhibited and this leads to reduction in blood pressure.

Another mechanism is the **renin-angiotensin** system. Renin is an enzyme produced in the kidney when there is a fall in blood pressure. The renin-angiotensinogen system operates to stimulate release of ADH from the pituitary and this leads to an increase in reabsorption of water, resulting in an increase in blood pressure.

Test yourself

1 Describe the process of ultrafiltration.
2 Describe how the loop of Henle assists in the reabsorption of water from the collecting duct.
3 Describe the role of ADH in osmoregulation.
4 Describe the role of the renin-angiotensin system in homeostasis.

B2.9 The integumentary system

If you were asked to name the organs of the human body you would probably focus on the *internal* organs and overlook the skin. However, as well as being the heaviest organ, the skin has a number of important functions. It is a part of the **integumentary system**, which also includes hair and nails.

Key terms

Integument: a tough outer protective layer.

Integumentary system: includes the skin, exocrine glands, hair and nails.

Components and organisation of the integumentary system

Skin

The strong surface layer of the skin is the **epidermis** (Figure 15.38) which consists of **squamous** (flattened) **epithelial** cells. These are continually worn away and so the epidermis is regenerated by division of **stem cells** in the lowest layer of the epidermis. There are no blood vessels in the epidermis, so it obtains nutrients from the underlying dermis. The protein **keratin** (the main fibrous protein of **hair** and **nails**) helps to waterproof the epidermis.

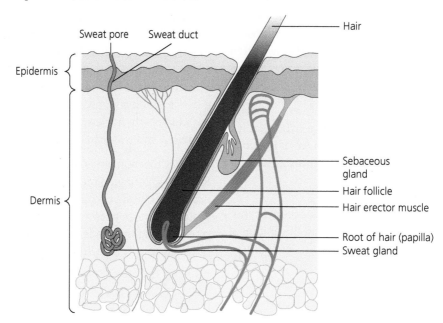

Sweat pore Sweat duct Hair
Epidermis
Dermis
Sebaceous gland
Hair follicle
Hair erector muscle
Root of hair (papilla)
Sweat gland

▲ Figure 15.38 Cross section of human skin

Lying below the epidermis is the **dermis**. This is a layer of connective tissue that helps to support the epidermis as well as making the skin elastic. There are many blood vessels and nerve endings in the dermis as well as the **hair follicles** and **exocrine glands** (**sweat glands** and **sebaceous glands**). See section B2.1 for a description of exocrine glands.

Hair consists of the fibrous protein **keratin** and grows outwards from **hair follicles** that are lined with epithelial cells.

Functions of the integumentary system

Protection

An essential function of the skin is to act as a physical barrier to infection. This was mentioned in section B1.30, page 255. However, the skin is not just a physical barrier. Antimicrobial peptides are produced by skin cells and exocrine glands and help to protect against infection by bacteria and fungi. In addition, we have a population of benign bacteria that live on our skin and help to prevent infection by pathogens such as other bacteria or fungi.

Temperature regulation

The importance of the **hypothalamus** in homeostasis was mentioned in section B2.1 and homeostasis will be discussed in more detail in section B2.12. Regulation of body temperature is controlled and coordinated by the hypothalamus, but the skin is an important **receptor** and **effector**.

The main **temperature receptors** are in the hypothalamus itself and monitor core body temperature (the temperature of the internal organs, which is often higher than the temperature of the body surface). However, **peripheral temperature receptors** are located in the skin and monitor the external temperature. The hypothalamus uses inputs from both types of receptor.

There are three main mechanisms under the control of the hypothalamus by which the skin helps to maintain an almost constant body temperature:

▶ **Sweat glands** release sweat when the body temperatures rises. Thermal energy from the skin and blood in capillaries close to the surface of the skin is transferred to the water in sweat, causing it to evaporate. This transfer of thermal energy cools the skin.

▶ **Arterioles** supplying the capillaries near the surface of the skin can constrict (**vasoconstriction**) or dilate (**vasodilation**), as shown in Figure 15.39.

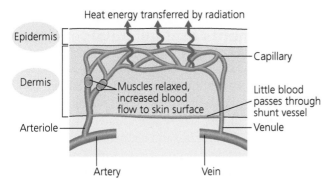

▲ Figure 15.39a Vasodilation in the skin

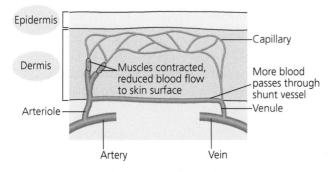

▲ Figure 15.39b Vasoconstriction in the skin

When the core body temperature rises, nerve impulses from the hypothalamus cause the muscles in the walls of the arterioles in the dermis to relax. This causes **vasodilation** – the diameter of the arterioles increases. As a result, more blood can flow through the capillaries close to the surface of the skin and so more thermal energy is transferred to the surroundings.

When the core body temperature falls, nerve impulses from the hypothalamus cause contraction of the muscles in the walls of the same arterioles. This causes vasoconstriction – the diameter of the arterioles decreases. As a result, less blood flows through the capillaries close to the surface of the skin and is diverted through the **shunt vessel** to a venule. A shunt vessel is a small

vessel connecting the arteriole to the venule, bypassing the capillaries. This means that less thermal energy is transferred by radiation.

The final mechanism involves **hairs** on the skin. A fall in core body temperature causes the hypothalamus to send nerve impulses to the **hair erector muscles**. This causes them to contract, which raises the hairs. As a result, a thicker layer of air is trapped next to the skin and forms an insulating layer, reducing heat loss. If the core body temperature rises, nerve impulses from the hypothalamus cause the erector muscles to **relax** and so the hair lies flat, reducing the thickness of the insulating layer. During human evolution, thick body hair has been replaced by clothes, so this mechanism is more important for other mammals than for us. We can still see the mechanism in action when we are cold and get 'goosebumps' – this is caused by contraction of the erector muscles.

Vitamin D synthesis

Vitamin D or **cholecalciferol** is, strictly speaking, not a vitamin. This is because it is made in the lower layers of the skin epidermis. This reaction is dependent on sunlight. Therefore, in the absence of sunlight, there can be a deficiency in vitamin D, meaning that it needs to be consumed in the diet. Vitamin D is fat soluble and relatively few foods contain significant levels of the vitamin. However, in many countries (including the UK) vitamin D is added to some foods such as milk and breakfast cereals.

Vitamin D works together with PTH and calcitonin to regulate the calcium balance of the body (see section B2.1).

Cutaneous sensation

Four different types of **mechanoreceptors** in the dermis respond to pressure and vibration. Between them they produce the sense of touch. The details are complex and not fully understood, but there are differences between the speed of nerve conduction that is related to the diameter and myelination of the neurones. Some of these respond to skin movement whereas others respond to static indentation of the skin. They have a large diameter and high degree of myelination and so conduct nerve signals most quickly. Another type is the most sensitive and these are responsible for rapid pain sensation. Finally, the most common type is the group known as C fibres. They are activated by mechanical and thermal stimuli as well as chemicals such as capsaicin (the chemical in chilli peppers that produces the burning sensation).

Excretion

Sweat glands (Figure 15.38) are an example of exocrine glands because they secrete their products onto a surface rather than into the blood. Although the main function of sweat is to help reduce body temperature, sweat contains inorganic ions and urea and so plays a part in excretion.

Sebaceous glands are another exocrine gland that excrete the oily substance sebum. This helps to lubricate the skin and hair. Sebum also keeps the skin slightly acidic, which helps protect against microbes.

> ### Test yourself
>
> 1 Describe two functions in the skin of the protein keratin.
> 2 Describe two functions of sweat glands.
> 3 Explain why vitamin D is often added to foods in northern European countries.

B2.10 Physiological measurements

So far in this chapter we have covered the key areas of human physiology, particularly how blood pressure, heart rate, respiratory (breathing) rate and body temperature are regulated. Therefore, in any situation where we are monitoring the health or disease state of an individual, we need to be able to measure those and compare them to the **normal** or **average range**.

Normal expected ranges for physiological measurements

The table shows the average range of the four key physiological measurement in adults. These ranges can be significantly different in children.

Physiological measurements	Average range for an adult
Blood pressure	systolic 90–120 mmHg diastolic 60–80 mmHg
Heart rate	60 to 100 beats per minute (bpm)
Respiratory rate (at rest)	12 to 20 breaths per minute (bpm)
Temperature	36 °C to 37.5 °C

Blood pressure is always shown as systolic then diastolic, for example, 120/80 mmHg. This is often referred to as '120 over 80'.

> ### Key terms
>
> **Blood pressure:** usually measured in mmHg (millimetres of mercury). Although the units of pressure are usually kPa, the unit mmHg relates to how blood pressure was (and often still is) measured – see section B2.11.
>
> **Systolic:** the pressure when the heart contracts.
>
> **Diastolic:** the pressure when the heart relaxes; always lower than the systolic pressure.

How to identify physiological measurements that fall outside of the normal range

If you have ever spent time in hospital, as a patient or otherwise, you will be aware of nurses taking regular **observations** (or **obs**). These will usually cover blood pressure, pulse (heart rate) and temperature, although other factors may be monitored in specific cases, such as **neurological observations** in patients who are unconscious or have a suspected neurological disorder. The frequency of these observations will depend on the status of the patient.

By regularly recording these physiological measurements it is possible to identify if any of them fall outside the normal range. More importantly, they can indicate a possible worsening in the patient's condition – or an improvement.

The techniques used are covered in section B2.11, but they can include manual measurements, electronic monitoring equipment used by the health practitioner or continuous automated monitoring equipment, often linked to a computer, of the type seen in an **intensive care unit** (**ICU**).

Factors that contribute to measurements outside of normal parameters

Age

Blood pressure in children is lower than in adults, increasing to the adult 'normal' of 120/80 mmHg by the age of 17–18 years. Blood pressure tends to increase with age as artery walls become less elastic.

In children, there are slight differences between boys and girls, with boys having a slightly higher normal blood pressure. Also, the height of a child more than actual age may determine blood pressure.

The normal resting heart rate for children is higher than for the typical adult. The normal resting heart rate for babies up to 3 months is 107–181 bpm.

Resting heart rate remains fairly constant in adults, with little change as we age. Other factors have more effect than age.

Weight

Excess weight (i.e. a higher BMI – see Chapter A9, page 163) can increase blood pressure above the typical level for the person's age. This can mean an increase in resting heart rate as the heart has to work harder to pump against the higher pressure.

At the same time, fat distribution is important. **Subcutaneous** fat lies in the lower level of the dermis (see Figure 15.38). However, **visceral fat**, which surrounds the internal organs such as heart and liver, is a bigger health risk and can lead to increased blood pressure and increased risk of **cardiovascular disease** and **Type 2 diabetes**.

Exercise

If you do regular weight training, your muscles become bigger and stronger. The same is true of the heart muscle if you regularly undertake **cardiovascular** or **cardio** exercise, such as running or cycling. The heart needs to pump harder to provide the body with oxygen and nutrients when doing strenuous exercise and responds by becoming larger. This means that it pumps more blood with each stroke – the **stroke volume** increases – and so it does not need to beat as fast when at rest. Therefore, the resting heart rate of a well-trained athlete will be below 60 bpm, perhaps even as low as 40 bpm.

Gender

It is only in recent years that sex-based differences in normal physiology have been fully recognised. The differences between **body mass** and **body composition** in men and women are well known. The sex hormones also have an obvious effect on the different development of men and women. However, there are also less obvious differences.

Men have larger lungs than women, even when adjusted for height differences. This means that the maximum exercise capacity in women may be limited by lung capacity, especially as they age.

Men also have larger left ventricles, which makes the stroke volume greater in men. There are even sex-related differences in the types of muscle proteins.

During pregnancy, the **functional residual capacity (FRC)** of the lungs can fall. FRC is the amount of air left in the lungs after a normal passive exhalation. This is due to the increased pressure on the diaphragm by the uterus and the reduction in FRC increases as pregnancy advances. However, there are other changes in the respiratory system during pregnancy, partly in response to increased levels of progesterone. These help to maintain the efficiency of the gas exchange system so that the foetus is given sufficient oxygen.

Pre-menopausal women tend to have a lower resting blood pressure and higher resting heart rate. However, blood pressure usually rises to equivalent levels to those of men after the **menopause**.

Summary

You will see that the overall state of health of an individual will contribute to whether their physiological measurements lie within or outside normal parameters. Therefore, a person who takes regular exercise, eats a balanced diet and has no underlying health conditions is likely to have physiological measurements within the normal range, whereas lack of exercise, poor diet or poor health can all lead to measurements outside the normal range.

Research

Think about what we have covered so far about human physiology and physiological measurements. Can you see any common themes emerging?

How do physiological measurements give a picture of a person's overall health and level of fitness?

Choose an area of interest to you – such as sport science, ageing, mental health or wellbeing – and research how understanding of physiology and use of physiological measurement can enable us to do things like:

▶ assess patients and/or healthy individuals
▶ monitor patients, athletes and others
▶ diagnose disease and predict outcomes.

You could use an internet search to help you, although you need to be careful – not everyone is giving impartial or even informed advice or information. There are many who have a product to sell or an agenda to promote.

One place to start is the Public Health Action Support Team (PHAST) website: www.healthknowledge.org.uk

This is part of the Department of Health and is aimed at supporting the continuing professional development of those working in the fields of health and social care.

1 For each of the following, explain whether the physiological measurements fall outside the normal range and would require further investigation:

   a an elderly woman with blood pressure of 120/80 mmHg, resting heart rate of 90 bpm and resting respiration rate of 30 bpm

   b a young child with a resting heart rate of 110 bpm

   c a middle-aged man with a sedentary lifestyle (i.e. takes very little exercise) who has a resting heart rate of 105 bpm and a blood pressure of 140/95 mmHg

   d a female athlete with a resting heart rate of 50 bpm and a blood pressure of 120/80 mmHg.

2 Describe two consequences of obesity (excess body mass).

B2.11 How physiological parameters are routinely measured

Blood pressure

Blood pressure has traditionally been measured using a **sphygmomanometer** and **stethoscope** (Figure 15.40). The measuring device shows the pressure in the cuff. The cuff is inflated to well above the expected systolic pressure. A valve on the cuff is opened and the cuff pressure slowly decreases. When the cuff pressure equals the systolic pressure, blood begins to flow past the cuff, causing sounds that can be heard with the stethoscope. These sounds continue until the cuff pressure falls below the diastolic pressure.

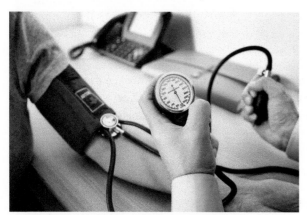

▲ Figure 15.40 Measuring blood pressure with a sphygmomanometer and stethoscope

An earlier type of sphygmomanometer used a column of mercury to measure the pressure – hence the units mmHg. Some practitioners still prefer these older types. Unlike the newer type, they do not need periodic recalibration to remain accurate.

More recently, electronic blood pressure monitors have become widespread. They require less skill to use, measure pulse rate at the same time and can also be used in continual monitoring, e.g. in the ICU. Some types are not very expensive and can be used to monitor your own blood pressure (Figure 15.41).

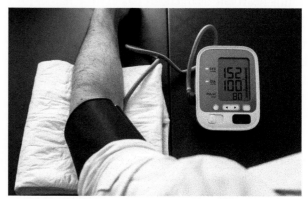

▲ Figure 15.41 A person using a blood pressure monitor to measure their own blood pressure

Pulse

The simplest way to measure heart rate is to measure the **pulse** (see section B2.6). The **radial pulse** is measured using two fingers placed on the wrist and a watch to count beats per minute. The **apical pulse** is measured using a stethoscope placed on the chest directly above the top of the heart. It is generally simpler to measure the radial pulse, although it can be difficult to measure in newborns and children under five. The apical pulse is therefore better used for individuals in this group.

Wristwatches are not usually allowed, for hygiene reasons, and so a fob watch worn on the uniform (Figure 15.42) is used instead.

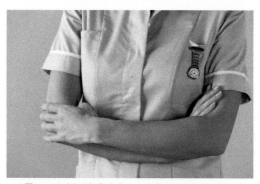

▲ Figure 15.42 A fob watch worn on the uniform

A more recent method to measure the heart rate is to use a **pulse oximeter**. This is typically placed on a finger and shines light through the skin. The oximeter measures how much light is absorbed and then uses this to calculate both pulse and the oxygen saturation of the blood.

▶ During each contraction of the heart, blood is forced through the capillaries. This increases their volume. The volume decreases between heartbeats. More light is absorbed when the volume increases and so the pulse can be detected and counted.

▶ Blood that is saturated with oxygen absorbs more red light than blood that is less saturated. This difference in absorbance is measured by the pulse oximeter and converted to a figure for percentage saturation.

Pulse oximeters have two advantages over manual pulse measurement:

▶ They give a measurement of oxygen saturation as well as heart rate.

▶ They can be connected to computers or data loggers to provide continual monitoring.

Practice point

Pulse oximeters have been widely used during the COVID-19 pandemic and have been given to patients infected with SARS-CoV-2 who are not sufficiently ill to need hospital treatment, to enable them to monitor their own condition from home. The normal range for oxygen saturation of the blood is 95–100 per cent. Patients are told to call 111 if the pulse oximeter reading falls to 94 per cent or 93 per cent and to call 999 if it falls to 92 per cent or less.

Arterial blood pressure can be monitored, for example, in the course of an electrocardiogram (ECG) or with a pulse oximeter. This makes it possible to observe the dicrotic notch and dicrotic wave (see section B2.6). As we age, these tend to come later after the peak arterial pressure. However, in some forms of cardiovascular disease, the dicrotic notch becomes less distinct. In severe cardiovascular disease this can be detected as a second or dicrotic pulse.

Temperature

Body temperature is measured using a clinical thermometer. Traditionally these were made of a long glass tube with a bulb of mercury at one end and marked in 0.1 °C divisions from 35 °C to 42 °C.

The thermometer is placed under the tongue, in the armpit or in the rectum. After a few minutes the temperature can be read. The disadvantage of this type of thermometer is that it requires sterilisation between patients (or each patient should have their own) and it can be difficult to read. Moreover, glass is easily broken and mercury is toxic.

This type of clinical thermometer has now been replaced almost completely by electronic versions, particularly ones that measure the temperature of the **tympanic membrane** (ear drum) as shown in Figure 15.43.

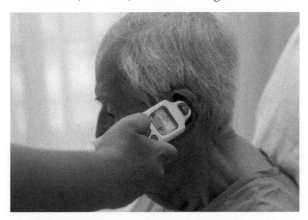

▲ Figure 15.43 A nurse using an electronic thermometer to measure a patient's body temperature

An electronic thermometer will give a much quicker reading than a traditional clinical thermometer. Another advantage of these is that they give a reading much closer to the core body temperature because the hypothalamus (which regulates body temperature) and the tympanic membrane share a blood supply. Other sites where temperature is measured give a reading that might be less accurate.

Electronic thermometers also need to be sterilised between patients, although it is possible to avoid this by using disposable single-use sleeves on the probe.

Respiratory rate

Like heart rate measured by taking the pulse, respiratory rate can be measured very simply by counting breaths per minute using a fob watch.

Essential recognition of any physiological deterioration

We mentioned the importance of regular **clinical observations** (obs) earlier in this section. Clinical obs measure and record the various physiological parameters or **vital signs**. It is essential that these are carried out regularly and recorded (for example, on a patient observation chart) so that it is possible to spot any deterioration in the patient's condition and then take appropriate action.

Test yourself

1 What are the units used to measure blood pressure?
2 Describe two ways of measuring heart rate.
3 Give two disadvantages of a traditional glass clinical thermometer.
4 Give one advantage of an electronic thermometer.
5 What precaution should be taken when using a thermometer for more than one patient?

B2.12 The principles of homeostasis and how this contributes to preserving a healthy body

In previous sections we have looked at several systems that play a part in regulating the function of the body. We will now see how the different physiological systems interconnect to maintain the healthy body.

Principles of homeostasis

Homeostasis is the maintenance of an **almost constant internal environment** despite fluctuations in the external environment.

By internal environment we mean the body temperature, concentration of the blood (e.g. water, glucose), levels of oxygen and carbon dioxide, among other physiological parameters. Note that we use the term 'almost constant' rather than 'constant'. The point about homeostasis is that the levels of all of these fluctuate, but they are maintained within a narrow range. This is because of the way in which negative feedback works (Figure 15.44).

For negative feedback to operate, there has to be a movement (however small) away from the normal level. Negative feedback works in a way that returns the factor to the normal level.

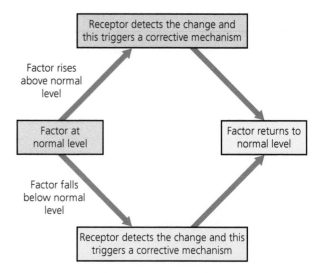

▲ Figure 15.44 Negative feedback

Homeostasis covers several components, most of which have already been discussed in earlier sections:

▶ **Receptors**, such as those that detect the blood concentration of glucose, carbon dioxide or oxygen or the core body temperature.
▶ **Effectors** – these are usually glands or muscles – that make changes such as secretion of hormones or constriction of blood vessels that return the factor to its normal level.
▶ **Feedback systems** usually involve a control or coordination centre, such as the hypothalamus, that receives inputs from receptors and sends signals (hormones or nerve impulses) to effectors.

Role of the nervous system

We saw how the nervous system is involved in the regulation of body temperature (section B2.9) or heart rate (section B2.6). Nerve impulses travel quickly and so the nervous system is usually involved in the most rapid feedback mechanisms.

Role of the endocrine system

The endocrine system is involved in the regulation of blood glucose (section B2.1) and the water balance of the body (section B2.8) among others. Because hormones are released into the blood and transported to effectors (target organs), the response can be slower than mechanisms involving the nervous system. Therefore, the endocrine system is usually involved in more long-term homeostasis.

However, it is important to understand how the two systems work together in many homeostatic mechanisms, as you will have seen in the various examples in this chapter.

How homeostasis contributes to preserving a healthy body

Bacteria that live in hot springs can survive perfectly well at temperatures close to the boiling point of water. Their enzymes seem remarkably heat-stable when compared to our own, which start to **denature** at temperatures above about 40 °C. This is because human enzymes have evolved alongside the development of a body temperature around 37 °C. Any significant variation above or below that temperature will affect the rate of enzyme-controlled reactions: too low and reactions are too slow; too high and the enzymes lose activity as they start to denature. This explains the need for **thermoregulation**, as described in section B2.9.

The same is true about the water balance in the body. If you observe erythrocytes under a microscope and add pure water, you will see the cells swell and burst as water enters by osmosis. Similarly, if you add a drop of salt solution, you will see the cells shrink and become crinkled as water leaves by osmosis. To function properly, our body cells need to be bathed in a fluid (called **tissue fluid**) that maintains a constant concentration of water. This explains the need for osmoregulation, as described in section B2.8.

Cells need a constant supply of glucose and oxygen for aerobic respiration – this is particularly true of brain cells. The brain is the organ with the highest consumption of glucose and the second highest consumption of oxygen. This explains the need for regulation of blood glucose concentration (section B2.1), breathing rate (section B2.2) and heart rate (section B2.6).

The regulation of the pH of the blood is also an important homeostatic mechanism as enzymes need a constant pH in order to function effectively. Carbon dioxide is an acidic gas and so the concentration of carbon dioxide in the blood is regulated by means of gas exchange in the lungs (section B2.2) and regulation of heart rate (section B2.6).

Test yourself

1 Explain why homeostasis is described as maintenance of an **almost constant** internal environment.
2 Name the two systems involved in homeostasis.
3 Explain the importance of maintaining the following within a narrow range:
   a body temperature
   b water balance
   c blood glucose concentration.

B2.13 How failure of homeostasis mechanisms can impact the body and the subsequent development of disorders

We have seen the importance of homeostasis and the correct operation of homeostasis mechanisms. Therefore, it is not surprising that failure of any of these mechanisms can lead to a number of disorders of different degrees of seriousness.

Failure of homeostasis mechanisms

Failure in a homeostasis mechanism can lead to cells being deprived of key nutrients or being exposed to toxic substances.

Disorders

Type 1 and Type 2 diabetes

Although they have different causes, both types of diabetes involve a breakdown in the homeostasis mechanisms regulating blood glucose concentrations.

Type 1 diabetes

In type 1 diabetes, the body attacks its own beta-cells within the pancreas. As these are the cells that produce insulin, this means that the body cannot produce insulin in response to a rise in blood glucose concentration, e.g. after a meal. This means that the liver and muscles will not take up glucose from the blood and so the blood glucose concentration rises sharply. This leads to excess glucose being excreted by the kidneys, which leads to a sudden fall in blood glucose concentration. These wide swings in blood glucose concentration can have short-term consequences (coma, even death) or long-term consequences such as nerve damage (**neuropathy**) or damage to blood vessels in the eye (**retinopathy**).

Treatment of Type 1 diabetes requires regular insulin injections to replace the insulin that the body does not produce.

Type 2 diabetes

Obesity is one risk factor for developing Type 2 diabetes (genetic factors can be another), with its associated high blood glucose concentration over many years. This can lead to liver and muscle cells becoming unresponsive to insulin and also to reduction in production of insulin meaning muscle and liver cells do not take up as much glucose. This means the normal homeostasis mechanism breaks down.

Treatment of Type 2 diabetes begins with diet – reduced intake of food rich in starch and sugars and increased intake of high-fibre foods – and increased exercise. If this is not successful, anti-diabetic drugs can be prescribed. In some cases, it might be necessary to prescribe insulin injections for Type 2 diabetes.

Heat stroke or hyperthermia

Hyperthermia occurs when the core body temperature rises above the normal range. **Heat stroke** is a sudden increase in body temperature. The normal thermoregulatory mechanisms described in section B2.9 can be overcome by a combination of excessive production of heat (strenuous exercise), high environmental temperatures and reduced heat loss, for example, when high humidity reduces the effectiveness of sweating as a cooling mechanism.

Hot, dry skin is typical in heat stroke as blood vessels dilate in an attempt to increase heat loss from the skin. Severe cases leads to:
- confusion and aggressive behaviour
- increased respiration rate and heart rate (**tachycardia**) as blood pressure drops and the heart tries to maintain adequate circulation
- eventually, organ failure, unconsciousness and possibly death.

Treatment of hyperthermia involves cooling the body, for example, in an ice bath.

Hypothermia occurs when the body temperature falls below the normal level – in humans this means a body temperature less than 35 °C. This is an example of **positive feedback** – where a movement away from the normal level leads to a change even further away from normal. In the case of body temperature, a fall in temperature reduces the rate of metabolic reactions, meaning less heat is generated. This causes the body temperature to fall even further. Positive feedback is not a part of homeostasis mechanisms as these are designed to return a factor to the normal level.

First-aid treatment of hypothermia involves passive warming, i.e. removing cold or wet clothing and keeping the patient insulated. Alcohol should never be given as this makes hypothermia worse. Severe hypothermia requires hospital treatment, often involving infusion of warm fluids to raise the body temperature gradually.

Renal failure

Renal failure is the result of chronic kidney disease, which is usually caused by other conditions that put a strain on the kidneys, such as:
- high blood pressure putting strain on the capillaries in the kidney
- diabetes, where high glucose concentrations damage the filtration mechanism
- high cholesterol leading to build-up of fatty deposits in the renal arteries
- inflammation or infection of the kidney.

We have seen that the kidney plays a key role in two important homeostasis mechanisms, which explains the key symptoms of kidney failure:
- The body retains water, leading to swollen ankles, and production of small volumes of urine as a result of a failure in osmoregulation.
- Accumulation of urea in the blood as a result of the failure of the kidney to excrete urea. As urea is toxic, this can lead to widespread organ damage.

Renal failure cannot be cured, other than by **kidney transplant**, although **renal dialysis** can control the disease by replicating some of the function of the kidney.

Graves' disease

Graves' disease is an autoimmune disease where the body's immune system creates antibodies that mimic TSH and so cause the thyroid gland to become overactive and over-produce thyroid hormones such as **thyroxine**.

Treatment of Graves' disease involves reducing the production of thyroid hormones. This can be done with drugs that interfere with the thyroid's ability to take in iodine, which is used in synthesis of thyroid hormones. Alternatively, radioactive iodine (^{131}I) can be administered. This is taken up by the thyroid and destroys the cells that produce thyroid hormones. The size of the thyroid is gradually reduced, after which the treatment can be stopped.

Sepsis

Sepsis occurs when the immune system over-reacts to an infection, usually in the blood rather than a localised infection. If sepsis is not treated, it can develop very quickly to **septic shock** involving damage to tissues throughout the body, causing multiple organ failure and, if not treated very quickly, death. Sepsis is more common than heart attack and causes more deaths than lung cancer and more than bowel, breast and prostate cancers combined.

Treatment of sepsis involves giving intravenous antibiotics (injected into the blood stream) as quickly as possible. Septic shock can be very difficult to treat as multiple organ failure occurs extremely rapidly.

Practice point

Sepsis illustrates the importance of regular monitoring and recording of clinical obs as these can be the first sign that a patient is deteriorating rapidly.

Test yourself

1 Describe the differences between Type 1 and Type 2 diabetes in terms of:
   a causes
   b treatments.
2 Describe the two types of homeostatic mechanism involved in hyperthermia and hypothermia.
3 Name two conditions that can lead to renal failure.
4 Suggest why injection of radioactive iodine is a more effective treatment of Graves' disease than other forms of radiation therapy.

B2.14–15 Different classification systems and their purpose; the most widely used classification systems of diseases and disorders

There is a saying in the world of business, 'what you can measure, you can manage', and the same is true in healthcare, which is why classification systems for different types of diseases or health conditions are important. The **World Health Organization (WHO)** is an agency of the United Nations that promotes health and monitors disease in an attempt to achieve good health for all. WHO has established a Family of International Classifications (FIC) to provide a common language for health information worldwide.

Classification systems

There are several different classification systems in use, but we will concentrate on just three, as shown in the table.

Type of classification	What conditions are classified under this classification type	Example
Topographic	bodily region	cardiovascular
Anatomic	organ or tissue	heart
Physiological	function or affect	angina

From the table you will see that angina is a symptom of heart disease, which is a type of cardiovascular disease.

Purpose

Good classification systems have multiple benefits:
▶ They provide a common language for reporting and monitoring of health and disease.
▶ They allow the sharing and comparing of data, making like-for-like comparison possible.
▶ The allow the rate and frequency of disease to be assessed.
▶ They support the development of possible treatments.

For example, COVID-19 is an illness caused by a respiratory virus (SARS-CoV-2) that infects the lungs. This means it can be compared with other respiratory illnesses such as flu. However, as we learned more about COVID-19 it became clear that there were differences between how the flu virus was transmitted and how SARS-CoV-2 was transmitted. One observation was that COVID-19 caused severe inflammation and this led to doctors trying the steroid dexamethasone. This cheap drug had been used for many years to treat inflammation and it was found to be effective in treating COVID-19.

There are other systems besides the three described, for example:
▶ **Pathological** classification is made according to the nature of the disease. For example, cancer is associated with uncontrolled cell growth, while some inflammatory diseases are related to autoimmunity.
▶ **Epidemiological** classification refers to the rate of occurrence and distribution of disease in a population – see sections B2.18 and B2.19.

B2.16 Examples of diseases and disorders and their relationship to the classification systems including the possible causes and symptoms

We are going to look at three examples of disease and how each one fits into the classification system.

Topographical

Diverticulitis is a type of **gastrointestinal disease** or disease of the gut. This is an example of classification according to the part of the body affected.

The symptoms of diverticulitis include abdominal pain. This comes on suddenly (we say it has **sudden onset**) but it can be prolonged.

Diverticula are small pouches that develop in the wall of the large intestine as you get older. Most people who develop diverticula do not have symptoms and may only become aware of them if they have a body scan for another reason.

When diverticula cause symptoms, it is described as **diverticular disease**. If the diverticula become inflamed or infected and cause more severe symptoms, it is known as **diverticulitis**.

Anatomical

Hepatitis (liver disease)

The term **hepatitis** is used to describe **inflammation** of the liver and so is an example of anatomical classification – disease linked to a particular organ. There are different types of hepatitis, some of which are more serious than others. This shows how an anatomical classification can cover a range of diseases.

The symptoms of hepatitis include:
▶ fatigue
▶ dark urine
▶ pale stools
▶ loss of appetite and unexplained weight loss.

Viral hepatitis is caused by five different types of virus (hepatitis viruses A to E).

Health and safety

Healthcare workers can be at risk from viral hepatitis, particularly hepatitis B and C, as these are spread by blood-to-blood contact. This could occur as a result of poor healthcare practice, unsafe injections or needle-stick injuries (i.e. when they are accidentally injected by used needles).

Vaccination against hepatitis B is recommended for people in high-risk groups such as healthcare workers.

There is currently no vaccine available for hepatitis C and it often causes no noticeable symptoms, although it can be successfully treated with anti-viral medication. About 25 per cent of people infected with hepatitis C will fight off the infection and remain virus-free. In the remaining 75 per cent, the virus will stay in the body for many years. This leads to chronic hepatitis C and can cause *cirrhosis* (scarring of the liver) and *liver failure*.

Antibody tests can show if you have been exposed to hepatitis C virus while PCR tests can show if the virus is still present.

Alcoholic hepatitis is caused by excess alcohol intake over a period of many years. The condition does not usually cause symptoms, although it can cause sudden jaundice and liver failure. Stopping drinking will usually allow the liver to recover, otherwise there is a risk of developing cirrhosis, liver failure or liver **cancer**.

Physiological

Chronic obstructive pulmonary disease (COPD)

Chronic obstructive pulmonary disease (**COPD**) is the name for a group of respiratory diseases caused by smoking, including:
▶ emphysema
▶ chronic bronchitis.

In individuals with **emphysema**, chemicals in cigarette smoke cause inflammation of the alveoli (see section B2.2), which leads to breakdown of **elastic tissue** and destruction of the **alveoli walls**. This reduces the surface area available for gas exchange in the lungs.

Chronic **bronchitis** is an infection of the bronchi that causes them to become irritated and inflamed, causing obstruction of airways, which also affects gas exchange.

The symptoms of COPD include:
▶ shortness of breath
▶ wheezing
▶ chest tightness
▶ chronic cough.

Unfortunately, there are several respiratory diseases that have superficially similar symptoms, so further investigation is usually necessary to provide a diagnosis.

Test yourself

1 Describe the two main types of hepatitis.
2 Suggest how physiological classification of various respiratory diseases can help in identifying causes and possible treatments.
3 Suggest what classification could be given to the following diseases:
   a Type 1 diabetes
   b coronary artery disease
   c irritable bowel syndrome.

B2.17 Injury and trauma

Injury is defined as **damage** to the body caused by external force. Injury and **trauma** differ only in degree; trauma is defined as an injury that has the potential to cause **disability** or **death**. The body responds initially in the same way but trauma is more severe so the response becomes greater.

How the body reacts as a response to injury

Some aspects of the body's response to injury are similar to the response to infection, namely the **inflammatory response**, which was described in section B1.30.

Involuntary inflammatory response

The initial response to injury involves an inflammatory response, similar to the response to infection:
▶ increased blood flow
▶ increased metabolic rate
▶ redness at the site of injury as a result of increased blood flow and rupture of blood vessels around the site of injury
▶ pain, caused by pressure on pain receptors as a result of accumulation of fluid
▶ swelling (**oedema**), caused by increased accumulation of tissue fluid around the site of injury.

Proliferation phase

This is the phase where tissue repair takes place. The goal of tissue repair is to remove damaged tissue and any associated toxins or waste products. The site of the injury is usually bridged by a **clot** (see section B2.6) that helps to reduce blood loss and prevent pathogens entering the wound. The clotting process also helps to bind the edges of the wound together and creates **scar tissue**.

Dead or damaged body cells are removed by **phagocytes** in a process similar to the removal of pathogens (see section B1.30).

The next stage is growth of new tissue to replace damaged tissue. This involves a type of cell known as **fibroblasts**. These replace the collagen lost by the injury. **Angiogenesis** (growth of new blood vessels) means that the new tissue is supplied with blood vessels (**vascularisation**).

The new tissue formed is known as **granulation** tissue. This results in the wound being remodelled as new connective tissue is formed.

The **maturation stage** is the final stage of wound healing. There is a reduction in vascularisation and the scar begins to fade. The collagen laid down begins to form cross links which increase the **tensile strength** of the wound. Tensile strength is a measure of the ability of the wound to resist pulling apart.

How the body reacts as a response to trauma

With trauma, the initial **inflammatory response** is the same as in injury. However, because of the greater severity of trauma, there will be several additional responses. These can include, depending on the nature of the trauma:
▶ loss of organ function (i.e. it stops working in some way or even totally)
▶ bone structure deformity, damage or loss of structure, e.g. a fracture
▶ haemorrhaging:
  – bleeding when the skin is broken and blood vessels are ruptured
  – skin bruising (caused by bleeding under intact skin).

The greater severity of trauma means that the inflammatory response is greater. Once it has begun, inflammation can become a disease process. This can lead to multi organ failure or even death.

Ischaemia

Ischaemia is known as 'going into shock'. Shock is not the same as having a fright – it is the medical term that describes the reduction in blood pressure following injury, excessive bleeding (**hypovolemic shock**), severe allergic reactions (**anaphylactic shock**) or infection of the blood (**septic shock** – see section B2.13).

As a result of the fall in blood pressure, there is a reduction in blood flow through organs or tissues – this is known as **hypoperfusion** or **ischaemia**. As a result, less oxygen and fewer nutrients can be delivered to the tissues – this is known as **circulatory shock**.

Proliferation phase

Provided the trauma or subsequent shock does not prove fatal, the body then goes through a similar recovery process to that described above under injury.

Test yourself

1 What are the two stages of the body's response to soft tissue injury?
2 Describe the role of phagocytes in the process of wound healing.
3 Describe the role of the blood in the response to injury.
4 State two possible causes of shock.

B2.18 Epidemiology

Having lived through a pandemic, we are probably all better informed now about epidemiology – as long as we have obtained our news and information from reliable sources!

The meaning of epidemiology

Epidemiology is the study and analysis of the distribution and patterns of disease in **populations** and why they occur. It also covers the application of this study and analysis to the control of health problems.

John Snow is sometimes called the 'father of the field of epidemiology' for his work in mid-1800s' London to discover the cause of cholera outbreaks and to prevent recurrence. This work was covered in the case study in section B1.27. The development of epidemiological methods continued in the late 19th and early 20th centuries, mostly focusing on infectious disease.

Epidemiology developed rapidly in the second half of the 20th century and has been extended to cover non-infectious diseases such as cardiovascular disease and lung cancer and its link with smoking.

Specific terminology used in epidemiology

Like so many fields in science and healthcare, epidemiology has its own set of terms that have specific meanings. It is important that we understand these terms and use them correctly.

Incidence

Incidence is the number of new cases within a specific time period. This means that it is a measure of the rate at which new cases occur. In the case of communicable/infectious disease you could think of it as being the risk of getting a particular disease.

Prevalence

Prevalence is the proportion of a population affected by a medical condition at a specific time. It is usually expressed as a percentage, fraction or number of cases per size of population. For example, at the end of December 2020 there were 81 520 recorded cases of COVID-19 in the UK, meaning a prevalence of 120 cases per 100 000 population. However, this is not an accurate figure for prevalence because it includes only those who had a positive test for COVID-19. The true figure for prevalence includes everyone with the disease, not just those who have been diagnosed.

Mortality and morbidity

The term **morbidity** refers to any physical or psychological state that is thought to be outside of the normal wellbeing. More simply, it describes illness or ill health. Morbidity is often used in describing **chronic** (long-lasting) or **age-related** illnesses. The greater a person's morbidity, the shorter their expected lifespan compared with healthy individuals. However, morbidity does not necessarily mean that the disease or illness is immediately life-threatening. The **morbidity rate** depends on the incidence **and** prevalence of a disease.

In the context of epidemiology, the term **mortality** means death caused by a particular disease. Like prevalence, mortality is often expressed per number of population. By the end of June 2021 the mortality from COVID-19 in the UK was 152 606 (deaths where COVID-19 was mentioned as cause of death on the death certificate). This equates to 225 per 100 000 of population.

The **mortality rate** is a measure of the frequency of death in a defined population within a specific time period.

> ### Test yourself
>
> 1 What is meant by epidemiology?
> 2 Explain the difference between the following terms:
>   a incidence and prevalence
>   b morbidity and mortality.

B2.19 How epidemiology is used to provide information to plan and evaluate strategies to prevent disease

Epidemiology is not just an academic exercise; its purpose is to help understand the cause and spread of the disease so that strategies can be developed to **prevent** disease.

In simple terms, epidemiology uses a systematic approach to:

1 count the number of cases of disease
2 calculate the rate of disease
3 compare rates, either over time or between different groups.

Identify the cause of disease

This may not be the starting point for an epidemiological study. We saw how John Snow used what we would now describe as epidemiology to identify the source (contaminated water), if not the actual cause (a bacterium), of cholera. More recently, epidemiology has led to acceptance of cigarette smoking as a cause of lung cancer.

Determine the extent of disease

By measuring **incidence** and **prevalence** of a disease, we get important insights into the extent of the disease – it gives us data to work with.

Identify trends and patterns

Equipped with data about the incidence and frequency of a disease we can then look for:

▶ **trends** – is the disease increasing or decreasing?
▶ **patterns** – does it affect mostly the elderly, is it related to factors such as poverty or living conditions?

Study the progression of disease

Looking for trends and patterns in a disease gives an insight into how the disease spreads and what type of action might be needed. Epidemiology helps track the mortality rate of a disease. This gives an indication of how many times the progression of the disease is fatal and also the effect of any therapeutics.

Plan and evaluate preventive and therapeutic measures

Once we have an understanding of the cause of a disease, how it spreads and how quickly it spreads, we can start to plan ways of treating it (**therapeutic measures** such as drug treatment) or ways to prevent it (**preventative measures** such as vaccination – see section B1.32).

Epidemiological methods also allow us to monitor the effectiveness of those measures so that we can **evaluate** and, if necessary, change or **improve** them.

Develop public health policy and preventative measures

Public health policy covers a wide range of issues, not just medical interventions like drug treatment or vaccination. Reduction in morbidity and mortality rates in the past 100 years has been due partly to medical advances such as the development of antibiotics or widespread vaccination campaigns. However, other factors that must be included in public health policy have also played an important part. These include:

▶ improved nutrition
▶ improved sanitation (availability of clean, fresh water and removal of sewage)
▶ improved housing – particularly reduction in overcrowding where infectious diseases are more likely to spread
▶ improved access to basic healthcare (rather than just advances in medical technology)
▶ greater education and health promotion.

> ### Test yourself
>
> 1 In an epidemiological study, once you have collected data about the incidence and prevalence of a disease, what would be the next steps?
> 2 Why is public health policy so important?

B2.20 How health promotion helps to control disease and disorder

We have just seen how education and health promotion have played a part in the reduction in morbidity and mortality rates over the past 100 years. Living through a pandemic, we have all seen how health promotion has helped to control the spread of the disease – to a greater or lesser extent in different countries. But health promotion is not just about infectious diseases – it applies equally, if not more, to the so-called **lifestyle** diseases of developed countries:

▶ obesity and related conditions, including Type 2 diabetes
▶ cardiovascular disease
▶ cirrhosis and other liver diseases
▶ some types of cancer.

Reflect

Is obesity a disease?

We have just listed obesity as a type of lifestyle disease, but is it actually a disease? In part, it depends on what we mean by 'disease'. One definition is 'a condition of the body or one of its parts that impairs normal functioning and has distinguishing signs and symptoms'.

On this basis, is obesity a disease? It is not a simple matter. Obesity is certainly a condition where the body develops excess fat. Measurements such as body mass, height and build can be used to define obesity. Obesity can be linked to increased risk of cardiovascular disease and Type 2 diabetes.

▶ Does this mean that obesity itself is a disease or simply a risk factor in developing other diseases?
▶ Does obesity always cause health problems?
▶ Does calling obesity a disease risk 'fat shaming' those who are obese?
▶ The World Health Organization (WHO) classifies obesity as a disease – do you agree?

Communication

Whether or not you think 'Hands – Face – Space' was the right approach to promoting ways to control the spread of COVID-19, you will almost certainly have heard it many times in recent months and years.

Case study

In 1986 the BBC showed a series of 'public information films' (adverts) on primetime TV to promote awareness of AIDS. The adverts were highly controversial at the time, featuring powerful tombstone images and the slogan 'Don't die of ignorance'. It was the first government-sponsored national AIDS awareness campaign and has been hailed as the most successful, with the approach being replicated worldwide.

At the time, about 90 per cent of the British public recognised the advert and many changed their behaviour because of it.

▶ Do you think it is justified to use powerful, even frightening, images in health promotion?
▶ What examples of health promotion campaigns (not just on TV) have you been aware of? Have they influenced you?

In the 1980s, radio, television, print media (newspapers and magazines) and posters were the main ways in which health promotion messages could be communicated. The advent of the internet and social media has changed this enormously. It has provided many more channels of communication. However, in some ways it has made communication more difficult because the audience is more fragmented.

Policy and systems

Government and public policy can play an important role in health promotion, particularly by changing procedures, regulations or laws to enforce required behaviour:

▶ restricted access to drugs of abuse
▶ restriction based on age on the sale of goods such as alcohol or cigarettes
▶ restricted movement of people, such as into and out of cities, regions or whole countries during the COVID-19 pandemic.

Education programmes

As mentioned in section B1.27, ignorance can be deadly. An important part of health promotion is improving knowledge and empowering individuals to adapt their behaviour.

People are increasingly turning to the internet to help diagnose their symptoms. Use of internet search engines is not an adequate substitute for visiting your doctor, however. Nevertheless, it shows how people are using the internet for information about all aspects of their lives, including health and wellbeing.

Many universities and other organisations are offering online courses (**e-Learning**). Many of these are aimed at health professionals, but others are suitable for the general public or non-specialists.

The NHS has a great deal of information on its website covering a range of topics:
- ▶ **Health A–Z** – this has articles on a huge number of medical conditions, symptoms and medicines, arranged alphabetically. This is where many internet searches will lead you.
- ▶ **Live Well** – this covers advice, tips and tools to help make informed choices about health and wellbeing.
- ▶ **Mental Health** – this has a great deal of information and support targeted at mental health issues.
- ▶ **Care and Support** – this is a guide to services for those who need help with day-to-day living because of illness or disability.

See also section A2.4 for various health apps which can support the work of healthcare professionals and help individuals to manage their health.

Health promotion for specific disease and disorders

Since early 2020, we have all been living through one of the biggest health promotion campaigns in this country. But COVID-19 is not the only threat to public health and wellbeing. Other examples of health promotion include targeted awareness raising and campaigns such as:
- ▶ Change4Life, a social marketing campaign by Public Health England aimed at reducing childhood obesity by giving parents the support and tools they need to make healthier choices for their families
- ▶ the annual flu vaccine, promoted through a range of media, including posters in GP surgeries, radio adverts, email and letters to vulnerable groups, as well as social media campaigns (Facebook, Twitter and Instagram).

See Chapter A9 for more on these and other health and wellbeing campaigns and initiatives.

Research

Change4Life and the flu vaccine campaigns are good examples of health promotion for specific diseases or disorders.

Search for 'PHE campaigns' to see more about all of the Public Health England health promotion campaigns (including Change4Life).

Responsibility for health matters is devolved to the four nations of the UK, so there are separate websites for Public Health Scotland, Public Health Wales and Public Health Agency (Northern Ireland).

How many of these campaigns are you aware of? Have any of them made you more aware of health and wellbeing issues? Have any of them made you change your behaviour? If not, what more needs to be done?

Test yourself

1 Describe the advantages of health promotion campaigns.
2 Describe two ways in which government policy can reduce disease.

Project practice

You are working as part of a multidisciplinary healthcare team and have been asked to prepare a report on the COVID-19 pandemic, focusing particularly on the lessons learned and how these could apply to potential pandemics in the future.

You need to carry out the following.

Background research

The NHS website aimed at patients (www.nhs.uk/conditions/coronavirus-covid-19/) may help. There is also information aimed at clinical staff (www.england.nhs.uk).

▶ What is known about the mechanism of transmission of the SARS-CoV-2 virus?
▶ How has epidemiology contributed to this understanding?
▶ SARS-CoV-2 is not simply a respiratory virus. What is known about the effects of COVID-19 on the main physiological systems in the body:
  – respiratory system
  – endocrine system
  – nervous system
  – cardiovascular system?
▶ Some people infected with SARS-CoV-2 develop a post-viral syndrome known as 'long COVID'.
  – How does 'long COVID' affect patients?
  – Is there a link between the severity of infection and the risk of 'long COVID'?

Health promotion

What were the policies and systems put in place to reduce spread of the disease? How well did they work?

Consider the different ways in which bodies such as Public Health England promoted awareness and understanding, including aspects such as:

▶ risk factors for severe disease (obesity, age, weakened immune system, etc.)
▶ precautions to reduce spread of the disease
▶ encouragement of vaccine take-up
▶ improving public awareness and countering misinformation.

Report

Prepare your report, either as a piece of extended writing or as a PowerPoint presentation. You should include the following points:

▶ how our understanding of COVID-19 developed
▶ the success, or otherwise, of health promotion campaigns
▶ what lessons can be learned and applied in future pandemics.

Group discussion

Have you given a balanced account? Are there any important areas that you have overlooked? Does the group feel that we will be better prepared for future pandemics?

Reflection

Write a reflective evaluation of your work.

Assessment practice

1 Patients with cardiovascular disease are sometimes prescribed exercise rather than medication. A middle-aged man recovering from a mild heart attack was recommended to monitor his heart rate while using a treadmill for walking at a moderate pace.

   a Suggest advantages and disadvantages of using a wrist heart rate monitor (e.g. a Fitbit or other exercise watch) or a pulse oximeter for monitoring heart rate.

   b Explain the physiological factors that the patient would experience if he exercised at too high an intensity.

2 In epidemiology, which of the following best describes the difference between morbidity and mortality?

   a Morbidity is a measure of the frequency of illness and mortality is a measure of the number of people who die from the disease.

   b Morbidity is a measure of the seriousness of illness and mortality is a measure of life expectancy.

   c Morbidity describes the state of ill health and mortality means death caused by a disease.

   d Morbidity measures the number of new cases of a disease and mortality measures the number of existing cases.

3 Of the three types of muscle (skeletal, smooth and cardiac), explain which has the highest and which has the lowest number of mitochondria.

4 Describe how the endocrine system contributes to chemical and mechanical digestion.

5 The table shows the concentrations of various substances in the blood plasma in glomerular capillaries, the glomerular filtrate and the urine.

Substance	Concentration in plasma of glomerular capillary (g/dm^3)	Concentration in glomerular filtrate (g/dm^3)	Concentration in urine (g/dm^3)
Proteins	80.0	0.005	Variable
Glucose	1.0	1.0	0.0
Urea	0.3	0.3	8–10
Mineral ions	7.2	7.2	3–4

a Explain what the figures for concentration in plasma and filtrate of these substances show about the process of ultrafiltration.

b Explain the difference in the concentration of glucose in the filtrate and in the urine.

c Describe how the endocrine system influences the concentration of urea in the urine.

d Type 1 diabetes is often diagnosed by the presence of glucose in the urine. Suggest why glucose might be present in the urine of someone with Type 1 diabetes.

6 The walls of the vagina secrete peptides that can destroy micro-organisms such as bacteria, yeasts and viruses. These antimicrobial peptides (AMPs) are produced all the time, although secretion of AMPs increases in response to inflammation. Secretion of some AMPs by the walls of the uterus and vagina also increases in response to progesterone during pregnancy. Suggest explanations for these facts.

7 The 'fight or flight' response to danger is controlled by both the endocrine and nervous systems. Cells in the sinoatrial node (SAN) have receptors for adrenalin on their plasma membranes.

a Explain how release of adrenalin will help prepare the body for 'fight or flight'.

b Suggest how the endocrine and nervous systems work together in the 'fight or flight' response.

8 Describe the similarities in the body's responses to injury and infection.

9 During the COVID-19 pandemic, the UK government was initially reluctant to make vaccination compulsory for care workers and healthcare staff. Suggest the reasons for this.

10 The UK birth rate and death rate have changed significantly in the period since 1700.

a Between 1700 and 1800 there were fluctuations in the death rate. Suggest **two** reasons why the death rate would fluctuate.

b The death rate declined steadily between 1800 and 1940. Explain reasons for this decline.

c There has been an increase in the death rate since 1980. Suggest **one** explanation for this.

Core skills

To pass the Employer Set Project and pass this qualification, you must demonstrate that you are able to apply core knowledge in context by demonstrating the following core skills.

CS1: Demonstrate person-centred care skills

CS1.1 Plan and develop person-centred care

Communicate with service users and their families

Adapt the communication style to meet the needs of the individual

Working in health professions, you will meet a variety of people. You may need to adapt the communication style to meet the needs of the individual, depending on their level of understanding. You may also need to adapt your language to make it simpler or more complex, depending on who you are talking to. For example, if you are talking to an individual with learning difficulties, your language will need to be easy to understand.

You should speak clearly and make an effort not to use medical jargon or acronyms, and be prepared to explain any technical terms. For instance, if you are discussing activities of daily living, you will have to say that (and explain what this means) rather than saying ADL. You may need to slow down your speech to allow the individual to absorb the information.

If necessary, you may have to use picture boards or photos to help the individual understand. You must show interest in what they are saying and not interrupt. Body language should be positive, with good eye contact throughout.

Gather information to inform the care plan

Views of the individual, their family, carers and healthcare professionals

When collecting information to produce a care plan, the healthcare professional must consider the views of the individual, their family, carers and healthcare professionals. Best practice involves gathering information from the individual and those who know them best so that they can build an accurate picture of the person. This information will include their likes and dislikes, their strengths and abilities, their interests, beliefs, culture, views and physical, emotional, social and intellectual needs. This is essential because the care plan must be designed and understood by the individual and all those involved in their lives. It will detail who is in charge or responsible, who will provide support, where and when it will be provided. A person-centred approach is to see the person as an individual, focusing on their personal wants, needs, goals and aspirations. The individual becomes central to the health and social care process.

Explore choices

Discuss options available

Individuals are entitled to have choices about their care, so to enable their preferences to be met as much as possible, there should be a discussion of the options available. One of the key aspects of person-centred care is for the carer to provide the individual with information so that they can make informed choices. Even if the individual cannot take part directly in the decision-making process (because of illness, disability or incapacity), they should be involved as much as they are able, and their family, carer or healthcare professional should be able to speak on their behalf and ensure that the person planning the care is aware of the wishes of the individual whose care is being decided.

Consider patient safety

Patient safety must always be considered, especially when designing a care plan, but this does not mean that individuals should not have a choice just because it may be risky if they do so. Many things are risky in life but these risks can be managed by putting measures in place to reduce the risk or prepare for any possible consequences. For example, when deciding on the course of treatment for the patient, the medical practitioner will choose the one that will be most beneficial for that patient. They will consider any allergies that the patient may have to medications and tailor the treatment to the individual to meet their needs, preferences and values.

Establish what is important to the individual and their family, encouraging their contribution

You need to establish what is important to the individual and their family by encouraging them to talk to you. You need to offer encouragement and support, ensuring that the individual and their family are not intimidated or do not lack the confidence to speak up if they are not happy. It is also important to listen carefully to what they have to say. This all allows them to take part in discussions and decision making so that they feel in control.

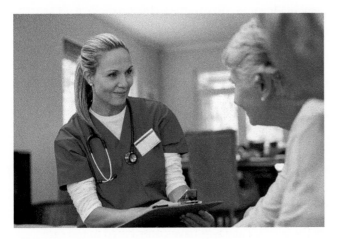

▲ Figure 16.1 Discussing a care plan

Discuss the possible outcome of different choices

You must make sure you have all the relevant information before you discuss the possible outcome of different choices with an individual. To do this, you must be well prepared. You must not choose the outcome for the individual or try to guide them towards the outcome you would like. Instead, you must present all the choices and their possible outcomes without any bias.

Establish mutual expectations for individuals, their families and carers

Be clear on your own expectations

Expectations that are set should be achievable and not out of the range of the individual. It is no good to anyone if you set unreasonable expectations – failure to succeed could cause the individual to become disillusioned with the care being offered.

Understand which areas of care require expectations to be set

The areas of care which need expectations to be set are the choices that are most important to the individual, so they must set the expectations as they are central to all the planning. Therefore, they will need to let the medical practitioner know exactly what they anticipate they will get from the service. The support the individual needs must be designed in partnership with the individual, their family and carers.

Discuss expectations of individuals, their families and carers by asking questions to establish understanding

To ensure you have the correct reading of the situation, you must ask questions about what you believe the individual wants. You should ask clear, unambiguous questions and give people time to think and answer. If you are then unsure about anything that has been said, you must clarify the situation so that there is no misunderstanding. If you ask a question and they reply, you can then paraphrase their reply back to them. For example, you could say, 'Have I got this right? You would like to …' They then have the opportunity to confirm or correct this impression.

Come to a mutual agreement and gain commitment

Having clarified the situation, both sides must agree a suitable way forward so that everyone is happy with what has been decided. This is so that everyone will be committed to making the plan work.

Record agreement processing and interpreting any data accurately

Once agreement has been reached on the way to proceed with the care plan, an accurate record of decisions should be made. This formal document can then be a source of reference so that everyone knows what should be happening and when. Everyone involved in the plan should have a copy so they can check that everything on the care plan is what has been agreed by everyone. It is a good idea that the professional completing the care plan goes through it step by step, patiently answering any questions and ensuring that everyone involved is happy and understands the outcome.

Set goals

Establish what they want to achieve and by when

This can be planned using SMART goals. These are goals that are:
▶ Specific – no vague goals, it must be definite what they mean
▶ Measurable – there must be a start and an end point – they must be measurable and it must be possible to state clearly when the goal has been met
▶ Achievable – what the individual wants and decides to attempt must be doable
▶ Realistic – takes into account the available resources and amount of work needed
▶ Timely – must have a clear start time and end date.

Establish who is responsible

All the healthcare professionals, carers, family, etc. involved in this person-centred care must be aware of what they are responsible for. All of them should have a copy of the completed plan so that there can be no misunderstandings.

Set a deadline for when the goals will be reviewed

When the goals are set there must be a review date agreed at the same time. This is because the individual will want to know that there is a finite date for their goals to be met.

Consider patient safety

When setting goals for the individual, the professional must consider patient safety. For example, if the patient has difficulty walking and is being discharged from hospital back to their own home, any necessary adaptations should be made to their house. If there are steps up to the house, perhaps a ramp could be installed to help the patient get into their home without any falls. Similarly, perhaps they may need a walker for support to help them get around.

Record plans, processing and interpreting any data accurately

Any changes to the person-centred plan must be recorded, e.g. if targets have not been met or the individual has changing needs. Any further information must be recorded accurately as this will affect future plans and funding. Data recorded on the individual's plan will help professionals be aware of important information which may need quick action – for example, if a patient reacts badly to a new medication, they will need to be prescribed a different one. If this is recorded on their care plan, the professionals will ensure that this medication is not prescribed in the future.

CS1.2 Provide person-centred care

In line with the care plan and patient's wishes

The care plan will have been devised with the patient as the focus. They will have contributed to the care plan and will have guided the healthcare professionals on what they want to happen. It is your job, therefore, to honour their wishes by following the plan.

Respect patient's and service user's rights and dignity

Without respect for them, it is unlikely that the care worker will be able to establish an effective relationship with the patient. Respect is about treating the patient as an individual and valuing them for themselves. This can be demonstrated by making sure you do the following.

Close doors and knock before entering when providing personal care

The healthcare worker should always knock on the patient's door and wait to be told they can come in before entering the room. This is common courtesy and shows respect for the patient – and they will feel that their privacy is respected. The worker should close the door as they leave to maintain the patient's privacy.

Ensure confidential discussions take place in an appropriate environment

The care worker must discuss confidential matters in a quiet, private area, making sure the door is closed so no one can overhear the conversation.

Where appropriate, ensure the patient consents to sharing information with family (for example, Gillick competence/Fraser guidelines)

Consent is required before any medical treatment can begin. The Gillick competence refers to the wider context of any medical treatment in that some children under 16 are mature and legally considered competent enough to consent to proposed treatment themselves, without parental involvement. The Fraser guidelines apply to advice/treatment relating to contraception and sexual health, where if certain criteria are met, the child does not need parental permission. In both cases, if a child is deemed competent and does not wish their parents to know their circumstances, the healthcare professional must respect their wishes and not share the information with their families.

Research

Research the origins of the Gillick competence and the Fraser guidelines. Explain why these guidelines came about. Then visit:

https://learning.nspcc.org.uk/child-protection-system/gillick-competence-fraser-guidelines#heading-top

Examine the Fraser guidelines and decide how easy/difficult it is for someone under the age of 16 to meet the guidelines.

Respect patients in line with equality, diversity and inclusion

Treat all patients fairly with the same access to services available

Healthcare services should reflect the individual's needs and preferences. This does not mean that everyone is treated the same, as individuals have different needs. However, everyone should have equal access and equal opportunities to make use of health services to get the best possible medical treatment. Individuals with physical and learning difficulties need to be supported to access services, so you will need to be equipped to do this.

Demonstrate compassion through language used and acknowledgement of patient's condition, asking questions about how they feel

Ask questions throughout and acknowledge how an individual might be feeling

A compassionate person will demonstrate sympathetic concern, kindness and understanding for an individual who may be feeling ill or suffering. After all, compassion is one of the core NHS values. To help the patient, the healthcare worker will ask questions about how they feel and how they can help, which make the patient feel reassured.

On your work placement, observe how a healthcare professional acts to show compassion towards a patient.

What did you learn? How could you use this knowledge to better your practice with patients?

Regular reviews of the plan

Ensure the plan still meets the needs of the individual

Regular reviews of the plan are essential as the individual's circumstances may change and areas of agreed support may no longer work for them. So the plan may need to be adapted as it no longer meets the needs of the patient. For example, their health may deteriorate and they could need more assistance with personal hygiene. Or a family member who has been giving informal care may no longer be able to do so. However, if the plan works for an individual and they are happy with it, then it can remain unchanged.

CS2: Communication skills

CS2.1 Communicate clearly and effectively with a variety of stakeholders

When communicating with other professionals, an interaction will probably be on a formal basis, either on a one-to-one basis or in a group situation. The group situation is more likely to occur when several professionals are consulting together or when they are in a case conference. Interactions with patients could be formal or informal. In both types of interaction, the message must be clear and unambiguous.

CS2.2 Communicate effectively with a variety of stakeholders within the health setting

Communicate in a clear and unambiguous way, tailoring language and technical information to the audience

The effectiveness of your communication skills may depend on how far your approach meets the needs of the other person. For example, you will have to approach a three-year-old child differently from the way you approach an older person. Language, posture, pace and tone all need to be adapted to the other person. You should not use technical language if you know the person would not understand you but should work to present the information in simpler terms.

Select the most appropriate way of presenting data

Use images and other tools (for example, visualisations or infographics) to clarify complex information

Visual aids such as objects, pictures, photographs or signs can offer alternative ways of communicating with individuals with speech, language and communication needs.

When presenting complicated information to an audience, it helps if the information is broken down into a simpler diagrammatic form to make it easier to understand. For example, the pictogram in Figure 16.2 is a simple way of presenting the number of students who owned a cat or a dog. You can see immediately what the pictogram represents and it is much simpler to follow than a bar chart or a graph.

Year	Cats	Dogs
2017		
2018		
2019		
2020		

Key:

= 5 dogs

= 5 cats

▲ Figure 16.2 Number of students owning dogs and cats

Augmentative and Alternative Communication (AAC) is often used by individuals who have communication difficulties. This system includes the use of communication boards and books, signing (such as British Sign Language) and Makaton, which uses signs, speech and symbols as well as **voice output communications (VOCAs)**. Comedian Lee Ridley ('the Lost Voice Guy'), who has cerebral palsy, uses an automated voice on his iPad to speak to his audience.

Ask appropriate questions to test understanding based on the task required

Use of probing questions to get further information

Questioning is a valuable tool when trying to establish whether the individual understands what is required. Questions are useful to clarify a point and are essential in reducing misunderstandings. Paraphrasing is a simple and effective way of testing understanding, so the questioner offers a summary of what they think the individual has said.

Actively and critically listen to the individual's contributions

Active listening is an important part of communication. If you do not give the speaker your full attention, you could miss important information which could put a different slant on the conversation.

Active and critical listening requires the listener to understand, interpret and evaluate what they hear through paraphrasing and summarising what the individual has said to them. **Paraphrasing** would be useful here as it captures the main points which the individual has made. Further questioning may be necessary to **clarify** or check points. Active and critical listening also involves watching body language and gestures and observing facial expressions as well as showing empathy by reflecting feelings.

Key terms

Paraphrasing: a repetition or summary of what has been said.

Clarify: to check for accuracy of understanding.

Respond to the individual's questions

Individuals who are in a health setting will usually have questions for the health professionals as they will be dealing with an unknown situation, so they may be stressed and upset. It is up to the healthcare professional to answer any questions honestly so that they build up a trusting relationship with the individual.

Speak clearly and confidently when talking to individual, their family and carers

Use appropriate tone and register that reflects the audience

A healthcare worker should offer reassurance to the individual and their family by speaking confidently and clearly. A calm, slow voice can indicate an unhurried and friendly approach to the individuals. The tone of voice together with facial expression and body language can show interest and concern for the patient.

Display appropriate body language

Demonstrating engagement

Communication can be enhanced by positive body language, which is also called non-verbal communication (see Figure 16.3). The healthcare worker can show through their body language whether they are friendly and responsive to the needs of the patient. For example, if a patient asks the healthcare worker a question and the worker looks at their watch and starts to move away, it demonstrates lack of engagement. To show engagement, the healthcare worker should make eye contact to demonstrate interest in the conversation.

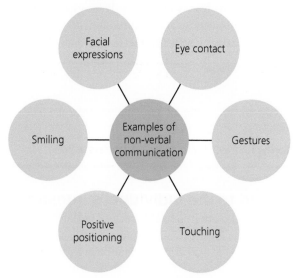

▲ Figure 16.3 Examples of non-verbal communication

Openness

One of the most significant forms of body language or non-verbal communication is a smile. Smiling shows warmth and openness and helps interactions to be positive. Good eye contact is also important for showing openness.

Answer the brief/research questions, providing supporting documentation in different formats

It is important to answer the brief and not wander off topic. If you have been asked a specific question, you must remind yourself what you are researching and not allow yourself to get distracted. Supporting documentation could be presented in the forms shown in Figure 16.4.

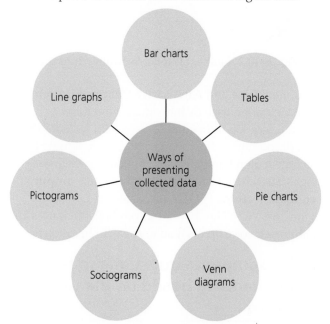

▲ Figure 16.4 Ways of presenting collected data

Case studies, clinical practice (i.e. the methods of delivering healthcare agreed upon by professionals such as doctors, nurses, physiotherapists), articles from professional journals, textbooks, etc. can also be used to give weight to the findings.

Highlight the commercial/business benefits to the individual

Use calculations, diagrams and data to support these assertions

As in Figure 16.4, the different diagrammatic presentations can be used to highlight commercial benefits, such as a good business relationship with suppliers. Even hospitals need to work with suppliers, such as companies which provide food for the hospital kitchen or with the company that removes their clinical waste products.

The hospital management have to get the best deal and the manager may need to present figures to the board of governors to reinforce the way the hospital budget is spent. This is done after careful research into the possible benefits of the preferred company. Figures presented must be accurate and honest; they must not be changed to fit the hoped-for outcome.

CS2.3 Use a range of techniques to overcome communication barriers

Succinctness

If you are succinct, you briefly and clearly express what you want to say without unnecessary words. This means that the person listening to the conversation does not have to pick out the main points among a lot of unnecessary speech.

Avoiding use of jargon/slang (for example, use non-clinical terminology where possible)

As a healthcare professional you will use medical jargon that would make no sense to a non-medical individual. For example, a medical practitioner might say to a colleague that the operation was iatrogenic. If that was repeated to a patient it would be meaningless as most people would not know that it meant that the operation did not go as planned. You could lose patient confidence if you speak to them using medical terminology and they misunderstand what you mean or what their condition or treatment involves.

Retaining awareness of cultural differences

To be able to communicate with individuals from different backgrounds, it is important to understand their cultural practices and religious beliefs. It is essential that individuals who are not fluent in English have access to interpreters and advocates to act on their behalf when using health services. Interpreters will interpret what they are saying so you can understand

and respond and advocates will help them gain access to services and will act on their behalf to obtain their rights within a service.

Family or friends can act as an advocate, so they speak up on the individual's behalf. However, if the person does not have family or friends to help them, the council (social services) must provide one free of charge. Lots of charities such as POhWER, Age UK or VoiceAbility will also provide advocates to help free of charge.

Use of assistive technology and other communication aids where appropriate

Any health setting may need to provide for individuals who have specialist communication needs. This could include individuals who have difficulty hearing, those who have poor eyesight, a physical disability or have had a stroke.

Examples of communication aids (see Figure 16.5) include:

▶ Braille – method of communication for individuals who have difficulty seeing
▶ hearing loop – special type of sound system for use by people with hearing aids
▶ digital voice recorder – records meetings, etc. with a light, portable recorder
▶ pen reader – portable pocket-sized reading pen that reads text out loud in a human-like voice.

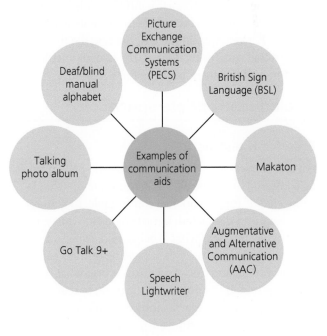

▲ Figure 16.5 Examples of communication aids

Knowing when to refer to a colleague (for example, if sign language or translation services are required)

It is a good idea to refer to a colleague as soon as you recognise you are out of your depth with a patient and need a signer or a translator to help you communicate. Rather than waste time and effort trying to communicate, it is better to admit you need assistance.

Use non-verbal communication such as gestures to imitate actions (for example, eating or drinking)

Gestures should be used to aid understanding but when they are used in a haphazard way and there are too many of them, this can cause confusion. It is important to be aware of what is acceptable for patients in different cultures. For example, in the UK, holding the thumb up is a sign that something is good, but in certain cultures this sign could be insulting or not understood.

Use an appropriate space

Free from distractions

For any conversation to be successful, the patient must be comfortable and be able to concentrate on what is being said. If they do not feel comfortable, they may be uneasy and distracted. If the room is too noisy, the patient may not hear what is being said, especially if they have problems with their hearing or their ability to concentrate, and they may misinterpret what they are being told. If the door is left open there may be lots of people going past, particularly in a busy hospital, so the patient may get distracted.

Consider positioning of the individual from the healthcare professional (for example, keep appropriate distance)

The space between people is called personal space. It is important that when talking to patients, the healthcare worker does not invade their personal space, meaning that they do not get too close to them unless they are carrying out a treatment or examining them. In this instance they would explain what they were going to need to do and seek permission from the patient.

Generally, there are four distinct zones:
▶ intimate zone – touching usually reserved for close family
▶ personal zone – less than 1 metre, reserved for friends
▶ social zone – 1–2 metres, usually for acquaintances
▶ public zone – 2+ metres, for strangers.

Ensure the space offers privacy when required

Being too far away from a patient can be problematic if you are trying to give them information – confidentiality would be difficult to maintain as you may have to speak very loudly so they can hear. It might be that they would not hear all the information and so would miss out on essential facts.

Practitioners must have privacy so that they can talk to the patient without anyone else overhearing. It may be upsetting news that the health practitioner wants to discuss with the patient, such as a diagnosis of a serious condition, and the patient could become upset and need reassurance.

The patient should also have a private space to get dressed if they have had a physical examination.

CS3: Team working

CS3.1 Identify the functions of teams/team members as well as their role within the wider team

Identify hierarchy within teams

It is a good idea for any worker to know the team **hierarchy** to see how the organisation is structured overall. This hierarchy is often displayed in a diagram in the staff room or on a document found on the staff intranet or website. It is useful because it gives the worker a clear reporting structure if there are any problems. Initially, however, the worker should always go to their line manager or supervisor if there is an issue.

Generally, a hierarchy will have a few skilled leaders at the top of the pyramid who direct the organisation's strategy. Below them are senior managers, managers and the rest of the workforce carrying out the leader's instructions. This means that everyone is working towards the same goal rather than just setting their own goals. If the individual at the top of the hierarchy fails to reach the targets they have set, they are accountable and could even lose their job. For example, in healthcare if the chief executive in a hospital trust fails to meet the targets of the waiting list, they will be called to account for their failure.

> ### Key term
>
> **Hierarchy:** a system in which workers are ranked in order of their role within the organisation, from the top down.

Ask and respond to questions for clarification

Always ask questions if you are unsure about anything. It is good practice to ask another team member/manager for advice if you are in doubt as they will be able to address your query and clear up your uncertainties. Managers should encourage staff to seek clarification as it demonstrates that staff are committed to getting the job completed correctly and avoids confusion and time wasting doing the wrong thing. It also ensures that there is no duplication of effort across the team with two members unknowingly carrying out the same task.

Establish the different expertise within the team

Everyone has different expertise and has a valuable contribution to make to the team. This is regardless of their role and status. It is important to know the different areas of expertise within your team so that if you require help in a certain area, you will know who will be able to assist you. Work should be allocated to team members by considering the knowledge, skills and understanding of the staff concerned.

Workload, too, should be considered so that individuals do not become overburdened or work is allocated unfairly.

Understand own responsibilities within the wider team

Tasks they are accountable for

Accountability means being answerable for something, primarily to your immediate boss, i.e. your line manager. To be accountable, the individual needs to be clear about what they need to do, then complete the tasks given to them within an agreed timeframe, then let the team or people involved know the task is finished.

Failure to complete the work could lead to disciplinary action. Obviously if there are extenuating circumstances, such as being absent through illness, then the deadline for the work would be extended. Similarly, if there is an unforeseen problem with the task, then a new timeline would be agreed, but this means the worker should sort this out as soon as it happened and not wait until the due date.

Everyone is accountable within an organisation, from the top down to the bottom.

Deliverables they are accountable for

A deliverable is a product or service created at the completion of any project or any smaller components of a project. For example, five Health students have been asked to take part in a Health Promotion event at a primary school. They have decided to give a presentation on healthy eating for Year 3 pupils.

In order to deliver this event, there are several components or tasks which have to be completed before the presentation can take place. One of the students needs to contact their local health promotion unit to obtain the latest resources. Another needs to write a questionnaire for the Year 3 pupils to fill out prior to the visit so the group can see what pupils already know about healthy eating. Another person has to book with the school for the initial visit. Then there is the actual presentation to design and write, and a slideshow presentation to produce.

These are all deliverables and every one of them depends on all the team members carrying out their agreed task for the event to go ahead. In other words, they all know which deliverables they are accountable for.

Direct reports (if applicable)

Direct reports are individual members of staff with a manager who is directly responsible for managing them. These individuals will have regular one-to-one meetings where the manager can build a supportive relationship with the individual who reports directly to them. These help staff to feel part of the organisation and therefore a valuable member of the team. It also allows the manager to give constructive feedback to the worker on any of their projects. The worker can discuss any issues they may have before they become a big problem. Praise, too, can be given for the successful completion of each project rather than waiting months for the annual review.

CS3.2 Undertake collaborative work demonstrating ability

Delegate work when appropriate

Delegation is when a manager/supervisor gives an individual, who is lower on the management hierarchy, responsibility for a task.

When a manager delegates, they must be sure that the worker is capable of carrying out the task, i.e. they must be competent. This will partly depend on how long they have been doing the job. If the staff member is new to the role, the manager may not know them well enough to delegate important tasks to them and may feel that they are too inexperienced. Smaller, less involved tasks could be delegated to these newer staff members to build up their confidence and demonstrate their competence.

Delegating can motivate staff as they enjoy the opportunity to take control and make decisions. Managers must set clear outcomes when delegating tasks so that staff know exactly what is required and when it is required by.

Work within the organisation's defined processes

Every organisation has its own processes in the form of guidelines, policies and procedures that set the tone for the workforce. These are to guide the behaviour and conduct of the team for day-to-day work. The idea is that if all staff follow these processes, they will carry out tasks in the same way to a similar standard and the organisation will run smoothly.

The processes give clear instructions in many areas, for example, health and safety, bullying, sexual harassment, risk assessment policy. Staff know what is expected of them and what they can expect from managers and other colleagues. It will increase their confidence that they are doing things correctly. For example, if they follow the health and safety policy, workplace accidents are less likely and everyone will feel safer. It is important that all staff adopt the processes as they will provide a clear framework for the team.

Encourage contributions from other participants

If individuals are encouraged to contribute to projects, they will work harder as they will feel that their contribution is valued. They will feel a sense of ownership of the project and want it to succeed. Everyone should be encouraged and have a chance to speak and meetings should be structured to create equal opportunities for every staff member to have their ideas heard.

It is a good management strategy to have a collaborative approach for projects rather than a hierarchical one. This allows every member of the team to have a leadership role, even if it is for a very small part of the project.

Demonstrate clear communication skills including making relevant and constructive contributions to move discussion forward

When working in a team, clear communication is vital. Good communication is needed to obtain information, to give information and to share ideas. All members of the team need to be kept up to date with any further developments for a project they may be working on. Failure to communicate can cause anger and a sense of mistrust. Poor communication can cause stress and anxiety as individuals may be unsure of what is happening.

To move things forward in discussions, it is a good idea to ask questions and give updates on progress after checking the latest status with other team members as they may have more up-to-date information. If you are the project leader for the part of the project being discussed, then the importance of clear communication cannot be over-emphasised. Everyone should be an active participant in the discussion, willing to share ideas and ready to help and support others in the team without monopolising the meeting.

Share thoughts, opinions and ideas

Sharing thoughts, opinions and ideas helps to develop a collaborative approach in the group as other team members should feel they can share theirs too. It also helps the group to bond and feel that they are all working towards the same goals. Sharing ideas can raise learning and creativity and help others to learn new skills and start to think outside the box. There is a better chance of solving issues quickly as the whole team can add their thinking power towards a solution if they are willing to share. This can enhance morale.

Sharing your ideas is a good way of demonstrating leadership skills, especially if it is a well-thought-through solution. The group must always respect other team members' ideas and give them a fair hearing without being dismissive.

Establish a common purpose or goal

A goal or purpose brings a team together as they are all working towards a common aim. Setting goals allows everyone the opportunity to demonstrate and develop their skills. Good communication and collaboration are necessary to meet these goals.

Once goals have been set, it is a good idea to draw up an action plan so everyone knows what is required from them and the dates they should aim for. It will also allow the organisation time to gather resources, etc. to meet the final objective or goal.

It might be advisable to follow the SMART targets system. That is:

▶ Specific goals or purpose – objectives should be specific about what you want to achieve
▶ Measurable – it should be able to measure whether objectives are being met or not
▶ Achievable – it should be possible to achieve the objectives set
▶ Realistic – not too ambitious given the resources available
▶ Timely – realistic time frame set with a clear end date.

Demonstrate adherence to relevant health and safety procedure

Managers must pay attention to health and safety because having and following an effective health and safety policy and procedure is in everyone's interest. Workers, too, have their duty to follow and obey any procedures laid down by the workplace.

The procedures provide a framework for keeping everyone safe from potential hazards and risks. For example, each workplace will have a fire evacuation policy, which is explained to all staff and practised regularly, so everyone knows when and how to leave the building in the event of a fire. However, this should also include ensuring that all workers are carrying out their duties in a clean, well-ventilated, heated and well-lit environment.

The health and safety policy (shortened version) should be on a notice board and should be published in any other relevant languages to make it accessible to all staff.

Follow standard operating procedure specific to the environment they are working in

Team members must follow standard operating procedures (SOPs; see page 104) specific to the environment that they are working in as there may be variation between different departments even for the same healthcare facility. If the healthcare worker has been moved to a different department, it is up to them to find out about the policies and procedures of the new department and make sure they note any similarities and differences. They must then ensure that they follow them; if they are unsure, they must ask another team member.

Make decisions

There should be a clear procedure within the team about decision-making, with everyone involved. If the team has decided that a majority decision will stand, then this should be followed wherever possible. If not, team members will feel missed out of the process and may consider that they do not have to follow the decision. This may alienate team members as they will not feel confident that the correct decision has been made and that their input is not valued. However, it should be noted that the manager may override a team decision if they feel it is in the best interests of the organisation.

Show reliability

Anyone in any job wants reliable team members, whom they can count on to turn up, do their share and get the job done. An individual who is reliable is consistent and delivers on time. If they set deadlines for themselves, they will meet them, and people can depend on them to play their part in the team.

Managers value reliability and reward members who demonstrate this. They are more likely to offer them the best opportunities for promotion and advancement. Regardless of their career, they will have the respect of the rest of the team.

Demonstrate respect and trust towards other team members

Team members need to respect other members as well. All partners are unique and bring their own knowledge, skills, creativity and understanding for the advantage of the group. Additionally, if team members are not acknowledged for their contribution to the group, they are less likely to be fully committed to team objectives.

Demonstrating respect and trust requires every member of the team to take responsibility for their actions. A team without trust is not really a team, and if trust is missing, they will not share information and might be reluctant to co-operate with one another, so reaching full potential is not possible.

Trust means relying on team members to perform every task with the best interests of the group in mind. Trust provides a sense of safety and individuals should not be afraid to open up, be honest and share their knowledge.

Work together to find solutions and problem solve

Teams have to problem solve every day using critical thinking skills and by working co-operatively with one another. Working together as a team improves the chances of coming up with a solution as the team can share ideas and bounce possible solutions off each other.

When a problem arises, it is a good idea to share this with the rest of the team sooner rather than later – if there is immediate action, there will be more time to solve the problem without it impacting the overall result of the project. Finding solutions and problem solving strengthen relationships and bonds within the group, building trust and respect between members.

CS4: Reflective practice

CS4.1 Undertake reflective practice and record reflections and experiences

Be able to identify what happened

Reflective practice is thinking about or reflecting on what you do. This involves the individual learning from what has happened and adapting their behaviour accordingly if things did not go well. It is about learning from experience. You think about what you did and therefore what happened and decide from that what you want to do differently next time, in order to improve the outcome. You do not repeat actions that did not go well.

It is useful to think about the situation as soon as possible after it has happened, otherwise you might forget some important details.

The approach taken

The approach taken very much depends on the individual. Schön (1987) identifies two concepts of reflection:

▶ reflection-in-action where the healthcare worker is thinking on their feet – thinking about the incident as it happens
▶ reflection-on-action where the healthcare worker thinks about the incident after it has happened – this could be spending time thinking it through on their own or discussing the incident with colleagues.

Schön's original book, *The Reflective Practitioner: How Professionals Think in Action* (1983), was written for health and social care practitioners. His model is praised for its simplicity and ease of use as it can be adopted during an event as well as after the event. It is also useful for the healthcare profession as individuals work in a highly charged atmosphere, often involving life-or-death situations, so they are expected to sum up a situation immediately and arrive at a satisfactory solution. This model emphasises the usefulness of reflecting immediately while in action.

Another possible model used by health, social care and childcare professionals is Gibbs (1988) reflective cycle. This is taken from Gibbs' 1988 book *Learning by Doing*. This model is also straightforward to use. It leads you through the different stages so that you can make sense of an experience and use it to improve your practice. It is a framework for examining experiences. See Figure 16.6.

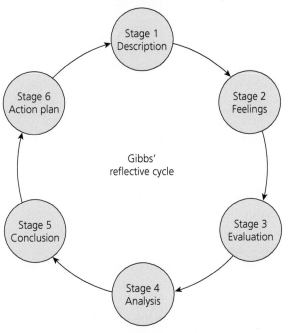

▲ Figure 16.6 Gibbs' reflective cycle

Stage 1 – a description of what happened.

Stage 2 – what did you think and feel? What was your reaction?

Stage 3 – what worked well and what did not?

Stage 4 – what happened and why?

Stage 5 – what else could be done? What have you learned?

Stage 6 – what would you do next time? What changes are you going to make?

Why that approach was taken

There is no right or wrong approach to take. Indeed, you may take either the Gibbs or the Schön approach and not necessarily stick to either one. It could be that you find Gibbs easier in the beginning as you may find it difficult to follow reflection-in-action when you start out. The reflection-on-action may not be as easy to follow when you are new to it as the Gibbs model, which guides you through each stage and gives you a clear pathway. Either way, it is down to the individual to choose a model that suits them.

The ability to understand and change develops over time as you become more confident in your own judgement. You will begin to reflect with speed and spontaneity required by the situation and make quick decisions when necessary.

What went well

It is just as important to record what went well so that those actions can be repeated and built on. This can boost morale and self-esteem. Even if more things went wrong than right, at least something went well! It is also a good idea to share things with colleagues that worked for you and went well. If, for example, you have had a thank-you card from a patient, it is good to share with other workers in the organisation as it will have been the result of a team effort.

What didn't go well

Obviously if things did not go well, they are going to have to be changed and you should not continue with them. However, what does not work on one occasion may work on another. You will just need to carefully analyse what happened to assess the situation in this instance. You could seek advice from your manager or you may speak to your colleagues who may have some helpful ideas. If several things did not go well, it may be an idea to address one or two areas at a time so you do not become overwhelmed by trying to do too much in one go and end up not doing anything well.

What could have been done better

There are always things that could have been done better. This is a common refrain when healthcare workers are rushed off their feet and have too many tasks to carry out. They may reflect on their day and feel they have let patients down. For example, they may feel they should have answered buzzers more quickly so they could have tended to patient needs faster but there were not the staff numbers to cope with a busy day. It is important to remember not to be too harsh on yourself and to realise that solving this issue would be a team effort and not down to an individual member of staff.

How things will be done differently in future to make improvements

Obviously all the positive and negative information will be gathered together and considered and a plan of action will be drawn up to address any negatives. Everyone learns from their mistakes and from their achievements, and when reflecting on any practice, they can see what was successful and what needed to be done differently. A good team ensures that mistakes lead to improvements as lessons will have been learned.

Use a range of methods to record reflections and experiences

Short communications

Reflective practice describes a way of working that involves keeping notes or a journal of what you do, your observations and ideas. Short communications can be all of these and in any format (notes on paper or digitally) as long as you can understand what your notes mean at a later date. This then becomes a resource for you to go back to, to think about and to ask questions about. It is usually informal and for the writer's use only.

Reports

A report is usually a formal, short, concise document written for the workplace. It is a factual document that needs to be clear, well structured and well written. It identifies a problem, then offers findings and research, recommendations and conclusions. An individual may be asked to produce one themselves or it could be a team effort. It would usually be distributed within the organisation.

Blogs

A blog is a regularly updated website or web page, often written in an informal, chatty style. It may be written by one person or by a small team of people. A healthcare worker could plot their daily work schedule, things that happen, etc., provided they made sure that the information is anonymised to comply with data protection legislation. They could still use the blog as their reflective diary as it would be the basis for a more serious document.

Creative writing

Creative writing does not have to be limited to fiction. It can include:

▶ journals
▶ diaries
▶ personal essays.

These can consist of personal thoughts, feelings and experiences. They can tell stories of real people in real situations. These would be ideal for reflective diaries as long as names and other details were changed so that patients were not recognisable and confidentiality was respected.

CS4.2 Make improvements to own practice

Be able to identify and seek out opportunities for continuous professional development and prevent future failings

If an individual undertakes reflective practice and discusses their progress with their line manager on a regular basis, they should know in what areas they need to upskill. They can then look out for courses that will help them to continue their professional development. If the individual seeks out courses, their employer will recognise that they are proactive in identifying knowledge gaps and then trying to fill those gaps.

Individuals need to refresh their academic and practical qualifications as they soon become out of date – this will allow the individual to constantly refresh their skills. It is up to the individual to keep a record of all their **continuous professional development (CPD)**, but this should be easy if they update their **curriculum vitae (CV)** with each course they take. If there are examples of CPD on the individual's CV, there is a better chance of promotion as it demonstrates interest and the will to improve. It also develops self-esteem and confidence.

> ### Key terms
>
> **Continuous professional development (CPD):** development of further skills and knowledge needed to do a professional job properly.
>
> **Curriculum vitae (CV):** brief account of an individual's education, qualifications and previous jobs sent with a job application.

Be able to request colleague feedback

If an individual is working with colleagues, they can always ask a manager or someone else to observe their performance and give them feedback. It does not have to be the manager – it could be a colleague who started the job at the same time, so it would be a peer observation. However, it is usually part of a manager's role to watch team members before performance management so they will have an idea of the worker's improvement.

The individual should ask the manager for feedback and to take part in their development. The manager will then have confidence that the individual is learning and developing the necessary skills to take them forward in the job. However, if an individual feels they are not performing well and they have had this confirmed by a manager, this could give weight to the individual requesting to go on a course.

Accept and act upon any performance-related feedback given

It is always a good idea to try to improve performance if an individual has had negative feedback. Usually when giving negative feedback, a manager will indicate what was wrong and how it could be improved. Always follow the advice and if unsure, ask for clarification. The individual should keep copies of any feedback so they can refer to it to help them improve their performance. They could ask a trusted colleague to observe them and see if their work has improved. Note, however, that many people find it difficult to accept criticism, even if it is supportive and constructive.

Seeking clarification where appropriate

It is important to check the individual's understanding of the feedback to make sure it is correct. Clarifying will resolve any areas of confusion or misunderstanding. This can be done by repeating what they think the speaker said and asking if that is right. The individual cannot expect to put right their performance if they are unsure about what needs to be corrected.

Self-evaluate

Consider own performance against job specification or objectives

The job specification is a good place for an individual to start when considering their own performance. They need to list all their achievements in meeting the job specification as well as the ones yet to be met. This will tell the individual how far they need to go to meet all

their objectives. They will need to develop a plan to help them achieve success in their weaker areas. If the plan does not work, they will need to revise it until it does work.

Monitor personal progress

An individual should monitor their performance regularly, looking back at targets and goals they have set themselves and taking into account regular feedback. They should change the way they work in line with new training recommendations and use feedback from colleagues, patients, etc. to develop their skills accordingly. Training courses can help an individual to look at improving their performance.

Set personal goals and milestones

Goals should be SMART (Specific, Measurable, Achievable, Realistic and Timely) – see page 356. The individual should be realistic and set small goals. If the goals are too big, it may seem as if they are not making any progress. The goals must be written down so that progress can be monitored. When the individual has achieved their first goal, they may find that their priorities have changed, so they may need to revise their original plan. Possibly they will have gained new skills and knowledge, leading to fresh opportunities that they may not have thought about, so they must adapt their goals.

CS5: Researching

CS5.1 Apply research skills

Be able to identify the need for change or improvement in relation to specific areas of practice

Utilise experience and clinical judgement

Newly qualified healthcare staff will probably find it difficult to make quick, sound clinical judgements as they lack the necessary experience to make a competent decision. Once they have two or three years' experience, their clinical judgement is faster as they begin to trust their own instincts. But making good clinical decisions is not left to the healthcare worker on their own – they can ask the opinion of more experienced colleagues who will be happy to share their knowledge. These colleagues should also be willing to share how they arrive at their decisions.

As new techniques develop, the staff will adapt their practice if they feel it would benefit their patient.

Consider risks to patient safety

An important aspect of clinical judgement is the safety of the patient. Newly qualified healthcare workers will find it difficult to make fast clinical judgements as their decision may affect the health of the patient. No professional healthcare worker should take an unnecessary risk with a patient's life. New techniques with possible risks would be considered only if the patient and their family agreed to the treatment, even if the treatment has been tested and proved to be effective in clinical trials.

Be able to carry out a detailed investigation into a specific problem by gathering information from independently sourced materials, originating from autonomous investigation

To investigate effectively, the researcher must be well organised and have a systematic approach to the topic under consideration. Choosing a sustainable, interesting, manageable topic is essential. The length of time available for the research will have a bearing on the final decision. Thorough planning is essential, whatever the research topic.

Carrying out a detailed investigation means collecting information from a wide variety of materials, so the individual must research thoroughly. The information could be gathered through primary research – that a researcher has carried out themselves (see Figure 16.7) – or secondary research – using existing material which has been produced by someone else (see Figure 16.8). The latter can make a researcher's job easier as it is useful to look at existing sources – they are a good starting point and can suggest useful ideas. However, it may not be as relevant as primary research.

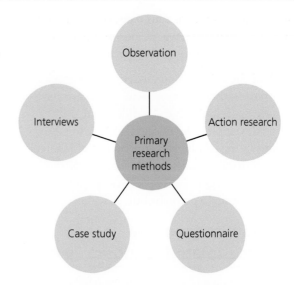

▲ Figure 16.7 Examples of primary research

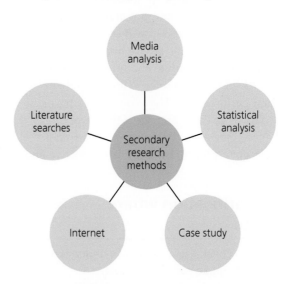

▲ Figure 16.8 Examples of secondary research

Be able to study sources, analyse data/information to draw conclusions

Research is exploring a topic to find out new information. In the health sector, practitioners have a duty to ensure they keep up to date with the latest research – for example, doctors have a duty to follow medical research into prescription drugs and their side effects so they can use this information to make the best decision for the treatment of their patients.

Drawing conclusions means that the researcher reflects on everything that has been done during the project. They weigh up facts from primary and secondary research and then come to a conclusion about how satisfactory the whole research project has been. They make decisions about the hypothesis, aims and objectives, time planning, methodology, presentation and analysis of results. Once they have drawn conclusions, it is the natural progression to make recommendations for future planning.

Be able to create and carry out a plan for research

Outline the scope of your research

Any researcher needs to plan, present and analyse their findings in a manner that is suitable for a research project. The process needs to include:

▶ choosing the subject area
▶ setting out the hypothesis, issue or research question
▶ writing the aims and objectives for the research
▶ selecting appropriate research methods
▶ identifying ethical considerations
▶ time management
▶ record keeping.

When selecting the subject area for a research project, it is good practice to choose a subject that interests the researcher. It is useful to make a list of possible topics. At this stage broad subject areas are fine; they can be narrowed down at the decision stage. A spider diagram is a useful tool when trying to decide on the focus of the research. Remember to consider the amount of time available for the research to be conducted.

Identify what you would like to achieve

Once the researcher has decided on the area of research, the hypothesis can be formulated. A hypothesis is a statement which is identified at the start of the chosen research. This statement makes a prediction about what the researcher will find evidence to support. The researcher tests the hypothesis by finding evidence that will either support or contradict it. However, the researcher need not always set a hypothesis – they might prefer to set an issue or research question for the subject area.

How to formulate questions to find further information in relation to a specific area

When setting the hypothesis, research question or statement, be sure the focus or end result of the project is clear, otherwise this could lead to data which does not relate to the original research idea and is difficult to explain. Be clear and specific and keep to the topic.

When researching, it is very important that the question remains foremost in the researcher's mind, which will ensure they will not go off target. It might mean, however, that after some weeks, the question will need to be adapted or narrowed down as the scope is too wide.

▶ Example of hypothesis: New mothers often feel pressured into breast feeding while in hospital but will start to bottle feed once they return home.
▶ Example of an issue: In today's society a lot of new mothers are concerned about going back to work and having issues with continuing to breastfeed their baby and hostility to breastfeeding in public.
▶ Example of a research question: To what extent have attitudes towards breastfeeding changed in the last 20 years?

Look into the background information around the specific area of practice

A sensible place to start with a research project is to gather background information. This will provide the reasons for the research paper and will help other healthcare professionals understand why this new study was carried out.

The researcher should summarise previous studies so readers will understand the context of the investigation. For instance, there may be gaps in previous findings which the researcher is attempting to address, or further data is required to establish the limits of effectiveness of a certain treatment.

Collate further relevant information using a range of independently gathered sources and materials

Independently gathered sources mean that the researcher has searched across a wide selection of documents and data, etc. that supply information relevant to their chosen research topic, without being influenced or directed by anyone else as to which to use.

The researcher must be able to collate information from a wide variety of primary and secondary sources. Information must be grouped together in relevant categories, which will depend on the topic chosen, so that the research is well organised and makes sense. The researcher must be careful to disregard any information which is not relevant to the hypothesis chosen so that they maintain focus and do not wander off topic.

Evaluate the information for reliability of the content source and currency

If the findings of research can be **replicated** or repeated (by a different researcher at a different time) with the same or similar results, then the data is said to be **reliable**. Reliability depends on the researcher using appropriate research methods. It is therefore important to choose the best method for the study. Could other methods have been used? Would they give similar results?

If the consumption of alcohol among teenagers was the topic, it is likely that interviewing different age groups of people (for example, 14–19 year olds and 45–50 year olds) would give very different results. Researchers must target participants who are representative of the group they wish to represent. If not, the results will be unreliable.

Make sure the information used is current and up to date. It is no good using a book from 1952 if the topic is latest medical advances for 2020! Check the age of the research and statistics in any book.

Use appropriate technology systems for the collection, processing and organisation of data in preparation for use

There are numerous commercial packages available for the collection of data. These systems allow data to be stored and to quickly move data ready for analysis and reporting.

Word-processing packages also come with features that can help with graphs and charts. For instance, Microsoft Excel or Google Sheets allow you to produce graphics and statistics from numerical data. Many educational establishments and home computers will have a licence for Microsoft Office software.

The ability to identify suitable data from research, professionals and patients to allow interpretation and analyse findings

The researcher must identify data which will be useful to their project. A lot of information from secondary research and from colleagues may be interesting but it may not address the issue they are examining in their project. They must ensure that they stick to the hypothesis they have set. It will take careful reading and sifting through the information available to relate it to their project – it is easy to wander off track and go off on a tangent.

> ## CS5.2 Apply principles for evidence-based practice to contribute to research and innovation within a specific area

Apply principles of evidence-based practice

Be able to combine research with clinical expertise and judgement

Combining research with clinical expertise for research purposes is not difficult for most practitioners as they take their job and excellence in it seriously. If they have an idea about researching a particular area, it will most likely have come from their evidence-based practice (EPB) initially. They will use their clinical expertise and judgement many times each day and will have ideas of how they could take this forward into research.

Their next step is to research their ideas in journals, books, on the internet, etc. to see if there is already research in this area. They will then search for similar themes before deciding whether this is a topic worth pursuing. Because they are working in the healthcare sector, they may have plenty of primary research to bring to the project.

Be able to use appropriate technology systems for the collection and processing of data in preparation for use

As the healthcare professional already works in a healthcare sector, they may find there is a lot of useful data, statistics, patient information, etc. stored on the healthcare technology system (this is unavailable to the general public). They will probably already have the ability and permission to access it as they will use the technology system in their everyday work. This will make the research easier if raw data is available; however, they may have to process it. They should, however, let their manager know that they intend to use the information if it is available. They will be able to download it and add their own data to it.

Be able to identify suitable data from research, professionals and patients to allow interpretation and analyse findings

The healthcare professional needs to keep the title of the hypothesis in mind all the time when looking for data from both primary and secondary research. When collecting primary data, the researcher will have had to devise questions, interviews and case studies with the outcome in mind.

Be able to articulate findings through a variety of methods

When presenting findings, the researcher must be sure that other people can access and understand the work. Any research projects must have a title page which gives the title of the research project (i.e. the hypothesis) and the name of the researcher producing the report. A contents page like the one below should follow the title page and it should list and give the page number of each section of the report.

Contents	Page
Abstract	1
Introduction	2
Methodology	3
Presentation of data	11
Analysis of results	19
Conclusion	25
Evaluation of design and conduct of research	30
Recommendations for future research	35
Bibliography	40

Any results from collected data need to be presented in the appropriate format. This could include:
▶ tables
▶ bar charts
▶ line graphs
▶ pie charts
▶ pictographs
▶ **sociograms**
▶ **Venn diagrams**.

The same information can be presented in different ways – it is often a matter of the personal preference of the researcher, but certain types of data are clearer in certain formats. These should be carefully labelled and presented in the same order as the analysis of results. Be very careful when changing raw data into percentages to ensure that figures are accurate.

Key terms

Abstract: a brief summary of the research project. It will contain the aim, research methods used and conclusions drawn.

Sociogram: can show the relationship between each group member or just one member of the group. A good way of representing a social structure within a group.

Venn diagram: consists of circles which interlink. The circles can be free standing or can overlap, demonstrating a link or relationship.

Demonstrate effective evaluation skills and draw conclusions to the research

In the conclusion to the research, all the findings of the report are pulled together and conclusions are drawn. The researcher should not add any new information in this section. Conclusions should only be made based on the information which has been presented in the project. The hypothesis should be referred to and the researcher should state whether the aims of the research have been met.

Be able to identify potential bias in results

When carrying out any research it is important that the researcher is objective. This means that they must examine any material that has been collected without any bias or prejudice. Research results must not be distorted by the researcher's feelings or preferences. They must report what they have found and must not add extra points which have not been demonstrated by their research. It is easy for personal opinions or views to affect research findings, therefore the researcher must try to be sure that any conclusions made are proven through the research, in order for their research to be valuable.

The facts as they appear should be analysed and presented. Recognising that personal opinions and views can affect objectivity will help the research to be as objective as possible. **Subjectivity** is when personal opinion and views are allowed to influence the conclusions of the research.

Be able to interrogate data

Interrogation simply means to get information from something. Once all the data has been collected, it is organised, analysed and put into bar charts, pie charts, etc. so that it can **interrogated** (examined).

The researcher must be able to understand what the data is telling them so that they can compare findings (with previous research) and draw conclusions in order that the research question/hypothesis can be met.

Be able to critically interoperate data

Interoperating data means being able to communicate and exchange data with another system or device. For example, a researcher could be working on a project in a hospital in Newcastle and be interoperating data from a colleague in Truro. This is because they are colleagues working together on the same research hypothesis and have access and permission to access each other's data. It could also happen within the same hospital trust but with colleagues from different departments.

Be able to make decisions based on findings

The idea of research is to help the decision-making process as there should be further evidence to help with making the decision. Making informed judgements is about the researcher measuring what they have found out in their research against any knowledge they already have. Their research may have confirmed what they thought would happen or may have changed their opinion.

Be able to make links between independent sources

Making links between different independent sources is straightforward if the researcher looks for key phrases or words so that they can see immediately if the information will be useful in their research. This is a quick way of finding useful links without spending time reading through the whole article. Obviously, if the work is not useful it can be quickly rejected.

Contribute to innovation within a specific area

Be able to apply findings

Improving existing practice

This is one of the main objectives for carrying out any research. For example, if a healthcare professional has been looking at lowering the incidents of Clostridium difficile (C. diff.) on their ward and has found out that certain practices work in other hospitals, it might be worth piloting the practice in their own hospital.

Introduce new or improved ways of working

Linked to improving practice, this may be small changes that have been introduced but they could have a big impact on the working practices of the organisation. They could also improve the wellbeing of the patients. For example, if the research helped to reduce the number of patients with C. diff. on the ward, it would most certainly improve the health of the patients. The staff would benefit also as they would be able to nurse the patients for their original complaint.

Investigate/introduce new and more effective treatment methods

Scientists constantly research new and more effective treatments for most diseases. For example, scientists developed several COVID-19 vaccines which were successful at helping to reduce the spread and effect of the virus on the population.

Treatments evolve all the time, with scientists trying to improve the outcome for patients. Most cancer patients now have a much better longer-term outlook with the advancement in cancer treatments.

CS6: Presenting

CS6.1 Present their project findings in a range of formats

Using digital formats

Video

Using a video adds variety and can complement a presentation. A video also gives the presenter a short break when they are not speaking to the audience. A short clip will add to the audience experience and can get large amounts of information across in a shorter timeframe.

Video clips can be stopped and started to facilitate discussion. They can also convey reality, particularly if they are clips from a workplace, for example. One disadvantage is the potential for technical problems, so it is a good idea to prepare an alternative.

PowerPoint

Digital slide presentations using software such as Microsoft PowerPoint can be prepared well in advance and are a simple way of presenting information in a professional way. The slides can be adapted and customised to suit the audience. For example, the researcher may want to put a slightly different slant on the information, depending on who they are presenting to. This is easy to achieve by changing one or two of the slides.

The presentation can easily be printed off to form handouts so that the audience can follow the presentation and make notes if they wish. This could work well for the presenter if there is a technical problem as everyone would have a copy of the slides. Adding animation can make the presentation more eye-catching.

Multimedia presentation

Multimedia presentation can include the internet, games, displays, film, television, radio, interactive videos and DVDs. This method of presentation is often more stimulating and engaging than traditional methods, such as a purely verbal delivery. Multimedia usually has high-quality video images and audio. However, it can be very time consuming to put together.

Using non-digital formats

The advantages and disadvantages of using non-digital formats are shown in the table.

Method	Advantages	Disadvantages
Verbal delivery	Cheap as no equipment needed. Can judge reactions and body language so address the issues before moving on	Can be less interesting Difficult to engage audience without any visual aids
Whiteboard	Cheap and usually available Good for highlighting main points Can be reused Won't break down	Limited use as if the group is too big, participants won't be able to read the board Must have correct pens or the board could be damaged
Flip chart	Can be prepared in advance Easily portable Nothing to break down Cheap and readily available Can share out paper for small groups to add their comments	Limited as people may not be able to read from a distance Paper easily damaged
Paper handout	Reduces need for note taking Information can be shared with colleagues back at work Cheap to produce People can read at their own pace later	Thrown away if not read Not durable Easily lost

Tools for the layout of information

Graphics

Graphics are an image or a visual representation of an object. Computer graphics are images displayed on a computer screen. They can be two or three dimensional. The term computer graphics includes almost everything on a computer that is not text or sound. Most computers can do some graphics.

Imagery/diagrams

Visual diagrams are better than just words for making a presentation effective and engaging to the audience.

There are many different types of diagrams and it can be difficult to know which one to use. Well-chosen diagrams help to draw in the audience and keep their attention. But any imagery/diagrams used must support the key messages, otherwise they become a distraction from the information being delivered.

Tables

Tables are very versatile and are a useful way of presenting information, especially in comparing data. The table below shows how many students opted for a vocational course in Year 12 at School X.

Course	2017		2018		2019		2020	
	Male	Female	Male	Female	Male	Female	Male	Female
Business	10	15	6	21	12	21	9	23
Engineering	10	0	15	1	18	2	20	6
Art and Design	0	15	4	8	6	12	4	5
Health and Social Care	2	23	0	29	4	27	2	31
Information Technology	20	5	23	8	24	7	29	8

Graphs

A bar chart is a type of graph. It is a popular method of presenting data because it is easy to understand and easy to draw. Bar charts are useful for presenting descriptive data such as how many students chose to follow a vocational course, as Figure 16.9 demonstrates.

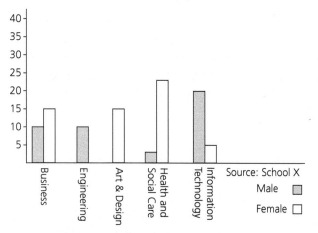

▲ Figure 16.9 Student choice of vocational course, 2017

A line graph is another type of graph. It is useful for showing changes over a period of time. If a meaningful line graph which does not distort facts is to be produced, then a large amount of data is needed. Line graphs can be used for comparisons between sets of figures.

Annotations

Annotations are notes that are added to a diagram as a way of explanation. When preparing PowerPoints there is a notation section at the bottom of the slide where the writer can add notes for themselves so they are prompted to highlight key aspects of their presentation.

Audio

Audio means sound and this can be added to a presentation to enhance it. For example, the presentation may start with a piece of uplifting or energetic music depending on what suits the topic. A recording of an interview with a patient could underline points made in the presentation. However, the participant must be asked, in advance, if they agree to this and **must** be given the option to refuse. Confidentiality must be respected at all times.

Visual

Visual aids can help the audience understand complicated ideas and recall the information much more quickly than just words. Visuals can simplify a complex concept because the brain uses visual information faster, as it processes the information faster than just words.

Animation

Animation is motion applied to pictures to create characters. Animation can enhance any presentation as it engages the audience and can have a positive impact on their ability to retain the information presented to them.

CS6.2 Present outcomes to a range of different stakeholders

Patients/service users

Usually an oral presentation will consist of the healthcare professional passing on information to the patient about their diagnosis and possible treatments. This will be informal. The healthcare professional will talk through and explain the different options available to the patient. They will need to explain the advantages and disadvantages of each course of treatment to help the patient have sufficient knowledge to make a decision. They should be able to answer questions to reassure the patient and offer advice if the patient asks for it, but they should not try to influence the patient's decision. They may have to adapt their language and technical terms so the patient can understand them.

Customers

It is important to build positive relationships with customers, so good communication is necessary. There should be a culture of trust and honesty. Customers should be encouraged to give feedback about the service they receive and the healthcare worker should make sure that any criticism is addressed. Communication needs to be regular and truthful, with a quick response to any issues. This would usually be a formal situation and may be on a one-to-one basis.

Carers

Similar to patient communication, the healthcare professional may find themselves advising the carer on the treatments available so that they can assist the patient in making a good decision. Communication could be informal, particularly if the patient and carer are well known to the healthcare worker. They may update the carer as a result of their research to help them assist the patient.

Other health and social care professionals

This would probably be a formal relationship, with the healthcare professional passing on information they have learned from their research. The other professionals would be keen to have facts and information which would help them to improve their practice and make things better for their patients. The language would be more technical as they are talking to fellow professionals.

CS6.3 Apply considerations for adapting presentation style when presenting to a range of stakeholders

Be able to adapt the presentation style to meet the needs of the target audience

Age

The best way to interact with young children is to keep things simple and visually interesting, for example, by using animations or plenty of colourful posters. It is important to use interactive activities to get children up and doing things, for example, the presenter could ask for volunteers to help them carry out certain tasks.

The presenter should connect with the children on a personal level, for example, asking how many of them have pets. The presentation should be short, with the presenter getting straight to the point. They should use short sentences with one-syllable words and not jargon or technical terms.

Gender

In terms of content, certain topics may be relevant to raise as regards reproductive health, for instance the effects of the menopause. However, there should be no difference between genders in terms of presentation style, otherwise the researcher could be accused of stereotyping. Unless there is a specific reason, most audiences will be mixed, with participants of a variety of genders, and there should be no discrimination between them.

Cultural differences

Understanding cultural differences is important for ensuring interpersonal communication is successful. If the presenter is culturally aware, it minimises the possibility of misunderstandings or causing unintentional offence. It is particularly important here that the speaker uses plain English, with no slang terms or phrases. They need to be careful with body language and gestures as some could be offensive to other cultures. It is a good idea to carry out research on this before a presentation.

Educational background

It is useful for the speaker to have an idea of the educational background of the participants and what their needs might be before starting to plan their presentation. It is not a successful presentation if the speaker talks down to the audience by underestimating their educational achievement. But it is equally unsuccessful if the speaker talks over their heads so that they do not understand what is being said to them. The speaker must ensure that they pitch the presentation at the right level for the audience.

Adapt presentation style to meet the needs of the stakeholder

Amend and tailor language appropriately

When amending and tailoring language appropriately, vocabulary should be adapted. Word choice will depend on the participants' rough age and educational level. For example, a child or a person educated to GCSE level may not be as familiar with more complex words as someone educated to degree level. So if it is a mixed audience with different levels of education, the speaker must use simple words that everyone can understand. Speak in plain English and avoid long sentences that participants might find difficult or confusing.

Set length of presentation to meet the purpose

People find it difficult to concentrate on presentations for long periods of time. Presentations should be short, well planned and structured and should stick to the points that need to be delivered. They should not be rushed but should focus on the content, with time left for questions and discussion. The length of the presentation depends on the information that needs to be disseminated – 20 minutes is usually long enough for people to maintain interest and to pay attention throughout.

Organise information and ideas in a coherent way to suit the length and purpose of the presentation

Information should be well organised and structured. There should be an introduction in which the presenter introduces the subject of the presentation. This should be followed by the main/key points, supported by evidence. Finally, there should be a summary in which the presenter sums up the key points they have made.

Summarise information where necessary

If you are producing a digital presentation, the information on the slides must be summarised to avoid too much information on a slide for the audience to read. A summary is a short and condensed version of the presentation. It should give a good idea about the substance of the presentation. The main points of the presentation should be in the summary. There should be no new information or points of view. The main point of a summary is to reinforce the main points and arguments made in the main body of the presentation.

Test understanding by asking and responding to questions

It is a good idea if the presenter plans for possible questions so that they are prepared and can answer quickly. It is also a good idea to ask the audience to save their questions for the end, otherwise the presenter may find it difficult to pick up where they left off before the interruption. Questions should be encouraged and answered in a concise way that people will understand. It would be useful to end the presentation with a recap and quick summary of the question and answer session.

Assessment

Assessment Overview

This qualification in assessed in the following ways:
- ▶ Core Component:
  - − Examination papers A and B
  - − Employer-set project (ESP).
- ▶ Occupational Specialism Component:
  - − Synoptic assessment.

Paper A

This is a written examination – you will have 2 hours 30 minutes to answer all of the questions.

The question types on Paper A are short answer or extended writing. The paper consists of four sections. Each section tests your knowledge of the content from two or three of the elements, each of which is covered by one chapter of this book. For instance, Element 2 is covered in Chapter A2.

Section A Working in the healthcare sector: 33 marks

Element 1: Working in the health and science sector

Element 2: The healthcare sector

Element 7: Good scientific and clinical practice

Section B Managing personal information and data in the health sector: 25 marks

Element 5: Managing information and data in the health and science sector

Element 6: Managing personal information

Section C Health and safety in the healthcare sector: 25 marks

Element 3: Health, safety and environmental regulations in the health and science sector

Element 4: Health and safety regulations applicable in the healthcare sector

Element 10: Infection prevention and control in health-specific settings

Section D Person-centred care in the healthcare sector: 33 marks

Element 8: Providing person-centred care

Element 9: Health and wellbeing

Element 11: Safeguarding health and wellbeing

Paper A is worth 104 marks plus an additional 12 marks for quality of written communication (QWC) – 116 marks in total.

Paper B

A written examination – you will have 2 hours 30 minutes to answer all of the questions.

100 marks inclusive of 6–10 marks for maths (plus 18 marks for quality of written communication (QWC)) = 118 marks in total.

The paper has four sections:
- ▶ **Section A:** multiple choice questions, short-answer and extended writing, 48 marks
- ▶ **Section B:** multiple choice questions, short-answer and extended writing, 23 marks
- ▶ **Section C:** multiple choice questions, short-answer and extended writing, 23 marks
- ▶ **Section D:** multiple choice questions, short-answer and extended writing, 24 marks

Paper B is worth 100 marks inclusive of 6–10 marks for maths (plus 18 marks for QWC)) = 118 marks in total.

ESP Tasks

In completing the employer-set project you will demonstrate six core skills, supported by underpinning knowledge and understanding from the core elements.

Core skills are covered in detail on pages 354–378

Task 1: 2 hours – Planning

You will have researched the individual and their situation and must now use the information from the case study, and your research from the pre-release brief preparation, to write a report that identifies how to best support the individual you have chosen in their outlined situation.

You should explain the support you propose for the individual, justifying your points with evidence.

Task 2a: 2 hours – Practical role play

For this task you will undertake a practical role play focusing on your chosen individual.

You will take the role of a supporting healthcare assistant. You have been asked by a senior colleague in the team to conduct a discussion with the individual you have chosen. You will discuss their case with them and ask questions to clarify points in the brief and to inform next steps for their care.

Task 2b: 2 hours 30 minutes – Create a healthcare plan for the chosen individual

Contribute to a healthcare plan for your chosen individual using your notes from Task 2a and your research from the preparation research. You should use the healthcare plan template provided.

Task 3a: 3 hours 30 minutes – Formative reflection task (peer feedback)

You must discuss your proposed healthcare plan with your peers to gain and offer feedback. Your tutor will put you into your peer discussion groups.

Task 3b: 2 hours 30 minutes – Produce and deliver a presentation

Produce and conduct a presentation for your tutor, who will assume the role of a senior colleague in the healthcare team who would be involved in your chosen individual's care.

Task 4: 2 hours – complete a reflective account.

You must now complete a reflective account that considers your approach to the overall project, including how well you feel you have achieved the expected outcomes.

Occupational Specialism Components

These are synoptic task-based assignments linked to your chosen occupational specialism. The components are:
- a case study assessment
- two practical activities assessments: one for the core Supporting Healthcare, and one for the occupational specialism
- a professional discussion

The Occupational Specialisms are:
- Supporting the Adult Nursing Team
- Supporting the Midwifery Team
- Supporting the Mental Health Team
- Supporting the Care of Children and Young People
- Supporting Therapy Teams

You will choose one of these and the assignments will be focused on this occupation. **Synoptic** means that it is an assessment of the overall specialism as a whole, rather than particular areas within it.

The assignments will include three types of assessment:
- Case Study Assessment (CSA)
- Practical Activity Assessment (PAA)
- Professional Discussion Assessment (PDA)

Time allowed to complete the assignments:

7 hours 45 minutes – 9 hours 15 minutes (plus 45 minutes preparation time)

Consisting of:
- Assignment 1: 4 hours 30 minutes
- Assignment 2 (Core): 1 hour to 1 hour 30 minutes
- Assignment 2 (Option): 1 hour 15 minutes to 2 hours 15 minutes
- Assignment 3: 1 hour (plus 45 minutes preparation time)

Question types

You can expect to find a range of different types of questions on the papers. These include:
- questions worth 1 mark requiring one-word answers or short sentences
- short-answer questions worth 2–4 marks
- medium-length answers worth 5–6 marks
- longer extended response questions worth 9 plus 3 QWC marks.

Paper B also includes some multiple choice questions worth 1 mark each where you must select the correct answer from four options.

Questions worth 1–2 marks will usually require factual knowledge-based, one-word or short sentence-type answers that 'name', 'identify' or 'state' the required information.

Medium-mark questions (4–6 marks) generally require a short description or short explanation with reasons, for example.

Three QWC marks are awarded based on your ability to produce answers for extended writing questions where you will:

▶ use a good standard of English
▶ express and organise ideas clearly and logically
▶ use a range of appropriate technical terms.

None of the individual parts of a question will be worth more than 12 marks – this is about your overall ability to write well.

Longer extended-response questions require answers that are well structured into paragraphs with developed reasoning. The information will need to be accurate and use appropriate terminology. Accurate use of grammar, punctuation and spelling in these longer questions will support the overall quality of your response, as well as earning you QWC marks.

Command verbs

T Level Technical Qualifications delivered by NCFE use the following command words at the start of questions. These tell you what you have to do to answer the question.

Command word	Use
Assess	Evaluate or estimate the quality of a given topic to make an informed judgement, may include advantages and disadvantages.
Analyse	Separate information into component parts. Make logical, evidence-based connections between the components.
Calculate	Work out the value of something, showing relevant working.
Choose	Select from a range of alternatives (MCQ).
Complete	Finish a task by adding to given information.
Consider	Review and respond to given information.
Define	Give a definition or specify meaning of an idea or concept.
Describe	Give an account of or set out characteristics or features.
Discuss	Present key points about different ideas or strengths and weaknesses of an idea. There should be some element of balance, although not necessarily equal weighting.
Evaluate	Review information and bring it together to make judgements and conclusions from available evidence. Students may also use their own understanding to consider evidence for and against.
Explain	Set out purposes or reasons or make something clear in relation to a particular situation. An explanation requires understanding to be demonstrated.
Explain how	Give a detailed account of a process or way of doing something.
Give examples	Answers should include relevant examples in the context of the question.
Identify	Name or otherwise characterise.
Justify	Support a case or idea with evidence. This might reasonably involve discussing and discounting alternative views or actions.
Label	Add names, indicating their correct position to an image or diagram.
List	Give a reasoned explanation for actions or decisions.
Name	Identify using a recognised technical term.
Outline	Set out main the characteristics or features.
Show	Provide structured evidence to reach a conclusion.
State	Express in clear, brief terms.
Summarise	Brief statement of the main points.
Suggest (what/why/how)	Present a possible cause or solution. Apply knowledge to a new situation to provide a reasoned explanation.

Command word	Use
Use or using **(Figure 1, Table 2, the information above/in the scenario, your own knowledge and understanding)**	Answer must be based on information given in the question. In some cases, students may be asked to use their own knowledge and understanding.
Work out	Perform one or a set of steps or calculations to arrive at an answer.

Source: https://www.qualhub.co.uk/media/22144/t-level-support-materials_command_verbs_v10.pdf

Always check the command verb carefully before answering a question. If you just describe something when an explanation is required, you will not be able to gain full marks because an explanation requires more detail than a description.

Preparing for the examinations

▶ Find the sample papers and mark schemes for this qualification on the T-Level website at the link below. Look at the type of questions included, have a go at a paper and mark it yourself using the mark scheme provided.

www.qualhub.co.uk/qualification-search/ qualification-detail/t-level-technical-qualification-in-health-level-3-delivered-by-ncfe-5045

▶ Use the 'Assessment Practice' questions at the end of each chapter to help with your revision.

▶ Always ask your tutor if you do not understand something or are not sure – they are there to help you.

▶ It is never too early to start revising. Begin your revision by going through your handouts and notes after each session – do not just file them away!

▶ Remember, the more times you go through a topic, the more you will remember.

▶ Make a revision plan, a timetable with dates – tick off each topic you have revised.

▶ Use the practice 'test yourself' questions and 'research' and 'reflect' activities suggested in this book as another way to revise and to extend your knowledge.

▶ Learn the key terms for each topic so that you are able to use specialist terminology correctly in your answers.

Exam technique

There is more to producing a good answer to an exam question than simply knowing the facts. The quality of your response, such as how you organise your answer and whether it is fully relevant to the question, will help you gain extra marks.

Top Tips

▶ Read each question carefully at least twice before you start your answer.

▶ Underline or highlight the command verb so that you are clear about what you have to do.

▶ Be guided by the number of marks and space provided for the length of your answer. The more marks available, the more space will be given.

▶ Many questions will include the number of points required – for instance, 'List **three** reasons'. Make sure you pay attention to this and provide enough information.

▶ If a question asks for 'ways' without saying how many ways, you must give a minimum of two as 'ways' is plural. The same applies to 'methods' 'reasons', etc.

▶ For higher-mark questions (for example, 6 or 12 marks), write your answer in paragraphs. Each paragraph should focus on a specific aspect of the answer. This ensures your answer is organised and logical.

▶ Make sure the information in your answer is accurate and relevant to the question – do not just write everything you know about a topic: answer the question.

▶ Do not leave any questions unanswered even if you feel you do not know the answer – have a go, you probably know more than you think you do.

Sample practice questions and commentaries

Extended response question

Helena is 87. She lives on her own, in rented accommodation. Helena had a minor stroke a few months ago and has been having daily visits from carers to assist her with daily living tasks such as bathing and preparing meals. Helena sometimes has difficulty communicating as a result of her stroke.

Helena has now decided to move nearer her daughter, but she still wants to live in her own home with the daily support visits. Helena's social worker is working with the local authority to help arrange this move.

Explain how a person-centred approach supports Helena's care in this situation.

Example medium-level response

A person-centred approach supports Helena because it promotes her rights and preferences, giving her choice and control. This means that together with her social worker, a personalised care plan that takes account of Helena's personal wishes and needs will be produced. For example, the social worker will liaise with the local authority and consult with Helena to find suitable living accommodation. This would be close to her daughter and provide for her needs (such as a bungalow) following her stroke. This puts Helena at the centre of her care. Suitability of living accommodation is one of the wellbeing principles of the Health and Social Care Act. The local authority is required by the Health and Social Care Act 2012 to promote individuals' wellbeing and this also supports Helena's rights and her desire for continued independence.

Having a person-centred care plan is very important for Helena as she cannot manage on her own any more. The social worker would make sure that Helena's care package continues in her new home. If Helena has difficulty communicating since her stroke, the social worker will ensure that someone is there to speak for her when planning her care and that her carers continue to look after her on a daily basis.

Commentary

Why it is a Band 2 (medium-level) response

The response is well developed, clear and logically structured and it demonstrates knowledge and understanding of how person-centred care supports Helena. The content of the answer is relevant to Helena's situation. The explanation accurately uses appropriate terminology such as 'person-centred approach', 'consult', 'personalised' and 'personal wishes and needs'. These are all relevant to supporting Helena. Knowledge and understanding of the relevant aspects of the HSC Act and person-centred care is clear, as shown by references to the local authority's responsibilities to promote the wellbeing principles, i.e. 'suitable living accommodation' and 'continuity of care'.

The second paragraph attempts an explanation with ensuring 'someone is there to speak for' Helena. However, the explanation here lacks precision and detail.

The answer gains mid-level marks for a sound response with reference to the HSC Act and to aspects of person-centred planning and care which are related to supporting Helena's choice of living alone. The quality of written communication is good, with no obvious errors of grammar, spelling or punctuation.

How it can become a Band 3 (higher-level) response

In order to become a high-level response, paragraph two needs to be developed with further detail in the explanation.

Additional and more accurate detail could be given where the answer suggests that the social worker will ensure that 'someone is there to speak for her when planning her care'. This is a vague reference to having an advocate to facilitate the involvement of an individual in their care planning – this could be Helena's daughter or another family member. However, the answer does not accurately describe the role of an advocate. An advocate does not 'speak for' someone, they speak on behalf of someone who is unable to speak up for themselves; they represent that person's best interests.

The response could also have referenced the fact that the HSC Act requires local authorities to ensure that there is no gap in the support being provided for an individual if they move to another area.

Extended-response question

A fire breaks out in a day centre for older adults.

Analyse ways that following health and safety legislation helps to minimise the risk of harm.

Your response should include:
- reference to appropriate legislation
- fire risk assessment
- evacuation procedures.

Example high-level response

The Regulatory Reform (Fire Safety) Order 2005 places legal responsibilities on employers to carry out a fire risk assessment. The Health and Safety at Work Act requires all organisations to have procedures in place for evacuation in the event of a fire, and evacuation should be practised. Working fire alarms, extinguishers and accessible fire doors should all be in place. All of these actions contribute to the safety of individuals in the event of a fire. Legislation ensures that employers and employees will know their responsibilities in the day centre.

Legislation ensures that regular fire risk assessments are carried out to ensure the safety of individuals. Fire hazards should be identified and dealt with, for example check for faulty electrical equipment; fabrics and textiles should be non-flammable. Also, for example, fire exits and corridors must be kept clear so that there is no delay in evacuating people. Fire risk assessments identify potential hazards such as obstructed exits which pose a risk to wheelchair users. A day centre with older adults would usually have some wheelchair users, so there should be a clear route for the wheelchair users, with wide fire exits, doorways and corridors, to use in the event of a fire breaking out, as any obstructions could cause a dangerous delay.

An evacuation procedure that is known by everyone is essential. Staff need to be trained so that they are aware of what to do, when and where. Designated members of staff need to be given specific responsibilities, checking particular areas or being responsible for giving assistance to a certain individual who would struggle to get out on their own. A fire warden should be appointed to stay back until everyone is evacuated and then check the building to see that everyone has been able to get out safely.

Commentary

This response achieved full marks.

The full 3 marks for QWC were awarded as the answer is clearly expressed and well structured. The answer is presented using three paragraphs to organise the analysis. Paragraph one focused on the impact of legislation, paragraph two focused on fire risk assessment and paragraph three covered evacuation procedures. This structure is to be recommended as it ensures all aspects of the question are covered in a structured and organised way. There were no noticeable errors of spelling, punctuation or grammar.

The response clearly and correctly references appropriate legislation and links it to the day centre scenario. The candidate goes on to provide a detailed analysis of how both fire risk assessment and evacuation procedures reduce the risk of harm. The answer is again explicitly related to the scenario as it explains the necessity of having designated staff members responsible for helping those with limited mobility and the need for fire exits being accessible for wheelchair users. A range of appropriate technical terminology is used confidently and effectively.

Short-answer question

A private residential care home which provides care and education for 15 children with physical and learning disabilities has recently been inspected by the regulatory body Ofsted. Following the inspection, the home has been graded as 'inadequate'.

Describe **two** ways that inspections and grading by regulatory bodies can help care settings to improve the standard of care they provide.

Response

1 Ofsted gives advice and information on how to improve the service provided by the care setting. The advice is presented in a report that highlights areas for improvement so that the setting knows what is not good enough.
2 Ofsted puts failing settings, rated 'inadequate', into 'special measures', which means they will be re-inspected and checked to monitor progress and improvements to the aspects of service that have been identified as unsatisfactory.

Commentary

This answer gains full marks, 2 marks for each 'way'. The first part of the answer gives a description of Ofsted providing advice and information about how to improve the standard of care and also references ld be produced which clearly identifies the areas requiring improvement.

The second part of the answer describes how the setting is given a low grade which results in repeat inspections to monitor improvements.

The candidate clearly understands the purpose of regulatory inspections and how they can provide information, advice and support to improve the standard of care.

Short-answer questions

1 Identify what the initials SOP stand for. (1 mark)
2 Describe the purpose of a SOP. (2 marks)

Response

1 Standard Operating Procedures.
2 The purpose of a SOP is to provide a set of step-by-step instructions for staff to follow when carrying out routine tasks.

Commentary

Answer 1 is correct. The command verb is 'identify' so no further information is required.

Answer 2 is also correct and provides enough detail to gain full marks. The command verb here is 'describe', so more information is required than for an 'identify' question. One mark is awarded for 'providing a set of standard instructions' and the second is for the point about informing staff about how to carry out routine tasks.

Employer-set project (ESP)

This project is specific to your chosen occupational specialism. It is an externally set project in conjunction with employers.

The purpose of the ESP is to ensure that you have the opportunity to apply care, knowledge and skills to develop a piece of work in response to an employer-set brief. You will have 14 hours 30 minutes to complete the ESP and an additiona l 2 hours for preparation research.

You will be given five pre-release briefs outlining the health contexts of five individuals. You must choose **one** of the five to research. The purpose of the pre-release is for you to carry out research into the situations and conditions of the individual you have chosen.

ESP tasks

Task 1: 2 hours – Planning

You will have researched the individual and must now use the information from the case study and your research from the pre-release brief preparation to write a report that identifies how to best support the individual you have chosen in their outlined situation.

You should explain the support you propose for the individual, justifying your points with evidence.

Task 2a: 2 hours – Practical role play

For this task you will undertake a practical role play focusing on your chosen individual.

You will take the role of a supporting healthcare assistant. You have been asked by a senior colleague in the team to conduct a discussion with the individual you have chosen. You will discuss their case with them and ask questions to clarify points in the brief and to inform next steps for their care.

Task 2b: 2 hours 30 minutes – Create a healthcare plan for the chosen individual

Contribute to a healthcare plan for your chosen individual using your notes from task 2a and your research from the preparation research. You should use the healthcare plan template provided.

Task 3a: 3 hours 30 minutes – Formative reflection task (peer feedback)

You must discuss your proposed healthcare plan with your peers to gain and offer feedback. Your tutor will put you into your peer discussion groups.

Task 3b: 2 hours 30 minutes – Produce and deliver a presentation

Produce and conduct a presentation for your tutor, who will assume the role of a senior colleague in the healthcare team that would be involved in your chosen individual's care.

Task 4: 2 hours – Complete a reflective account

You must now complete a reflective account that considers your approach to the overall project, including how well you feel you have achieved the expected outcomes.

In completing the employer-set project you will demonstrate six core skills, supported by underpinning knowledge and understanding from the core elements.

Core skills are covered in detail on pages 354–378.

Occupational specialism component: synoptic assessment

These are synoptic task-based assignments linked to your chosen occupational specialism.

The occupational specialisms are:
- Supporting the Adult Nursing Team
- Supporting the Midwifery Team
- Supporting the Mental Health Team
- Supporting the Care of Children and Young People
- Supporting Therapy Teams

You will choose one of these and the assignments will be focused on this occupation. Synoptic means that it is an assessment of the overall specialism as a whole rather than particular areas within it.

The assignments will include three types of assessment:
- Case Study Assessment (CSA)
- Practical Activity Assessment (PAA)
- Professional Discussion Assessment (PDA).

There are four assignments in total for the Occupational Specialisms, including two separate Assignments for Assignment 2. The assignments and their durations are as follows:
- Assignment 1 (case study assessment CSA): 4 hours 30 minutes
- Assignment 2 (practical activity assessment (PAA) core): 1 hour to 1 hour 30 minutes
- Assignment 2 (practical activity assessment (PAA) option): 1 hour 15 minutes to 2 hours 15 minutes
- Assignment 3 (professional discussion assessment (PDA)): 1 hour (plus 45 minutes of preparation time).

Glossary

Abstract A brief summary of the research project. It will contain the aim, research methods used and conclusions drawn.

Accident A separate, identifiable, unintended incident, which causes physical injury. This specifically includes acts of violence to people at work.

Accuracy Measurements that are close to the true value.

Acid A proton (H^+ ion) donor. An acidic solution contains H^+ ions.

Activity The rate at which a radioactive source decays. The unit of activity is the becquerel (Bq) where $1\,Bq = 1$ decay per second. Count-rate is the number of radioactive decays recorded each second. You can see that activity and count-rate can be used interchangeably.

Adsorbent Often used to describe the stationary phase in chromatography because substances become adsorbed to it during separation.

Adsorption When a substance (e.g. a gas, liquid or solute) binds to or attaches to another, usually solid.

Adverse Harmful or unfavourable.

Advocate Someone who speaks on behalf of an individual who is unable to speak up for themselves.

AI Stands for artificial intelligence.

Algorithm A computer process that dictates a way of doing things or a set of rules to follow.

Alkali A water-soluble base, such as sodium hydroxide. An alkaline solution contains hydroxide (OH^-) ions.

Allele A variant of a gene.

Ammeter Measures the flow of current; always connected in series. Voltmeters measure the potential difference in a circuit and are always connected in parallel.

Amplitude The maximum displacement of any point from the equilibrium position.

Analyte The solution of unknown concentration in a titration.

Ancillary roles Roles not specific to the care sector and not involving the provision of direct care. However, they are vital to providing a high-quality service to service users. Roles within the ancillary category may include administration staff, domestic/housekeeping/cleaning staff, catering assistant/cook/chef, driver/transport manager, maintenance worker/gardener.

Antibody A blood protein that is produced in response to a specific antigen. An antibody binds specifically to an antigen in a similar way to an enzyme binding specifically to its substrate.

Antigen A substance that is recognised by the immune system as self (the body's own cells) or non-self (foreign cells and pathogens) and stimulates an immune response. Antigens are found on pathogens but also on the surfaces of all body cells.

Antimicrobial or antibiotic stewardship The effort to measure and improve how antibiotics are prescribed by clinicians and used by patients. Improving antibiotic prescribing and use is critical in continuing to effectively treat infections.

Appropriate adult Their role is to protect the wellbeing and best interests of a young person aged 17 or younger, or someone of any age with a learning disability, when they are interviewed or attend a meeting. Usually this will be a parent or guardian, or alternatively a social worker or someone who has been trained as an appropriate adult.

Aseptic Free from contamination caused by harmful bacteria, viruses or other micro-organisms; surgically sterile or sterilised.

Atomic number Refers to the number of protons in the nucleus.

Autonomic nervous system Part of the peripheral nervous system that controls many of the processes in the body over which we have no conscious control.

Autonomous Able to act independently, having control; not being forced to do something.

Autonomy In the case of safeguarding an adult, staff must respect the competent decisions made by an individual as they have the right to make these independently. Staff should not act without consulting the adult at risk unless the adult does not have the mental capacity for this.

Base A proton (H^+ ion) acceptor. Examples include hydroxides as well as ammonia and amines.

Beri-beri Vitamin B1 deficiency that leads to a nervous system disorder.

Biomarkers Found by laboratory testing of blood, other body fluids or tissue, provide a measurable indicator of a biological state or condition, e.g. indicating the progress of a disease. They can help to determine the most effective therapy for a condition and establish the likelihood of recurrence of a condition such as cancer.

Biosecurity Refers to procedures or measures designed to protect the population against harmful biological or biochemical substances.

Blood pressure Usually measured in mmHg (millimetres of mercury). Although the units of pressure are usually kPa, the unit mmHg relates to how blood pressure was (and often still is) measured.

Burette A long glass tube that has a tap at the bottom and is marked in $0.1\,cm^3$ divisions. It is used to deliver an accurate volume of liquid (the titre) to reach the end point.

CAD/CAM Computer-aided design/computer-aided manufacture.

Calibration The process of comparing measurements, usually against a reference standard.

Carbon monoxide Odourless, colourless, tasteless toxic gas.

Cardiovascular Relating to the heart and blood vessels.

Cardiovascular disease General term that describes a disease of the heart or blood vessels.

Caring roles Directly involved in providing care for individuals, roles such as nursing, midwifery, GP or a surgeon.

Cartilage Another type of connective tissue that contains, among other components, collagen and the elastic protein elastin. Cartilage is more flexible than ligaments and muscles, but not as hard and rigid as bone.

Categorical data Is divided into groups or categories, such as male and female, ethnic group, city or country of residence.

Cell-signalling The process by which cells communicate with each other, usually by release of chemicals such as histamine, cytokines and interleukins.

Charge A fundamental property of many subatomic particles. Electrons, by convention, have a negative charge. The unit of charge is the coulomb (C) and the symbol is Q.

Chromatography The separation of the components of a mixture dissolved in a liquid or gas (the mobile phase) carrying it through a structure holding the stationary phase.

Chronic An illness or condition that lasts longer than three months and is ongoing. It can be controlled but not cured.

Chronic obstructive pulmonary disease (COPD) The name for a collection of lung diseases which make breathing increasingly difficult.

Cilia Hair-like structures found on the plasma membranes of epithelial cells. These are known as ciliated epithelial cells.

Clarify To check for accuracy of understanding.

Clinical Related to the observation and treatment of patients.

Clinical Commissioning Group (CCG) Most of the NHS commissioning budget is now managed by 209 CCGs. These are groups of general practices which come together in each area to commission the best services for their patients and the local population.

Cognitive Relating to the processes of perception, memory, judgement and reasoning.

Cognitive behaviour therapy (CBT) Talking and listening therapy which examines how an individual behaves and thinks in order to help change the behaviour that is an issue and ultimately improve mental health.

Commissioning The process of planning and agreeing health services that are needed in a local area.

Compulsory required by law or by other regulations.

Confidentiality Limits access or places restrictions on sharing certain types of sensitive information, such as medical records, so that it is kept private and available only to those who need to be aware of it.

Constipation Infrequent, irregular or difficulty with defecating.

Consumables Items that are used and then disposed of. They are mostly single-use but might be re-used in some circumstances.

Continence The ability to control the bladder and bowel.

Continuous data Is numerical and can be measured. It is possible to have any intermediate value, for example, height, mass, length.

Continuous professional development (CPD) Development of further skills and knowledge needed to do a professional job properly.

Contraindication A reason that makes it inadvisable to combine certain foods with particular drugs.

Control measures Actions that can be taken to reduce the risks posed by a hazard or to remove the hazard altogether.

Corrosion The process where metals react with substances in the air to form oxides, carbonates, hydroxides or other compounds.

Cosmic radiation (Also called cosmic rays) originates from the sun as well as from outside the solar system. It is a mixture of high energy protons (hydrogen nuclei), alpha particles (helium nuclei) and beta particles (electrons).

Coulomb (C) The unit of charge. Current is the rate of flow of charge past a given point in a circuit, i.e. how fast it flows past. The unit of current is the ampere (A), often shortened to 'amp', and the symbol is I.

Cross infection The process by which bacteria or other micro-organisms are unintentionally transferred from one person to another, with harmful effect.

Curriculum vitae (CV) Brief account of an individual's education, qualifications and previous jobs sent with a job application.

Defecation Final act of digestion which removes solid or semi-solid waste material from the digestive tract via the anus.

Dehydration When the body loses more fluids than it takes in.

Delocalised electrons 'Free' electrons that are not associated with any single atom.

Demographics The study of the changing characteristics of populations over time, for example, the proportion in each age group, gender balance.

Denaturing Protein structures are disrupted and changed so that they are no longer able to cause infection.

Dependent variable (Often denoted by y) a variable whose value depends on that of another variable. In an experiment, we usually count or measure the dependent variable.

Depolarisation The reversal of the charge difference. Polarisation: of a nerve or muscle cell refers to the different electrical charges on either side of the plasma membrane caused by active transport of ions.

Detergent Purifying or cleansing agent which increases the ability of water to break down grease or dirt. Detergents act like soap but unlike soap they are derived from organic acids rather than fatty acids. Common examples are laundry detergent, e.g. soap powder or liquid, and dish detergent, e.g. washing-up liquid.

Diastole Refers to the relaxation of either atrium or ventricle.

Diastolic The pressure when the heart relaxes; always lower than the systolic pressure.

Discrete data Is numerical and can be counted. For example, number of patients (you cannot have half a patient). This is sometimes referred to as integer (only whole numbers).

Disinfectant A substance that destroys, inactivates or significantly reduces the concentration of pathogens such as bacteria, viruses or fungi.

Domiciliary care Care offered to any individuals living in their own homes to help them stay there rather than go into residential care. This can include help with personal tasks such as bathing, getting out of bed, dressing, and breakfast and other meals.

Ducts Tubes that lead from an exocrine gland to the place where the products are used or needed. Examples include tear ducts in the eye, or salivary and pancreatic ducts in the digestive system.

Dynavox Speech-generating software. A person touches a screen that contains text, pictures and symbols, then the software converts those symbols into speech.

Electromagnet Produced when a current flows through a coil of wire.

Electromagnetic spectrum Describes all the different types of electromagnetic waves. The properties of the different types of waves varies considerably, so we usually consider the spectrum as seven groups, with slight overlaps.

Electromagnetic waves Include gamma rays, X-rays, visible light, microwaves and radio waves. Their energy is carried by oscillating electric and magnetic fields.

Electromotive force (emf) Like potential difference, except that it refers to power supplies such as cells (batteries), generators or mains power supplies. These transfer other forms of energy, such as light energy or kinetic energy, into electrical energy. The unit of emf is also the volt (V).

Eluate The mobile phase, containing dissolved substances, as it emerges from a column.

Eluent The solvent (mobile phase) used to wash substances out of a column.

Elution To wash out. In column chromatography this means 'washing out' a substance that has become adsorbed to the column (stationary phase).

Empathy The ability to understand and share the feelings of an individual.

Employment tribunals Responsible for hearing claims from people who think an employer has treated them unlawfully, for example, through unfair dismissal or discrimination.

Empower To give someone the authority or control to do something; the way a health worker encourages an individual to make decisions and to take control of their own life.

End point The point in a titration where the indicator changes colour.

Endocrine Glands release (secrete) their products directly into the blood. Examples are the alpha (α) and beta (β) cells in the pancreas that secrete the hormones glucagon and insulin respectively.

Endocrine system A system of hormones that control many aspects of physiology (the normal functioning of the body).

Epithelial Cells line structures in the body and are usually thin, single layers.

Equivalence point The point of neutralisation where the number of moles of acid and base are equal. This should ideally be the same as the end point.

Ethics Concerned with what is morally right or wrong.

Evidence-based approach Making better decisions by considering all the facts, statistics, etc. and using them as a basis for making a decision.

Exocrine Glands release (secrete) their products into ducts or onto the body surface.

Fertilisation Involves fusion of haploid gametes (sperm and egg) to form the diploid zygote with the full number of chromosomes.

Fluid mosaic model Describes the structure of the plasma membrane and how its components are arranged. The proteins, lipids and carbohydrates that are found in the plasma membrane vary in shape, size and location which creates the mosaic pattern. Due to the relatively weak forces between phospholipids, the membrane can be considered to be fluid as these components can move throughout the membrane.

Frequency In Hz, the number of complete waves that pass a given point in one second. One complete wave is a cycle, so a frequency of 1 Hz corresponds to one cycle per second. This is a very low frequency, so you will often see frequency measured in kHz (kilohertz, 10^3 Hz), MHz (megahertz, 10^6 Hz) or GHz (gigahertz, 10^9 Hz).

Gametes Haploid cells (half the number of chromosomes) that are produced by meiosis, a type of cell division that halves the number of chromosomes.

Gamma radiation A penetrating form of electromagnetic radiation arising from the radioactive decay of atomic nuclei.

Gene A sequence of bases in DNA that codes for (contains the information to make) a polypeptide, or, in some cases, functional RNA (this is involved in regulating how genes are expressed).

Genetics The study of how single genes, or a small group of genes, function and how they affect the appearance and functioning of the organism.

Genitalia The male and female sex organs.

Genome The entire genetic material of an organism. This includes DNA that does not code for proteins as well as the coding DNA (genes).

Genomics The study of how all the genes in an organism interact, as well as the role of non-coding sequences of DNA.

Gland A group of cells that make chemicals such as hormones or enzymes.

GP General practitioner. This is the doctor in the local community and is usually based in a health centre or surgery. GPs deliver primary care and will provide initial diagnosis and treatment or will refer the individual to a specialist.

Grievance Any concern, problem or complaint you may have at work. If you take this up with your employer, it is called 'raising a grievance'.

Group Refers to the rows in the periodic table. Elements in each group have the same number of outer shell electrons. Period refers to the rows in the periodic table. Elements in each period have the same number of shells.

Half-life The time taken for half the unstable nuclei in a sample to decay.

Hazard Something that has the potential to cause harm.

Healthcare-associated infections (HCAIs) Infections which can occur as a result of having treatment in hospital or after surgical or medical treatment.

Healthcare professional (HCP) Someone who looks after the health and welfare of individuals who have been arrested and are kept in custody.

Healthwatch The national consumer champion in health and care. It has significant statutory powers to ensure the voice of the consumer is strengthened and heard by those who commission, deliver and regulate health and care services.

Hearing loop A special type of sound system to assist people with hearing aids. The hearing loop provides a magnetic wireless signal that is picked up by the hearing aid and can greatly improve the quality of sound while reducing background noise.

HEPA (high-efficiency particulate air) filter A type of filter that can trap tiny particles that other vacuum cleaners would simply recirculate back into the air. HEPA vacuums are recommended for minimising dust and other common allergens.

Hierarchy (I) an arrangement of things in order of importance. (II) a system in which workers are ranked in order of their role within the organisation, from the top down.

Holistic approach A way of approaching the delivery of healthcare that considers the whole person, not just the part that requires physical treatment. It also takes into account an individual's intellectual, emotional and social needs.

Horizontal gene transfer The transfer of genetic material directly from one organism to another by various processes, without reproduction.

Hormone A chemical messenger released into the blood by an endocrine gland that acts on target tissues elsewhere in the body.

Hospice Provides support and end of life care to individuals and their families. Hospice care can be provided where individuals choose, for example, at home, in a hospice room at a hospital, in a nursing home or at a Marie Curie hospice.

Immunodeficiency A condition in which the body has difficulty protecting itself against disease.

Incision A cut made through the skin and soft tissue for a surgical procedure.

Independent variable (Often denoted by x) a variable whose value does not depend on that of another variable. In an experiment, the independent variable is usually what we change.

Indicator A substance that changes from one colour to another or from coloured to colourless depending on whether it is in acidic or basic solution.

Induced magnet An object that can become a magnet when it is placed in a magnetic field.

Infection The process of bacteria, viruses or other micro-organisms (such as fungi or parasites) invading the body, making someone ill or diseased.

Inflammation A local response to injury and infection.

Innate immunity The non-specific mechanisms, present from birth, that protect against a wide range of pathogens. These mechanisms, including inflammation, phagocytosis and antimicrobial proteins work quickly, but are not always very effective.

Inpatient Patient who receives medical treatment, tests, etc. while staying in hospital.

Inspection The process of observing and carrying out checks to see whether services provided meet the required standards.

Integrated care Provides people with the support they need across local councils, the NHS and other partners. The idea is that barriers between GPs, hospitals and council services have been removed, meaning people no longer have disjointed care.

Integument A tough outer protective layer.

Integumentary system Includes the skin, hair and nails.

Ionisation The formation of charged particles from neutral molecules or atoms by adding or removing electrons.

Ionising radiation Any form of radiation that interacts with matter, resulting in ionisation of that matter.

Ions Atoms that have lost electrons (negative ions) or gained electrons (positive ions).

Irradiation When objects are exposed to different types of radiation. It may be used to penetrate various materials and can be used to sterilise surgical instruments.

Isotopes Atoms of the same element (they have the same number of protons) but with different number of neutrons.

IVF In vitro fertilisation. A fertility treatment in which an egg is fertilised by sperm in a test tube and then the fertilised egg is implanted in the uterus.

Joint The area where two or more bones connect.

Judicial healthcare Healthcare provided for those individuals detained in prison and detainees who are kept in police custody before being charged with an offence. Also involves the Youth Offending Team which aims to engage young people in health education, and reduce drugs and alcohol misuse in the local area.

Lack capacity Unable to use and understand information to make a decision. This is a term with a specific meaning in law and should not be applied without meeting certain criteria.

Laws (legislation) Passed by Parliament. They state the rights and entitlements of individuals and provide legal rules that have to be followed. The law is upheld through the courts. If an individual or care setting breaks the law by, for example, inappropriately sharing or inaccurately recording information, they can, in certain circumstances, be fined, dismissed or given a prison sentence.

Legislation A collection of laws passed by Parliament which state the rights and entitlements of the individual. Law is upheld through the courts.

Levels In this context, a way of grading a qualification or set of skills and the corresponding occupations. The levels used today are based on the National Vocational Qualifications (NVQ) levels 1 to 5 developed in the 1980s. Over time, more emphasis has been given to the degree of difficulty or challenge of the qualification rather than the level of occupational competence in the workplace. There are now eight levels, and they cover academic qualifications such as GCSEs, A Levels and undergraduate and graduate degrees, as well as vocational qualifications such as T Levels and apprenticeships.

Ligaments Made of connective tissue containing the protein collagen. Their function is to join bones together and to strengthen joints.

Lightwriter A text-to-speech device. A message is typed on a keyboard, displayed on a screen and then converted into speech.

Lines of magnetic flux Indicate the direction and strength of a magnetic field.

Lymphocytes Small white blood cells. B lymphocytes, or B cells, are responsible for antibody production. Different types of T lymphocytes, or T cells, play different roles in the immune response.

Machine learning The study of computer algorithms that improve in validity automatically through experience over time and by the use of huge amounts of data. Machine learning algorithms build a model based on sample data, known as 'training data', in order to make predictions or decisions without being explicitly programmed to do so.

Magnet A material or object that produces a magnetic field.

Magnetic field A region where a magnet exerts a force on other magnets or magnetic materials.

Magnetic materials Such as iron, steel, nickel and cobalt will experience an attractive force when placed in a magnetic field.

Magnetism The force experienced by some types of metals in the earth's magnetic field or in a magnetic field of a magnet. It is also defined as the attractive or repulsive force produced by a moving electric charge.

Magnification How much bigger the image is than the actual object we are viewing. It should not be confused with resolution.

Management roles Involve the leadership, monitoring and supervision of staff and the organisation.

Manual handling Using the correct procedures when physically moving any load by lifting, putting down, pushing or pulling.

MAR A medicine administration record that is updated every time any medication is given to a patient in a healthcare setting, i.e. a hospital, nursing or care home, etc. It contains a list of what has been administered and when, and can be an electronic or paper-based record.

Materials Include items such as ingredients or components used in the manufacture of a product.

Medical device A healthcare product or piece of equipment that someone uses for a medical purpose. Medical devices can diagnose, monitor or treat disease and help people with physical impairments become more independent.

Medicine Any substance (or combination of substances) that is claimed to be able to prevent or treat human disease. Medicines are often referred to as (medical) drugs or pharmaceuticals. Medicines do not include food supplements, herbal products or cosmetics and so companies are not legally allowed to claim that these can be used to prevent or treat disease.

Mental capacity The ability to make a decision. It involves being able to understand information and remember it for long enough to make a decision and to be able to communicate it to others.

Mole An amount of substance. This helps us to work out the reacting proportions in any reaction. We can also use the mole to work out reacting masses or volumes. The abbreviation is mol.

Monitor The sector regulator for health services in England. Monitor's job is to make the health sector work better for patients by continually improving the service and getting good value for money.

Motor effect When a current-carrying wire is placed between magnetic poles. The magnetic field around the wire interacts with the magnetic field it is placed in. This causes the wire and magnet to exert a force on each other and can cause the wire to move.

Multidisciplinary team A team of professionals from different specialisms who work together for the good of the patient, e.g. a physiotherapist working with a dietician and an orthopaedic surgeon after someone has had a traffic accident.

Mutation A change in the sequence of bases in DNA. This can occur in a number of ways. When a mutation occurs within a coding region of DNA a new allele can be formed.

Need-to-know basis Information is only shared with those directly involved with the care and support of an individual. They need the information to enable them to provide appropriate care.

Nerves Usually bundles of many neurones.

Neural growth Refers to any growth of the nervous system.

Neurological Relating to a disorder of the nerves and nervous system.

Neurone A nerve cell.

NHS Improvement Works with the NHS to help improve care for patients and provides leadership and support for the NHS.

NICE The National Institute for Health and Care Excellence. This organisation provides guidelines and information on standards and effectiveness of care.

Norovirus Very infectious virus common in the winter which causes diarrhoea and vomiting.

Orthotist Someone who makes splints or braces for weakened limbs for patients who require support due to an accident, injury or disease.

Osteoporosis Causes a loss of bone density which weakens them and as a result they fracture easily.

Outpatient Patient who visits a hospital or clinic to have treatment, tests and investigations, but does not have to stay there.

Oxygen saturation Level of oxygen delivered to red blood cells through arteries and delivered to internal organs.

Palliative care Aims to achieve the best quality of life possible, as actively as possible, until the individual's death from a terminal illness. It is a holistic approach and supports the individual and their family.

Pancreatitis Pancreas becomes inflamed over a short period of time.

Parallel circuits Where the components are each connected separately to the positive and negative terminals of the power supply.

Paraphrasing A repetition or summary of what has been said.

PECS Stands for 'picture exchange communication system'; developed for use with children who have autism, it helps them learn to start communicating by exchanging a picture for the item they want.

Permanent magnet Produces its own magnetic field.

Person-centred care To see the person as an individual, focusing on their needs, wants, goals and aspirations.

Phagocytes Produced in the bone marrow and circulate in the blood. Some leave the blood and are present in the tissues.

Phagocytosis The process of a phagocyte engulfing a pathogen or other foreign material.

Photosynthesis The process that plants use to make complex organic compounds such as sugars from carbon dioxide and water using light energy.

Physiological Anything to do with the body and its systems.

Plant Any equipment used in the workplace, e.g. laboratory equipment.

Polar A polar (hydrophilic) substance will dissolve in or mix with water.

Polarisation Of a nerve or muscle cell refers to the different electrical charges on either side of the plasma membrane caused by active transport of ions.

Practice nurse Based at the GP surgery, offers a range of services including immunisations, diabetes monitoring, cervical smears and general health checks.

Precise Measurements that are close to each other, but they may be inaccurate.

Primary care The first tier of healthcare, usually consisting of professionals with day-to-day responsibility for the health of patients. This includes the GP, midwife, health visitor, etc.

Prosthetics Artificial replacements for missing limbs such as a leg, foot, hand or arm.

Prosthetist Specialist in prosthetics, which are artificial replacements for a missing limb such as a leg, foot, hand or arm.

Psychological Relating to a person's mental and emotional state.

Qualitative data Is descriptive, for example, a patient's medical history.

Quantitative data Is numerical, for example, the results from a laboratory experiment.

Radioactive decay The random process that occurs when an unstable nucleus loses energy by giving out alpha or beta particles or gamma radiation.

Radiocarbon dating The process that uses a radioactive isotope of carbon, carbon-14, to determine the age of an object containing organic material.

Radioisotopes Unstable isotopes that undergo radioactive decay emitting radioactivity as they do so.

Radiologist A medical practitioner who diagnoses, using X-rays, CT and MRI scans, and treats illness or injury with therapeutic radiography.

Radiopharmaceuticals Therapeutic drugs (medicines) that incorporate radioisotopes. Some radiopharmaceuticals are used to treat disease whereas diagnostic radiopharmaceuticals are used to help in diagnosis of disease.

Recoil The process where elastic tissues or fibres return to their original length after having been stretched or expanded. This is what happens to an elastic band when you stretch it and then let go. Be careful not to use the term contraction to describe this process. Contraction is what muscles do, whereas elastic tissues recoil.

Reference standard Something of known size, mass, concentration, etc. that we can use to calibrate equipment or methods.

Regulator Independent organisation that carries out inspections to monitor and rate the quality of services provided.

Repolarisation The restoration of the original charge difference.

Reportable injuries The following injuries are reportable under RIDDOR when they result from a work-related accident:

▶ the death of any person
▶ specified injuries to workers (see the HSE website for more information)
▶ injuries to workers which result in them being unable to work for more than seven days
▶ injuries to non-workers which result in them being taken directly to hospital for treatment, or specified injuries to non-workers which occur on the premises.

Residential care setting Where long-term care is given to adults or children who live in a residential (designed for people to live in) setting rather than their own home.

Resolution The ability of a microscope to distinguish between two adjacent points. The resolution of a microscope is the smallest distance between two points that can be seen as separate. A high resolution microscope can show a clearer image. You have probably encountered resolution when using a camera phone. An old phone will probably have quite a low resolution. If you take a photo you may be able to enlarge the image to the same size as one taken with the latest high-resolution camera phone, but the modern phone will give a much clearer, sharper image.

Respiratory Related to breathing.

Respite care Offers a break for carers from caring responsibilities, while the person they care for is looked after by someone else. Increasingly known as 'short breaks' care because of negative implications of 'respite', i.e. that the cared-for person is a burden.

Risk How likely a hazard is to cause that harm.

Risk assessment The process of evaluating the likelihood of a hazard actually causing harm.

Safeguarding Actions taken to protect individuals, reduce the risks of harm and abuse, and provide a safe and healthy environment.

Scurvy Vitamin C deficiency which causes tooth loss, poor skin healing with sores, anaemia.

Semi-conservative replication When DNA replicates two new double helix molecules are formed, but each one consists of one of the original strands and one newly synthesised strand.

Series Circuits where the components are connected in line, end to end between the positive and negative terminals of the power supply.

Skeletal The main type of muscle involved in movement because it is attached to the skeleton.

Smooth (or involuntary) muscle Is not under conscious control. It is controlled by the autonomic nervous system and hormones.

Social health The ability to form friendships and meaningful personal relationships with other people.

Social prescribing When individuals are referred to support and help from the community in order to improve their health and wellbeing. Sometimes referred to as 'community referral', it involves a range of local, non-clinical services. Examples include local support groups where meeting people with the same problems provides peer support; local activity groups such as for walking, knitting, swimming to improve mental health and general health and wellbeing.

Sociogram Can show the relationship between each group member or just one member of the group. A good way of representing a social structure within a group.

Spiritual health Having a sense of purpose, a clear set of morals and values, and living life according to those morals and values. This is different for different people. It is not religion.

Sputum Mucus or coughed-up material (phlegm) from lower airways (trachea and bronchi).

Standard solution The solution of known concentration in a titration.

Stem cells Unspecialised cells that are able to divide, to allow growth or to repair or replace worn-out cells.

STI or **sexually transmitted infection** Caused by a pathogen that is passed from person to person during sexual contact.

Stroke Serious and life-threatening medical event that occurs when the blood supply to part of the brain is cut off.

Systole Refers to the contraction of either atrium or ventricle. Hence the terms atrial systole and ventricular systole respectively.

Systolic The pressure when the heart contracts.

Tendons Similar in structure and composition to ligaments. Their function is to attach the muscles to the bones that make up the skeleton.

Therapeutics The different treatments for symptoms, a disease or condition.

Third sector Also called the voluntary sector. An umbrella term for non-profit making organisations and other organisations that are not public (i.e. state-run) or private, such as non-governmental organisations (NGOs) and charities.

Titre The volume of standard solution needed to neutralise the analyte (i.e. to reach the end point of the titration).

Transparency Nothing is concealed, hidden or covered up, the inspections show things exactly as they are, whether good or not.

Triage Screening of individuals by a medical professional to decide the order in which patients are treated, or the type of care required, depending on the urgency and nature of symptoms, wounds or illness.

Ultraviolet light A form of radiation not visible to the human eye but present in sunlight.

Venn diagram Consists of circles which interlink. The circles can be free standing or can overlap, demonstrating a link or relationship.

Wavelength The distance between the same point in successive cycles. The standard unit of wavelength is the metre, m. However, electromagnetic waves can have wavelengths from 10^4 m to 10^{-15} m, so you will often see wavelengths expressed in units such as nanometres, nm. ($1 \, \text{nm} = 1 \times 10^{-9}$ m.)

Whistleblowing When someone reveals serious wrongdoing within an organisation to an outside authority such as the Care Quality Commission, so that it can be investigated.

Work-related An accident in the workplace does not always mean that the accident is work-related – the work activity itself must contribute to the accident. An accident is 'work-related' if any of the following played a significant role: the way the work was carried out; any machinery, plant, substances or equipment used for the work; the condition of the site or premises where the accident happened.

X-ray An electromagnetic wave of high energy and very short wavelength, which is able to pass through many materials, opaque to light.

Index